MIDDLE RANGE THEORY DEVELOPMENT
USING KING'S CONCEPTUAL SYSTEM

Christina Leibold Sieloff, PhD, RN, CNA, BC, is an associate professor at Montana State University, College of Nursing, Billings Campus, where she teaches both undergraduate and graduate nursing courses with an emphasis on nursing theory and management. Sieloff received her BSN from Wayne State University, Detroit, Michigan; her MSN with a major in nursing administration and a minor in child and adolescent psychiatric nursing; and her doctorate in nursing with a cognate in management. Sieloff's past honors have included the Faculty Research Award from Oakland University in 1994; the Faculty Recognition award in 1996; the early awarding of tenure in 2000; and Featured Faculty Recognition by the Board of Trustees in 2003. Sieloff has authored or collaborated with others on 19 publications and 17 presentations related to her theoretical studies. Her primary program of research focuses on the testing of her middle range theory, the theory of group power within organizations, and the related instrument, the Sieloff–King Assessment of Group Power Within Organizations. Her most recent research involved the development of the Collaborative Research Group of nursing faculty. The first research project from this group is a pilot study examining the relationship of nursing group power to the attainment of positive patient outcomes.

Sieloff is a member of the American Nurses Association (ANA), American Psychiatric Nurses Association, and Sigma Theta Tau International, and she has been active in a variety of positions, including serving on the ANA Board of Directors.

Maureen A. Frey, PhD, RN, is a research associate at Wayne State University School of Medicine, in Detroit, Michigan, and is coordinator of the Collaborative Pediatric Critical Care Medicine Research Network. Frey received her MSN and doctorate (PhD in nursing) from Wayne State University. She is a pioneer in developing and testing middle range theory derived from King's conceptual system. Her theoretical formulation of families, children, chronic conditions, and health outcomes has been tested among youth with diabetes, asthma, and HIV/AIDS. Her focus is on understanding interactions that influence behavior and the relationship between behavioral change and improved health status. Frey is a strong advocate for the utility of King's conceptual system outside of nursing and currently works with a multidisciplinary team. She has implemented theory-based research in both academic and service settings.

Middle Range Theory Development Using King's Conceptual System

Christina Leibold Sieloff, PhD, RN,
CNA, BC
and
Maureen A. Frey, PhD, RN
Editors

SPRINGER PUBLISHING COMPANY
New York

Springer Publishing Company, LLC
11 West 42nd Street
New York, NY 10036
www.springerpub.com

Acquisitions Editor: Sally J. Barhydt
Production Editor: Shana Meyer
Cover Design: Joanne E. Honigman
Composition: TechBooks

07 08 09 10/5 4 3 2 1

Library of Congress Cataloging-in-Publication Data

Middle range theory development using King's conceptual system / [edited by] Christina Leibold Sieloff and Maureen A. Frey.
    p. cm.
    Includes bibliographical references and index.
    ISBN-13: 978-0-8261-0238-6 (pbk.)
    ISBN-10: 0-8261-0238-7 (pbk.)
   1. Nursing—Philosophy. 2. Nursing models. I. Sieloff, Christina L. II. Frey, Maureen A. III. King, Imogene M.
[DNLM: 1. Nursing Theory. 2. Goals. 3. Philosophy, Nursing. 4. Systems Theory. WY 86 M627 2007]

RT84.5.M5365   2007
610.73—dc22

                     2006036137

Printed in the United States of America by Bang Printing.

This book is dedicated to Imogene King. As a pioneer in nursing theory, Dr. King was the first to develop a framework and a middle range theory related to that framework. Dr. King has consistently encouraged other nurse scholars and researchers to extend the ideas and ideals to which she is committed. We are honored by Dr. King's trust and her support in our efforts to make nursing knowledge development related to her work more visible. We continue to respect and admire her for the work she has done on behalf of nursing.

Contents

Part III   Post–Middle Range Theory Development

Contributors

Martha Raile Alligood, RN, PhD
Professor and Director of PhD
  Program
School of Nursing
East Carolina University
Greenville, North Carolina

**Mary Molewyk Doornbos,
PhD, RN**
Chairperson and Professor of
  Nursing
Calvin College
Science Building
Grand Rapids, Michigan

Phyllis du Mont, PhD, RN
Assistant Clinical Professor
Coordinator of Psychiatric Mental
  Health Concentration
College of Nursing
University of Tennessee, Knoxville
Knoxville, Tennessee

**Heidi E. Ehrenberger, PhD, RN,
AOCN**
Assistant Professor and Program
  Director
Clinical Research Management
University of Maryland School of
  Nursing
Baltimore, Maryland

Deborah A. Ellis, PhD
Assistant Professor
Carman and Ann Adams
  Department of Pediatrics
Wayne State University
Detroit, Michigan

Jenecia Fairfax, PhD, RN
Chief Nurse Executive
BVI Health Services Authority
East Carolina University
Tortola, British Virgin Islands

Jacqueline Fawcett, PhD, FAAN
Professor
College of Nursing and Health
  Sciences
University of Massachusetts,
  Boston

Naomi Funashima, RN, DNSc
Professor
Chiba University
Chiba, Japan

**Cheri Ann Hernandez, RN, PhD,
CDE**
Associate Professor
Faculty of Nursing, University of
  Windsor
Windsor, Ontario, Canada

Tomomi Kameoka, RN, DNSc
Professor
National College of Nursing
Tokyo, Japan

**Mary B. Killeen, PhD, RN,
CNAA, BC**
Research Fellow
The University of Michigan
School of Nursing
Ann Arbor, Michigan

Imogene King, EdD, RN, FAAN
Professor Emeritus
University of South Florida
Tampa, Florida
South Pasadena, Florida

**Cynthia M. Licavoli, RN,
BSN, MA**
Clinical Research Nurse
    Manager
ARCH Medical Groups
St. John's Mercy Medical
    Center
St. Louis, Missouri

Barbara A. May, PhD, RN
Assistant Professor
Department of Nursing
Lamar University
Beaumont, Texas

Sylvie Naar-King, PhD
Assistant Professor
Carmen and Ann Adams
    Department of Pediatrics
Wayne State University
Detroit, Michigan

Janice E. Fries Reed, RN, PhD
University of Phoenix, Cleveland
    Campus
North Central State College
Mansfield, Ohio

Muriel C. Rice, PhD, APRN
Assistant Professor
University of Tennessee Health
    Science Center
College of Nursing
Memphis, Tennessee

**Nancy C. Sharts-Hopko, PhD,
RN, FAAN**
Professor and Director, Doctoral
    Program
Villanova University College of
    Nursing
Villanova, Pennsylvania

Midori Sugimori, RN, BLL
President
Gunma Prefectural College of
    Health Science
Gunma, Japan

Costellia H. Talley, PhD, RN
Staff Nurse
Veteran's Administration Medical
    Center
Memphis, Tennessee

**Sandra P. Thomas, RN, PhD,
FAAN**
Professor
College of Nursing
The University of Tennessee
Knoxville, Tennessee

Debra C. Wallace, RN, PhD
Professor
School of Nursing
The University of North Carolina,
    Greensboro

**Beverly J. B. Whelton, PhD,
MSN, RN**
Assistant Professor of Philosophy
Associate Director of the WJU
    Center for Applied Ethics
Wheeling Jesuit University
Wheeling, West Virginia

Mona Newsome Wicks, PhD, RN
Professor and Director, PhD
   Nursing Program
Director, Office of Research and
   Grant Support
University of Tennessee Health
   Science Center
College of Nursing
Memphis, Tennessee

**Tamara L. Zurakowski, PhD,
CRNP**
Practice Assistant Professor
University of Pennsylvania
School of Nursing
Gerontological Nurse Practitioner
   Penn LIFE
Philadelphia, Pennsylvania

Preface

Developing and testing propositions and formulations from nursing theory are critical for the development of nursing science. This process is also one of the most difficult approaches to knowledge building to establish and maintain. A primary reason for this may be the lack of support for nursing theories within the discipline. Exposure to nursing theory is variable across all educational programs, and the explicit use of nursing theory in the practice setting is almost nonexistent. In addition, doctoral level programs, the educational level primarily responsible for developing the science of nursing, rarely require the use of an explicit nursing theory for dissertation work. The purpose of this text is to highlight significant work in extending and testing King's conceptual system and theory of goal attainment. The primary focus is on middle range theory development, but this text also includes other seminal chapters, including one that advances philosophical understanding.

To identify the state of middle range theory development from within King's conceptual system, several sources were reviewed. The initial sources were the theorists we identified in our first text (Frey & Sieloff, 1995). Each theorist was contacted and asked to update the development and testing of the middle range theory described in the 1995 publication. Several researchers continued to work within King's conceptual system, whereas other researchers had changed directions for various reasons.

Second, the authors did a literature review of several databases to identify new references in refereed publications as well as master's theses and doctoral dissertations. Additional sources of new material were book chapters and articles that provided summaries of work related to King's conceptual system or the theory of goal attainment, such as Frey, Sieloff, and Norris (2002); Frey, Roose, Sieloff, Messmer, and Kameoka (1995); Sieloff (2006); Sieloff, Frey, and Killeen (2006); and Frey (2005). Authors were contacted to determine whether they had, indeed, developed a middle range theory from within King's conceptual system and whether that theory had been tested. Criteria for inclusion in this text were that the middle range theory had to have been based within King's conceptual system or have been the result of knowledge-building efforts based within King's conceptual system. The middle range theories included here represent a wide variety of geographic locations, including a theory from Japan.

Middle Range Theory Development Using King's Conceptual System is divided into three sections in order to capture the variety of knowledge development work occurring in relation to middle range theory. Part I includes chapters that provide an overview of the foundations on which middle range theories are built from within King's conceptual system (King, 1981). In this section, Dr. King provides her perspective on knowledge development in the 21st century. In Chapter 2, Whelton offers a philosophical analysis of King's conceptual system that can serve as a way to view ongoing knowledge development efforts related to King's conceptual system.

The chapters in Part II cover a variety of middle range theories, all of which have their basis in King's conceptual system. These theories can be applied to individuals (personal system), groups and families (interpersonal systems), and organizations (social systems). The ages of individuals addressed by these theories vary from children to the elderly. Each author was asked to follow a consistent format that would enable readers to compare knowledge-building efforts across the chapters.

The final section, Part III, challenges the reader to think beyond the initial development and testing of a single middle range theory. Kameoka, Funashima, & Sugimori's chapter highlights the testing of King's middle range Theory of Goal Attainment in a non-Western culture. Frey, Ellis, & Naar-King address the use of interventions research to develop and test middle range theories derived from King's conceptual system and, in doing so, raise the critical issues of congruency, specification, and fidelity. Programs of research can also be established as a result of one theory, as shown in Alligood's chapter. Finally, Fawcett offers her commentary on the status of middle range theory development as explored in this book and challenges nurses to design, implement, and report additional theory development efforts.

Overall, this text presents the "state of the science" based on King's conceptual system and Theory of Goal Attainment. As such, it is a pivotal text to accompany King's original text and other work. Students and graduates of nursing education courses at the master's and doctoral level will find it useful in order to understand the foundational work conducted by others. Practicing nurses will also gain an appreciation as to how King's conceptual system and new middle range theories can be applied to clinical practice questions. It is also hoped that this text will encourage other nurses to begin the work of developing and testing middle range theories.

This might involve testing an already developed middle range theory, developing a new middle range theory to address current gaps in nursing knowledge, or further refining an existing middle range theory into a practice theory that addresses specific patient and nursing concerns within a particular nursing situation. Whatever actions are taken by the readers, the editors believe that the base of nursing knowledge will be strengthened, providing the foundation for evidence-based practice decisions.

Finally, it is hoped that this text will encourage those who are presently engaged in such work to publish in order to increase both the visibility of the knowledge, as well as the sharing of such knowledge between colleagues. The editors wish to thank all the authors for their contributions to this text and for their patience as the manuscript came to fruition.

CHRISTINA LEIBOLD SIELOFF
MAUREEN A. FREY

REFERENCES

Frey, M. A., Roose, L., Sieloff, C. L., Messmer, P., & Kameoka, T. (1995). King's framework and theory in Japan, Sweden, and the United States. *IMAGE: Journal of Nursing Scholarship, 27,* 127–130.

Frey, M. A., & Sieloff, C. L. (Eds.). (1995). *Advancing King's systems framework and theory of nursing.* Thousand Oaks, CA: Sage.

Frey, M. A., Sieloff, C. L., & Norris, D. M. (2002). King's conceptual system and theory of goal attainment: Past, present, and future. *Nursing Science Quarterly, 15,* 107–112.

King, I. (1981). *A theory for nursing: Systems, concepts, process.* New York: Wiley.

Sieloff, C. L. (2006). Imogene King: Systems framework and theory of goal attainment. In A. Marriner-Tomey & M. R. Alligood (Eds.), *Nursing theorists and their work* (6th ed.) (pp. 297–317). St. Louis, MO: Mosby.

Sieloff, C. L., Frey, M. A., & Killeen, M. (2006). Application of King's theory of goal attainment. In M. Parker (Ed.), *Nursing theorists and their application in practice* (2nd ed.) (pp. 244–267). Philadelphia: F. A. Davis.

Acknowledgments

I thank Imogene King, who continues to be a mentor in my ongoing efforts to revise and test my middle range theory and instrument. I would also like to recognize the support of Mildred, Louis, and Doris Sieloff who shared in my goals and dreams. Finally, I thank my husband, Ronald Leibold, for his untiring support of the refinement of this manuscript.

CHRISTINA LEIBOLD SIELOFF

This book would not be possible without the ongoing support, friendship, and trust of Imogene King and Christina's dedication to seeking out others who share our interest in developing and testing middle range theory. As in all other endeavors, I am grateful for the support of my family.

MAUREEN A. FREY

PART I

Foundations

CHAPTER ONE

King's Structure, Process, and Outcome in the 21st Century

Imogene King

In the last half of the 20th century, advances in science brought about an explosion of knowledge ruled by technology. Scientists recognized the need to find ways to study complex systems. A *system* is defined as a set of components connected by communication links that exhibit goal-directed purposeful behavior (King, 1997). Some scientists indicated that the only way to study human beings and environments is to study these phenomena as a system of mutually interdependent variables and concepts. Von Bertalanffy (1968) identified a scientific approach to study "organized wholes" called general systems theory. Nurses recognized the need to identify scientific knowledge to cope with increasing diversity in nursing practice and health care. The general systems theory movement in science influenced me to use this approach to study the complexity of nursing by identifying and studying mutually interdependent variables and concepts.

Systems have been designed to provide access to data, information, and knowledge for use by nurses in a culturally diverse world society. Nursing informatics has provided a framework that is "a combination of computer science, information science, and nursing science designed to assist in the management and processing of nursing data, information, and knowledge to support the practice of nursing and delivery of nursing care" (Graves & Corcoran, 1989, p. 227).

Language is the method used to label the categories of these systems and to describe the characteristics of the concepts. The words we use represent concepts that identify substantive knowledge such as growth and development, communication, interaction, and stress. A concept is the basic unit of the mind just as the cell is the basic unit of the body. Concepts structure the domain of knowledge in a discipline and a profession. Knowledge is a synthesis of information that identifies relationships of distinct phenomena in nursing. Data represent specific information that describe phenomena in nursing. Knowledge deals with relationships that connect the elements of data and result in decisions. Data are organized and structured and provide information to help nurses group similar ideas and facts in nursing practice. Knowledge is the cognitive representation of things in our real world.

The diverse phenomena that nurses encounter in the complex world of nursing have been presented in classification systems, conceptual systems, and theories. Three classification systems, NANDA (North American Nursing Diagnosis Association), NIC (Nursing Interventions Classification), and NOC (Nursing Outcomes Classification), have provided the beginning of a universal language for nursing (McCloskey-Dochterman & Jones, 2003). In addition, the Home Health Care Classification system (Saba, 1992), the Omaha System in Community Health (Martin, 1996), and the Ozbolt System (Ozbolt, 1993) are published systems for specific areas in nursing that have provided further unification of nursing languages.

Simultaneously, another relevant factor in the identification and use of knowledge has been the development of conceptual systems and theories. A conceptual system is a set of defined concepts that represent essential knowledge in a field of study such as nursing. The exploration of knowledge requires that a number of abstract and relevant concepts are identified to capture the knowledge of a domain. Concepts and their explanation in facts represent scientific knowledge in a field of study. We know our world through human perceptions. Knowledge is the cognitive representation of things in the real world. The explosion of knowledge and its use in complex health care systems have demanded a way to provide quality care for individuals, families, and communities.

One approach in the organization and management of systems, such as nursing and health care, has been to propose a structure to explain "organized wholes." A conceptual system demonstrates the relationship of individuals and small and large groups of human beings. Process demonstrates the use of technology in communication and interactions among individuals in various environments to achieve goals which represent outcomes. One example that provides structure, process, and outcome in nursing is King's conceptual system, theory of goal attainment, and transaction process model (1981).

STRUCTURE

Structure identifies the relationship of multiple factors in an organization. A systems approach to deal with changes and complexity in the environment was highlighted more than 50 years ago (Howland, 1976; Von Bertalanffy, 1968; Wiener, 1967). After studying systems research, an approach was identified to study the complexity of nursing as a "whole system" interacting with other whole systems to achieve goals to maintain and attain health for individuals, families, and communities.

King's conceptual system demonstrates structure that identifies the interrelationship between individuals and small and large groups that make up a society. These three interacting systems define the physical and social environments in which human beings function (King, 1981) (see Figure 1.1). This structure shows the interrelationships of three complex systems that make up the world in which all individuals and groups interact in their daily lives. Husting (1997) noted that the focus on relationships appears to allow response to cultural issues. Although cultural issues are not identified specifically as a line item in King's model, cultural issues are implicit variables within each of the three primary systems. For example, the values and priorities of the society will influence interpersonal groups. The cultural beliefs, roles, and behaviors of the groups will, in turn, have an impact on individuals.

In an exploration of general systems theory for nursing, concepts that consistently appeared in nursing literature, in research findings, and in speeches by nurses and that were observable in the real world of nursing practice were identified and synthesized into a conceptual system. The term *person* (human being) is the central focus for the system. The term *environment,* in both its internal and external contexts, is an essential factor in one's adaptation to life and health.

In King's conceptual system, individuals are called personal systems. Concepts identified as relevant for understanding human beings as persons are (a) self, (b) perception, (c) growth and development, (d) time, (e) personal space, and (f) coping. Several kinds of interpersonal systems exist, for example, two interacting individuals (a *dyad;* e.g., nurse–patient); three interacting individuals (*triad;* e.g., nurse–patient–physician); and various small groups of individuals (e.g., a family interacting with a nurse in a health care system). Concepts that help one understand interactions of human beings are roles such as the self in the role of a professional

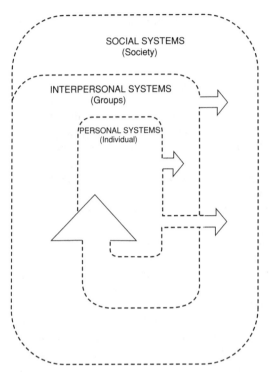

Figure 1.1. A conceptual system for nursing. (From King, I. M. (1981) *A Theory for Nursing: Systems, Concepts, Process*, p. 11. Reprinted with permission of Dr. King.)

health care provider called a nurse or the self in the role of a health care consumer called the patient or client, and concepts of communication, interaction, transaction, and stress. Groups with common interests and goals that make up a community or a society are called social systems. These systems represent the various environments within which individuals live and work. Examples of social systems are (a) family system, (b) religious or belief systems, (c) educational systems, (d) work systems, and (e) health care systems. Several concepts that provide knowledge to help nurses function in a variety of social systems are (a) organization, (b) authority, (c) power, (d) status, and (e) decision making. Age is a critical variable in all systems.

Professional nurses deal with behaviors of individuals and groups in potentially stressful situations pertaining to health, to illness and crises, and to helping individuals cope with changes in daily activities in various environments. Human beings function in social systems through interpersonal relationships in terms of their perceptions, which influence their life and health. Groups of individuals join together in a network of social relationships to achieve common goals developed about a system of values. Structural and functional characteristics, such as values, behavior patterns, prescribed roles, status, authority, and age, are found in all social systems.

An understanding of the ways that human beings interact with their environment to maintain health is essential for nurses because this enables professionals to promote health, to prevent disease, and to care for ill and disabled individuals. The goal of nursing is to help individuals maintain their health so that they can function in their roles. The domain of nursing includes promotion of health, maintenance and restoration of health, care of the sick and injured, and care of the dying. A concept of health is essential for nurses if they are expected to help individuals achieve the goal of health. "Health has been defined as dynamic life experiences of a human being, which implies continuous adjustment to stressors in the internal and external environment through optimum use of one's resources to achieve maximum potential for daily living" (King, 1981, p. 5). Health relates to the way individuals deal with the stress of growth and development while functioning within the cultural pattern in which they were born and to which they attempt to conform. Environment is mentioned throughout this systems framework. For example, King's definition of the nursing situation is "the immediate environment, spatial and temporal reality, in which nurse and client establish a relationship to cope with health states and adapt to changes in activities of daily living if the situation demands adjustment" (King, 1981, p. 2). Nursing is a dynamic system related to other systems.

King's conceptual system is one example of a basic structure not only for nursing practice but also for use in health care systems for the 21st century in a high-tech world society. This system explains "organized wholes." A theory of goal attainment has been developed from this conceptual system.

> Although personal systems and social systems influence quality of care, the major elements in a theory of goal attainment are discovered in the interpersonal systems in which two people who are usually strangers come together in a health care organization to help and to be helped to maintain a state of health that permits functioning in roles. (King, 1981, p. 142)

From the 15 concepts identified in the conceptual system, 10 were selected, and a theory of goal attainment was developed.

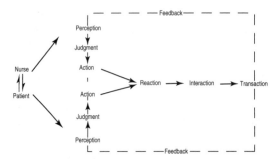

Figure 1.2. A process of human interactions that leads to transactions. (From King, I. M. (1981) *A Theory for Nursing: Systems, Concepts, Process*, p. 145. Reprinted with permission of Dr. King.)

PROCESS

A personal philosophy of human beings influenced the development of the theory of goal attainment within which a transaction process model is described (see Figure 1.2). Nursing is a process of human interactions between nurse and client whereby each perceives the other and the situation, and, through communication, they set goals, explore, and agree to the means to achieve the goals (King, 1981). The concepts selected represent essential knowledge to understand two or more persons interacting in concrete situations. These concepts are perception, communication, interaction, transaction, role, stress, and time. Communication is the informational component of human interactions. Transaction represents the valuation component of human interactions. Role knowledge is essential to understand nurse–client interactions. These concepts offer one approach to understanding the interactive process and the relation of individuals and groups in any environment (King, 1971).

The world comprises human beings who function in a variety of interpersonal systems. Nursing is a dynamic system related to other systems. The physical and social environments provide support for individuals to grow and develop as human beings and to move from a state of dependency in childhood to independence and interdependence in adulthood. The boundaries perceived in the life space of individuals give structure to their interpersonal field. Perception is the means through which individuals experience direct contact with other human beings and things in the environment. The concepts in the transaction process present a standard that describes the nature of nurse–patient interactions—namely, that nurses purposefully interact mutually with clients to set goals, explore, and agree to the means to achieve goals. The critical variable in this

Table 1.1. Comparison of nursing process theory (King, 1981) and nursing process method (Yura & Walsh, 1983)

Nursing Process Theory (King)	Nursing Process Method (Yura & Walsh)
A System of Interrelated Concepts	A System of Interrelated Action
Perception	Assess
Communication	Nursing Diagnosis
Interaction	Plan
Transaction	Implement
Goal Attainment	Evaluate

transaction process is *mutual goal setting.* The concepts in this process—perception, communication, interaction, transaction, and role—represent theoretical knowledge that should be used to implement the nursing process method (Yura & Walsh, 1983) (see Table 1.1). The concepts of perception, communication, and interaction are used to assess clients, a nursing diagnosis (NANDA) is made, and transactions represent a plan and its implementation (interventions; NIC), evaluation highlights the goals achieved or determines why they were not achieved. Goal achievement is a category of outcomes.

OUTCOME

Process criteria are the focus of nursing actions that lead to outcomes. King's transaction process presents a set of concepts that identify theoretical knowledge to implement actions described in the nursing process, which is a standard method used internationally. When nurses gather information from the assessment of individuals, they use NANDA to make a nursing diagnosis. From the data and information, nurses design a plan of care and use knowledge from NIC to implement the plan. The transaction process is used mutually to set goals, explore, and agree to means to implement the plan. Evaluation of the plan indicates whether the goals set were achieved. In most instances, goals mutually set are attained, and this represents outcomes (NOC). Outcomes not only demonstrate effective nursing care but also evidence-based practice. When goals are noted in the client's record, the information provides continuous data for research.

King's law of human interaction states that two or more human beings in mutual presence, face-to-face or via technology, interacting purposefully, make transactions in real-world nursing situations that lead to goal attainment, which represent outcomes. Outcomes provide evidence-based nursing practice.

SUMMARY

In any discussion of the nature of nursing, the central theme revolves around human beings and their physical and social environments, with the goal of health. Although personal and social systems influence the quality of health care, the major elements in the theory of goal attainment are identified in the interpersonal systems in which two persons, usually strangers, come together in a health care system to help or be helped to maintain or regain a state of health that permits one to function in role. The transaction process, designed within the theory of goal attainment, identifies a critical variable—mutual goal setting—that leads to outcomes in human interactions.

In the information-processing world of the 21st century, systems have been designed to provide access to data, information, and knowledge for nurses to use. Unifying languages such as classification systems, conceptual systems, and theories provide information, data, and knowledge. One approach in the organization and management of systems such as nursing and health care has revolved around structure, process, and outcome. King's conceptual system was presented in this chapter as one example of structure for nursing and health care systems. The basic concepts of the system are individual human beings interacting in various environments that help them to maintain health. Basic concepts in the transaction process provide a process that leads to goal attainment. Use of the process leads to outcomes that represent evidence-based practice.

REFERENCES

Graves, J., & Corcoran, S. (1989). The study of nursing informatics. *Image: The Journal of Nursing Scholarship, 21*, 227–231.

Howland, D. (1976). An adaptive health system model. In H. Werley, A. Zuzich, M. Zajkowski, & D. Zagornik (Eds.), *Health research: The systems approach* (pp. 109–122). New York: Springer Publishing Company.

Husting, P. (1997). A transcultural critique of Imogene King's theory of goal attainment. *Journal of Multicultural Nursing and Health, 3*(3), 15–21.

King, I. M. (1971). *Toward a theory for nursing.* New York: Wiley.

King, I. M. (1981). *A theory for nursing: Systems, concepts, process.* New York: Wiley.

King, I. M. (1997). King's theory of goal attainment for research and practice. *Nursing Science Quarterly, 9*, 61–66.

Martin, R. S. (1996). The Omaha system: A model for describing holistic nursing practice. *Holistic Nursing Practice, 11*, 75–83.

McCloskey-Dochterman, J., & Jones, D. (Eds.). (2003). *Unifying nursing language: The harmonizing of NANDA, NIC, and NOC.* Washington, DC: Nursing Books.

Ozbolt, J. (1993). *Nursing informatics: Enhancing patient care: A report for the NCNR priority expert panel on nursing informatics.* Bethesda, MD: U.S. Department of Health and Human Services.

Saba, V. K. (1992). Home health care classification. *Caring, 11*(5), 58–60.

Von Bertalanffy, L. (1968). *General systems theory.* New York: Brazilier.

Wiener, N. (1967). *The human use of human beings.* New York: Avon.

Yura, H., & Walsh, M. (1983). *The nursing process.* Norwalk, CT: Appleton-Century-Crofts.

CHAPTER TWO

The Nursing Act Is an Excellent Human Act

A Philosophical Analysis Derived From Classical Philosophy and the Conceptual System and Theory of Imogene King

Beverly J. B. Whelton

This chapter values Imogene King's conceptual system and theory of goal attainment for their historical depth. The 2,000-year-old tradition of Greek philosophy is significant external validation of King's work. Whelton (1996, 1999b, 2000) previously showed that King was grounded in the Aristotelian–Thomistic, realist perspective on nature, knowledge, and humanity. In personal conversation (October 29, 1996) and at the Philosophy in the Nurses World Biannual Conference in Banff, Canada (May 11, 1999), King affirmed that she studied the philosophy of St. Thomas Aquinas as an undergraduate at St. Louis University and that this view of humanity was at the core of the personal system. Without elaborating on the origin of her ideas, King (1971) had simply said, "Man, the human organism, is the central focus for the framework" (p. 24).

Aquinas is the 13th-century philosopher whose commentaries made Aristotelian philosophy accessible to the European West after recovery of Aristotle's original manuscripts in the Middle East, where they were preserved after the fall of the Roman Empire. Although King studied Aristotle through the eyes of Aquinas, the Christian focus of Medieval Europe has faded. Thus, this chapter returns to the work of Aristotle, the third-century B.C. pagan philosopher who more easily speaks to today's multicultural community. William A. Wallace (1996) updated the Aristotelian–Thomistic perspective of the human person with the findings of contemporary science. Insight into Wallace will allow us to complete King's personal system with a description of the capacities of the individual, the core of King's conceptual framework (Whelton, 1999b).

After each summary overview of Aristotelian–Thomistic philosophical realism (*Nature and Knowledge* and *Human Nature and Human Action*), this chapter turns to consider how King wove this traditional wisdom into a foundation for nursing theory and practice. The chapter also extends King's work by an analysis of the nursing act, revealing that it is an excellent human act. King's early text, *Toward a Theory for Nursing: General Concepts of Human Behavior* (1971), anticipated this philosophical exposition of the nursing act by referencing *"human acts, the behavior of individuals," "purposeful action* implies that an individual has control over and is responsible for the events," and *"nursing acts* are goal-directed toward health" (p. 90). This chapter uses human behavior for the broadest level of human actions. Human acts are what King called purposeful actions. Actions are described by King as "*a sequence of behaviors of interacting persons which includes (1) recognition of presenting conditions; (2) operations or activities related to the condition or situation; and (3) motivation to exert some control over the events to achieve goals*" (italics in original, p. 90). As recently as 2004, King expressed regret that she was unable to do an exposition of human action and the nursing act (personal communication, February 24, 2004).

In *A Theory for Nursing: Systems, Concepts, Processes* (1981), King wrote, "In the hospital, the nurse brings self to the role. The nurse also brings special knowledge, skills, and professional values to provide nursing care for the patients" (p. 3). In this way, nursing is the healing action of one coming into the presence of a person in need with the knowledge, skills and values of a nurse. It is suggested that the nursing act is a healing act at the heart of King's interpersonal system.

The nursing act is a class of excellent human actions called healing acts in this chapter. The healing act is a moment of communication in the interpersonal space between two persons. They both are enriched and aided in their life's journey by this moment. The recipients of nursing receive the care they need, and the nurse is affirmed in his or her vocation as nurse. This reciprocity of human action is described in *Person and Being* (Clarke, 1993).

What is provided in the later portion of this chapter is this philosophical description of nursing as a healing moment between the recipient of nursing care and the nurse. Although the discipline of nursing includes multiple complex sets of activities, it is believed there is an identifiable interpersonal healing phenomenon that emerges between nurse and patient. This temporarily exaggerated view of nursing as the nursing act will facilitate a foundational understanding of nursing within King's interpersonal system.

This chapter is divided into two parts. The first provides the Aristotelian philosophical foundations of King's conceptual system and theory of goal attainment. The other is an original extension of King's work to consider the nursing act within a typology of human behavior. This is a magnified look at a moment within nursing that has implications for what it means to be a nurse.

I. PHILOSOPHICAL FOUNDATIONS

This first section provides a description of the Aristotelian–Thomistic view of nature and knowledge. From nature and knowing, the chapter moves to a discussion of human nature and human actions to build a foundation within which one can understand the philosophical depth of King's conceptual system and theory.

Nature and Knowledge

The worldview that King adopts (realism) holds that items and events in the external world have shared content that makes them capable of being known beyond the empirical data associated with them (Aristotle, 1941c, 1941d). This intelligible content can be grasped by the human intellect as concepts. This capacity to grasp the world in a universal way is part of what it means to be human. As a result of (a) particular individual items having shared content that unites them as being of the same kind and (b) the human capacity to grasp this sameness in a universal way, concepts bear a direct relationship to the world outside the mind. Once these concepts are abstracted from particular items or experiences, they can be used to identify and understand similar things, persons, or events. When fully grasped by the intellect, concepts can be used to state something true about the extramental world of experience (Wallace, 1996).

In addition to the intelligibility of the world and the intellectual acquisition of concepts about the world, the realist holds that reason can form verifiable statements that can be checked against the extramental world to judge whether the attribution of predicate(s) to the subject(s) has been accurate (Aristotle, 1941c; Wallace 1996). Because concepts, and thus statements, may be expressed either verbally or mathematically, research methodology may be either qualitative or quantitative depending on the question and the subject being investigated. Insight into effects and their causal sources allows for either verification or falsification of hypotheses. The critical issue for a realist is that the actual extramental existent world forms the basis of judgments about human experiences of the world.

Thus, theory statements are informative when founded on this extramental world. In 1971, King wrote, "theoretical models organize sets of concepts that are related and provide methodology for gathering information that is essential for decision making in nursing" (p. 120). Concepts are grasped from the shared content in the world that can then be used to describe other similar items or experiences. The relationships among things in the world give rise to the relationships among concepts.

This account asserts that King's theory of goal attainment expresses something real about the world that can be confirmed by research. Although respecting individual responses to events, this perspective prevents one from asserting that everything is subjective and relative. An individual's experience is always truly his or her experience (subjective reality), but the truth and falsity of a statement about the world outside of the individual can be checked to see whether it matches with what actually happened (objective reality). For the realist, the world outside the mind is the standard of truth and falsity, rather than the individual or a consensus of individuals. King's theory can be validated as grounded in human life—that is, something real that is shared among humans. This shared human form, or human nature, can be known as that which gives rise to characteristically human actions, such as the attainment of conceptual knowledge and having the freedom to choose based on that knowledge. Because there is something that it is to be a human, there can be moral and practice standards based on needs and the meaning of human life (Whelton, 2002a, 2002b).

Within King's perspective, the clinical nurse interviewing a patient will confirm with that patient what he or she intended to communicate with verbal and nonverbal behaviors. This confirmation is not done simply because the manual says to do so but because the patient in the extramental world gives rise to the nurse's interpretation and is thus the source for confirming that interpretation.

Additionally, although humans are individuals with insight into nature, we each remain hidden in our desires and ideas unless we choose to share these through verbal or nonverbal communications. This leads to King's emphasis on listening and perception. King wrote, "Health professionals have a responsibility to gather relevant information about the perceptions of the client so that their goals and the goals of the client are congruent" (1981, p. 144). In this simple sketch, the patient's intent and behavioral responses are the standard for evaluation of the nurses' clinical judgment. This means that although the nurse's feelings are an important part of assessments and interactions, they are not determinate of nursing behavior. Professional interventions are determined by knowledge of principles related to human life in health and illness (King's personal system), communication (King's interpersonal system), and society (King's social system) as well as the specific information of individual circumstances.

As an Aristotelian–Thomistic realist, King has suggested that patients, family members, nurses, and all health care providers, in fact, all humans hold in common that which makes them human: human nature. The intellect has the capacity to grasp concepts from this shared reality and form propositions that can be tested as true or false. Because there is something that it is to be human, the way humans ought to be treated, morally or clinically, arises from an understanding of humanity.

Human Nature and Human Action

The Aristotelian–Thomistic tradition holds that items in nature can be known as they really are because individuals are a unified composite of materials (that out of which they are made) and energizing forms (that which makes them be what they are). Matter accounts for the concrete individual, whereas form accounts for all individuals of the same kind being what they are as tree, cow, or human. In living things, form is energizing. It is the form of the tree that powers the transitions from acorn to sapling to oak. Scientists can construct a kernel of corn by replicating DNA structures and cellular components, but the corn does not germinate. This artificial corn has the form of corn as shape and structure but not the energizing principle of life that is required for growth. This internal actualizing principle is also called nature and is the source of activity and rest, giving rise to characteristic properties that allow us to identify individuals as a kind of being or person. An entity has this internal principle of activity and rest the moment it comes into existence. The moment its genome activates, the individual begins making proteins and mRNA specific to what it is. For humans, this embryonic genome activation occurs after two cleavages of the zygote, at the four-cell stage. From that moment the embryo makes human proteins, giving rise to the knowledge that it is human because something is as it behaves (Aristotle, 1941c; Whelton, 1998, 1999a).

It is this shared actualizing unifying form that is grasped by the intellect as the concept. This concept may be of tree, dog, or human or of a state of being, such as being beautiful or in pain. Knowledge of our world is achieved when the intellect grasps this actualizing form or nature as it is, the state of affairs. Nature, as in the phrase *human nature*, refers to this form shared by all humans that makes them human and recognizable as human and with which we interact to form a concept of human (Wallace, 1996; Whelton, 1996, 2002a, 2002b)

As a part of the natural world, humans share with plants and animals the bodily activities characteristic of living things: nutrition, growth and development, reproduction, and dynamic interactions with the environment. To interact effectively in the world as mobile, humans share with all animals capacities for sensation and perception. Sensation is the receipt of stimuli through the five outer senses. Perception, in this technical sense, includes coordination of sensations into an image, comparing that image with past experience, and using imagination to complete missing details. This sensory knowledge is concerned with the immediate environment and is critical to an animal's ability to solve problems.

Human nature entails intellectual capacities that go beyond the particulars of the environment to a grasp of the universal, immaterial concepts spoken of earlier. Whereas sensitive animals experience fear, humans experience fear and also consider what fear is and what it means to be afraid. These immaterial concepts make reasoning and language possible.

Having concepts and language is not enough, however. To navigate the world of human society, one must also choose to speak and to act. This capacity of choosing is the will, the appetite of the intellect. The will chooses from among options provided by the intellect, which means one has to know what his or her options are. This requires information, highlighting the role of nursing in health education. Additionally, as the advertising industry shows, having knowledge generates an appetite or desire for the known.

Choosing well requires both knowledge and a habit of careful reasoning. In addition, acting well requires the excellent habits called virtues. Patterns of reasoning include the logic of inquiry and proof, techniques of art, and the deliberations characteristic of practical life and practice disciplines (Aristotle, 1941b). These ideas about humanity led King (1981) to state that "Individuals are characterized as social beings who are rational and sentient" (p. 19). In 1971, she had written, "nursing involves thinking, relating, judging, and acting relative to the health status manifested in the behavior of individuals and groups" (p. 97). Further, "nurses, who structure communication and information, tend to guide individuals to recognize their health needs, to express their feelings about meeting them, and to share in decisions about the means and the goals to be achieved" (p. 99).

King operationalized within a nursing context what Aristotle taught about being human. Passages expressing the importance of empowering patients to make decisions and participate in mutual goal setting reflect the uniquely human capacity of conceptual knowledge and the capacity of making choices based on that knowledge.

Mobility, appetites, and many emotions are shared with other animals. However, the desire for knowledge and goodness (excellent living) are uniquely human as appetites of the intellect. These are capacities of the will. Human freedom is making choices based on knowledge of situations and principles or laws within the situations. Without knowledge, there is no real freedom. The capacity for shared knowledge, requiring immaterial concepts and language, is unique to human life.

An action based on emotion or appetite is voluntary, the individual is still responsible for what was done, but the behavior was not freely chosen unless the person decided earlier to follow emotion or appetite. In the face of strong emotion, principles that normally guide an individual's action can fade. Intense feelings tend to cloud the intellect (Aristotle, 1941b). This distinction guides the courts to distinguish between manslaughter and first-degree murder. It is also important in issues of informed consent. An individual confronted with a fear-filled situation has difficulty making a decision. To obtain informed consent, one must first support the individual and reduce anxiety so information can be processed and a reasoned decision can be made. One must also assess individuals' ability to learn and participate in their care, given their perception of stressors in their present environment (King, 1981). Simply reacting to a situation or desire is very different from responding and choosing an action based on knowledge.

A treatment plan with mutually set goals respects the humanity and, thus, the inherent dignity of the human person (Whelton, 1996, 1999b). In 1971, King wrote, "nursing practice at its best is based on an understanding of man [humans], from conception to old age, in health and in illness" (p. 1). In 1981, she wrote, "a basic assumption is made that the focus of nursing is the care of human beings" (p. 10). As a student of human nature, King recognized that human action requires knowledge and freedom: "health professionals have a responsibility to share information that helps individuals make informed decisions about their health" (King, 1981, p. 144). Notice that the caregiver has the responsibility to share knowledge with the client and to develop options in a treatment plan with the client. This mutuality of knowledge and shared vision is critical for therapeutic transactions in King's theory of goal attainment. In 1981, King wrote, "working together they [the nurse and patient] experience a new kind of relationship in the health care system, one in which the patient is recognized as having a part in making decisions that affect him now and in the future and is recognized as a person whose participation gives him some independence and control in the situation" (p. 86).

Human Action and Human Excellence

Human responses go beyond interaction with the physical environment because the intellect has the capacity to reason to new ideas from known concepts. Concepts may originate from within the physical world, but they may also be totally immaterial, such as kindness, culture, spirit, charity, goodness, and hope. Humans can contemplate life, existence, self, thought, and even a Supreme Being. For Aristotle, the highest human activity was contemplation that brought insight into the universe. Inner peace and happiness accompany this contemplative state.

Aristotle emphasized that the integrity of the individual is the intimate union of body (materials) and soul (energizing principle of nature, the form) from the beginning of life through to death. Yet for him this capacity to reflect on immaterial thought was evidence of the spiritual nature of the human soul and the potential of existence after death (1941b, 1941c).

Anything that is living requires homeostatic environmental interactions—food and energy conversions, cell differentiation and growth. Being healthy means more than being alive. Health goes beyond the proper functioning of the organ systems that allow an individual to live to the well working of the organism as a whole. In addition to a well-working body, the excellence that is human health requires the proper use of intellect and will, that is, concept formation, judgment, reasoning, and the intellectual and moral virtues (Aristotle, 1941b; Wallace, 1996; Whelton, 1996, 1999b). In this understanding of health, being healthy requires the development of virtuous habits of acting and being. The virtues of the intellect are science, practical reason, and good judgment (Aristotle, 1941a, 1941b).

Social and spiritual health, involving the will, requires the development of good judgment in making decisions about actions (wisdom) and the moral virtues to follow through with decisions made. Moral virtues include justice to guide one's relationships with others; courage to control the dramatic emotions such as fear, rage, and lust; and moderation to curb the appetites for food and drink. For Aristotle, one could not lead a happy life without virtue. Human excellence was moral excellence.

II. THE MORAL ACT, THE HEALING ACT, THE NURSING ACT

Overview

If one were to use a set of circles to develop a typology of human actions (see Figure 2.1), the outer sphere that incorporates all the others would represent all human behaviors, the conscious and unconscious biological,

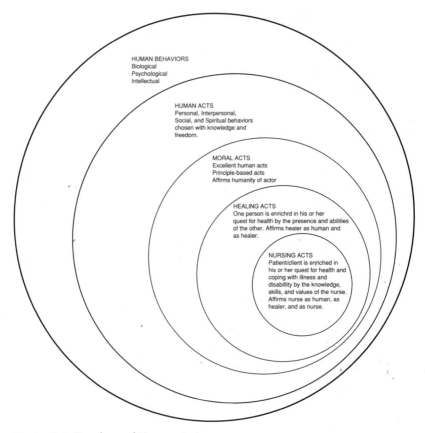

HUMAN BEHAVIORS
Biological
Psychological
Intellectual

HUMAN ACTS
Personal, Interpersonal,
Social, and Spiritual behaviors
chosen with knowledge and
freedom.

MORAL ACTS
Excellent human acts
Principle-based acts
Affirms humanity of actor

HEALING ACTS
One person is enrichrd in his or her
quest for health by the presence and abilities
of the other. Affirms healer as human and
as healer.

NURSING ACTS
Patient/client is enriched in
his or her quest for health and
coping with illness and
disabillity by the knowledge,
skills, and values of the nurse.
Affirms nurse as human, as
healer, and as nurse.

Figure 2.1. Typology of Human Action.

psychological, and intellectual actions and responses that continue from
the beginning to the end of life. Inside human behaviors, as a portion
of them, would be those personal, interpersonal, social, and spiritual behaviors chosen with knowledge and freedom. These uniquely human behaviors requiring knowledge of the world, personal insight, and choice
based on that knowledge are human acts. Inside human acts would be the
excellent principle-based human actions called moral acts, performed as
good for the recipient and as the actor's own good. They affirm the acting
person in their humanity.

Among the multiple moral acts that can be performed is the healing
act. In this healing moment, one person is enriched in his or her quest
for health by the presence, skills, and abilities of the other. The healing
act affirms the healer as human and as healer. Among all of the activities
that fall within the responsibilities of nurses is the potential for nurses to

be healers. This aspect of nursing care recalls the therapeutic use of self (Travelbee, 1969). Thus, within the domain of healing acts is the nursing act in which the patient or client is enriched in his or her quest for health and coping with illness and disability by the nurse's knowledge, skills, and values. Nursing acts affirm the nurse as human, as healer, and as nurse.

The Moral Act

In the foregoing brief analysis, human acts are contrasted with behaviors humans do such as eating, breathing, sleeping, and walking. Although human behaviors are usually within King's personal system, human actions usually become interpersonal. Human acts require knowledge, freedom, and, in some cases, enough discipline to place this chosen action ahead of personal desire. Human excellence is based in discerning the best action to be done in a situation, deciding to take that action, and having the discipline actually to do that chosen good action. This excellent human act is a moral act, a principle-based action performed as good for another and as the agent's own good (Sokolowski, 1989). Thus, what I do that is good for you is, in fact, good for me. In this context, *good* means the action moves the individual toward his or her proper end, living the fullness of a healthy human life.

Speaking of virtue or discipline opposes the contemporary position that the world is value-neutral and that all preferences are equally valid. Aristotle asserted that there is something it means to be a human and to live this excellent human life. If this is true, and King thought it was, then one can identify kinds of human actions that lead to inner peace and happiness, to human flourishing. These actions that promote the proper human end were summarized by Aquinas as preserving human life, educating the young, and living in peace (Pegis, 1948).

The Healing Act as Moral Act

As emerging from the humanity of the practitioner, the healing act is a human act. The healing act is also a moral act requiring that one be disposed to see the good to be done and have the discipline to do it. The healing act is an interpersonal interaction that focuses directly on the individual patient's well-being. As a healing moment, the healing act is good in itself, valuable here and now, but the action also points beyond itself toward the end of health for this individual and to the fulfillment of the professional as healer. In his treatment of ethics, Aristotle (1941b) taught that moral action is good in itself as the right thing to do, in its outcomes toward the recipient of the action and its impact on the one acting. Acting virtuously makes one virtuous.

Robert Sokolowski (1989), in his analysis *The Moral Act: A Phenomenological Study*, stressed the interpersonal character of moral action. A moral act is an interaction in which another's good becomes my good in the given circumstances. It is essential, however, that the actor be disposed to see both the truth of the need and his or her responsibility to act. The actor must also have the virtue to do what is now known to be required as the moral action, fulfilling the good of the other. It is experienced as the actor's own good.

One of Sokolowski's important insights is the reflexivity of the moral act. Morality is not just giving of oneself. When one acts for another's good, it is also good for the actor.

The Nursing Act as Moral Excellence

The nursing act is within but distinct from the multiple behaviors requiring the knowledge, skills, and values characteristic of nursing. The whole nursing process is carried out with the intent to bring about, improve, maintain, or restore health of individuals, families, and social systems. Within this process, however, are unique interpersonal exchanges that in themselves enrich and enhance the patient and the nurse. These healing moments are called the nursing act.

The following was written in a course paper about the nursing act: "the nursing act is the nurse acting for the good of the patient as his or her good for the patient" (Whelton, 1986). Sokolowski crossed through "for the patient." Thinking about this puzzling change leads one to see that if nurses act only for the good of the patient, they will feel drained by their practice. They are apt to experience burnout. My good for the other must also be good for me as the fulfillment of who I am.

If the nursing act is a specification of the healing act, which is a moral act, as here proposed, it is an excellence, the fulfillment of oneself as human as well as the fulfillment of oneself as healer and nurse. When actions done for the good of the other—in this case, for the other's health—are also good for the nurse because they fulfill who the person is as nurse, the nurse is energized rather than fatigued. At the end of the day, nurses may be physically exhausted, but when their actions have expressed who they are, there will also be an energized satisfaction, even joy, at having served well.

The synthesis of being and acting found in the healing act is seen in Sokolowski's (1985) description of medicine and the physician:

> Because the art of medicine aims at something that is a good for the patient, the doctor, in the exercise of his art, seeks the medical good of the patient as his own good.... The nature of his art, with the perspectives

it provides on the medical good, gives the physician this harmony, and it makes him, in the good exercise of his art, not only a good doctor but also essentially a good moral agent, one who seeks the good of another formally as his own. The doctor's profession essentially makes him a good man, provided he is true to his art and follows its insistence. (p. 269)

This virtuous formation of the physician as the profession making him or her a good person need not be unique to medicine. Nurses who are true to the good practice of nursing also become, by the demands of the profession, good persons. For nursing we can paraphrase: because the art of nursing aims at something that is a good for the patient, the nurse, in the exercise of his or her art, seeks the nursing good of the patient as his or her own good.... The nature of nursing art, with the perspectives it provides on the nursing good, gives the nursing practitioner this harmony of being and doing, and it makes him or her, in the good exercise of nursing art, not only a good nurse but also essentially a good moral agent, one who seeks the good of another formally as his or her own. In this way, the nurse's profession essentially makes a person good, provided the nurse is true to his or her art and follows its insistence.

Of nursing acts, King (1971) wrote:

> Nursing acts are goal-directed toward health and can be observed as a process of interaction between nurses and clients in specific situations; they may be influenced by the situation and by interaction with the family, the physician, and other persons and events ... [Nursing] action is a sequence of behaviors of *interacting persons* which includes (1) recognition of presenting conditions; (2) operations or activities related to the condition or situation; and (3) motivation to exert some control over the events to achieve goals. (p. 90; italics added)

Notice the phrase *interacting persons*. This designates that nursing is within the interpersonal system. It also highlights that both the nurse and patient or client are persons, making humanity—and thus, human actions—foundational to nursing practice.

Nursing activities are not the nursing act but the opportunity for it. Activities performed by a nurse are not nursing acts unless there is a human transaction in which the nurse and patient connect person to person. As the nurse acts toward formation or fulfillment of mutually set goals, the healing moment becomes fulfillment of the nurse as nurse, not as technician, moneymaker, or manager. The skeptic and naysayer claim the nurse was just performing a skill to fulfill the role description and make money. This reduces the nurse to a mechanic and the human person to a body, a machine in need of repair. This is a disservice to them both.

Health Care Is Healing

In all its complexity, health care is about healing. The healing agent is the person who gives of him or herself to the patient as the agent's own good. In acting for the good of the patient as the agent's own good, the agent enriches and fulfills the meaning of being a healer, a provider of "health" and "care" in their richest sense. The kind of professional practitioner one is and one's presentation of self as that professional enables the patient to be a client of that discipline, be it nursing, physical therapy, dentistry, or medicine, to name only a few of the health care professions.

Ideally, this unity of being and doing is achieved; however, this is one of the tensions in health care when it is managed as a business rather than a human service. If a nurse or other practitioner is acting only for his or her own benefit, it is still a human action chosen with knowledge of what is involved, but it is not a healing act. The healing in this case is incidental. Health is a side effect rather than an end. This may be a part of the emptiness that patients and staff feel when health care providers are on the job only to earn money. This perspective is evident in the emotional distance maintained and the disinterested services provided.

Clearly, much of the health care enterprise does not fall within the conception of the healing act and the nursing act presented in this chapter. Many interventions are removing impediments or making a way for nature to restore itself within the patient. Personal healing interactions may not be required, or patients get better despite their absence.

A number of activities of health care providers are not directly related to healing. In addition to managing human resources, there is much technology to manage and there are businesses to run. These are intended for the end of health; but in themselves, they do not heal. They are maintaining the health care establishment.

The paradigm of health care is in the moment when the nurse or other health care professional interacts in a significant way specifically for the good health of the patient, and this transaction is the good fulfillment of the individual professional as healer.

Health care is a uniquely human activity required by the vulnerability of humans to disease, injury, and other illness states. It is also made possible by human capacities to reason beyond current experience to new knowledge and new opportunities. According to the physician and ethicist Edmund Pellegrino (2001), this vulnerability of the patient and the physician's knowledge and abilities impose on the physician a duty to heal. It is the basis of the physician–patient relationship. In this relationship, one member is vulnerable because of illness or injury (be that physical, intellectual, spiritual, or emotional). This infirmity leads the one person to be receptive to what the other has to give of the self and of his or her knowledge and skills. As a healing profession, the same is true of nursing and nurse–patient relationships. Clearly, the healing that is the core of the nurse–patient relationship is not exclusive to nursing or medicine or even to the healing professions. The use practitioners make of their knowledge and experience makes the difference in whether the patient is a patient of nursing, physical therapy, or medicine (King, 1971).

It is commonly said that bartenders are the best therapists. They are an informal healer, if what is needed is a listening ear and someone who acknowledges the personal pain of the patron. (Of course, the difficulty with this scenario is the mix with alcohol can generate more pain rather than healing.) Another setting is the nurturance of maternal caring. A nurturing mother detects her child's need as an opportunity to give of herself for the child's good, and this is the fulfillment of herself as person and as mother. King (1981) used this maternal example to express the mutual benefit in nursing interactions. Sometimes the chaplain is the most important healer, resolving conflicts and strengthening the individual so that his or her energy can be focused on becoming healthy again or living peacefully until death occurs.

These healing actions are unique interpersonal transactions. They are not acts of friendship. They are not actions among equals, and there is not a mutual sharing of stories; one person needs to have the capacity to meet the need of the other. Pellegrino (2001) had noted that need becomes vulnerability in the recipient, and the capacity to meet this need awakens responsibility in the healer and is also a source of power. This power differential is an inequality in the relationship. However, not all aspects of the caregiver–patient relationship and not all behaviors of health care providers are healing actions. The healing actions we are considering are unique interpersonal transactions epitomized by moments of intense exchange in which the patient is energized toward health and the caregiver is energized and affirmed in his or her vocation as healer.

Nursing as a Moral Art

According to Aristotle (1941c) in the *Nicomachean Ethics*, the best in human living, that is, moral action, requires that one do the right action, at the right time, for the right reasons, toward the right person, in the right way. A virtuous upbringing is required to fulfill these five aspects of every virtuous action. Today, nearly 25 centuries later, everyone educated as a health care professional has been trained in these five "rights." They came to my attention in medication administration: the right medication, at the right time, for the right patient, by the right route, in the right amount. As a nurse, I have a moral and legal obligation to fulfill them.

The art of nursing is the skillful, experienced application of nursing knowledge within particular nursing situations (Blondeau, 2002). Practitioners require good judgment (wisdom) in the use of principles acquired from learning the accepted body of knowledge. These principles are used in the composition of interventions toward reaching the end state of health. Nursing principles may be acquired from speculative, productive, and practical disciplines or from primary research within the discipline itself. Research inquiring into principles from other disciplines, such as cellular biology, appropriates these principles into the organized body of nursing knowledge, but only if their explanatory and prescriptive value within nursing is confirmed (Whelton, 2002a).

A professional nurse has available the body of knowledge learned as disciplinary science. In a particular patient interaction, principles are selected, applied, and even modified to compose a response to intervene in the patient situation. This composition of a healing situation is the practitioner's art. The healing art of nursing practice is the nurse seeing and meeting the needs of the individual as the nurse's good for this patient in this situation. This interpersonal interaction is the setting within which the nursing act occurs. The nursing act, as a healing act, is a moral transaction grounded in the humanity of both nurse and patient, and the professional nurse's good practice.

If the nursing act carries the attributes and responsibilities of a moral act, there are significant implications for understanding effective health care interventions as requiring the practitioner to be virtuously disposed toward the patient's good in order to grasp both the principles and particulars in a situation requiring intervention. Without a virtuous disposition, an individual would not see the good of the other as his or her own good, bringing self-fulfillment as an individual and as a practitioner. This interpersonal core makes the practice of the nurse professional a moral art and makes nursing science a practical science.

CONCLUSION

This chapter has provided the Aristotelian–Thomistic foundation of King's philosophical perspectives. Human nature is at the core of King's personal system and is the source of human actions within the interpersonal system between nurse and patient. Nursing was acknowledged here as multifaceted, but in the healing moment called the nursing act, nursing is a human excellence requiring virtue. Virtue is required to perceive the good of the patient as a desirable good. If they strive to be healers, nurses must practice nursing as who they are rather than as what they do.

Nursing is the healing act of one person with the knowledge, skills, and values of a nurse coming into the presence of a person in need.'

The significance of seeing the nursing act as a moral act is the requirement of virtue to see the good end of the patient's health as one's own good. There is also a requirement for virtue in decision making and action. The healing act is a moment of communication in the interpersonal space between two persons. They both are enriched and aided in their life's journey by this moment. The recipients of nursing receive the care they need, and the nurse is affirmed and fulfilled in his or her vocation as nurse. This chapter ends with the words of King (1971): "In conclusion, it is the nurses who weave human skills, technical equipment, and administrative structure into a unified approach for delivering nursing and health care within the social systems" (p. 63).

ACKNOWLEDGMENTS

This research is part of a larger project funded by a 2004 West Virginia Humanities Council Summer Fellowship.

REFERENCES

Aristotle. (1941a). *Metaphysics*. In R. McKeon (Ed.), *The basic works of Aristotle* (pp. 689–926). New York: Random House.

Aristotle. (1941b). *Nicomachean ethics*. In R. McKeon (Ed.), *The basic works of Aristotle* (pp. 935–1112). New York: Random House.

Aristotle. (1941c). *On the soul*. In R. McKeon (Ed.), *The basic works of Aristotle* (pp. 535–603). New York: Random House.

Aristotle. (1941d). *Physics*. In R. McKeon (Ed.), *The basic works of Aristotle* (pp. 217–394). New York: Random House.

Blondeau, D. (2002). Nursing art as a practical art: The necessary relationship between nursing art and nursing ethics. *Nursing Philosophy, 3*, 252–259.

Clarke, W. N. (1993). *Person and being*. Milwaukee, WI: Marquette University Press.

King, I. M. (1971). *Toward a theory for nursing: General concepts of human behavior*. New York: Wiley.

King, I. M. (1981). *A theory for nursing: Systems, concepts, processes*. New York: Wiley.

Pegis, A. C. (1948). *Introduction to Saint Thomas Aquinas*. New York: Random House.

Pellegrino, E. (2001). The internal morality of clinical medicine: A paradigm for the ethics of the helping and healing professions. *Journal of Medicine and Philosophy, 26*, 559–579.

Sokolowski, R. (1985). *The moral act: A phenomenological study*. Bloomington: Indiana University Press.

Sokolowski, R. (1989). The art and science of medicine. In E. D. Pellegrino, J. P. Langan, & J. C. Harvey (Eds.), *Catholic perspectives on medical morals: Foundational issues* (pp. 263–275). Dordrecht, The Netherlands: Kluwer Academic.

Travelbee, J. (1969). *Intervention in psychiatric nursing: Process in the one-to-one relationship*. Philadelphia: Davis.

Wallace, W. A. (1996). *The modeling of nature: Philosophy of science and philosophy of nature in synthesis*. Washington, DC: Catholic University of America Press.

Whelton, B. J. (1986). The nursing act. Unpublished course paper. The Catholic University of America.

Whelton, B. J. B. (1996). A philosophy of nursing practice: An application of the Thomistic–Aristotelian concept of nature to the science of nursing (Doctoral dissertation, Catholic University of America, Washington, DC). *Dissertation Abstracts International*, A57103, 1176.

Whelton, B. J. B. (1998). On the beginning of human life. *Linacre Quarterly, 65*, 51–65.

Whelton, B. J. B. (1999a). Human nature, substantial change, and modern science: Rethinking when a new human life begins. *Proceedings of The American Catholic Philosophical Association*, LXXII, 305–313.

Whelton, B. J. B. (1999b). The philosophical core of Imogene King's behavioral system. *Nursing Science Quarterly, 12*(2), 158–163.

Whelton, B. J. B. (2000). Nursing as a practical science: Some insights from classical Aristotelian science. *Nursing Philosophy, 1*(1), 57–63.

Whelton, B. J. B. (2002a). Human nature as a source of practical truth: Aristotelian-Thomistic realism and the practical science of nursing. *Nursing Philosophy, 3*(1), 35–46.

Whelton, B. J. B. (2002b). Human life as a foundation for ethical health-care decisions: A synthesis of the work of E. D. Pellegrino and W. A. Wallace. *Linacre Quarterly, 69*(4), 271–299.

PART II

Middle Range Theories

King's Conceptual System and Family Health Theory in the Families of Adults With Persistent Mental Illnesses—An Evolving Conceptualization

Mary Molewyk Doornbos

The New Freedom Commission on Mental Health (2003) estimated that in any given year, 5% to 7% of U.S. adults have serious, diagnosable mental illnesses. Of that number, approximately 2.2 million have schizophrenia, and another 2.3 million have bipolar disorder (National Institute of Mental Health, 2001). The President's New Freedom Commission issued an interim report in October of 2002 stating that "America's mental health service delivery system is in shambles ... and it is often impossible for families and consumers to find the care that they urgently need" (cover letter, p. 1) The final report of this commission, issued in July 2003, supported this initial contention as well and asserted "the system presents barriers that all too often add to the burden of mental illnesses for individuals, their families and our communities" (cover letter, p. 1).

The burden experienced by the families of those who struggle with persistent mental illnesses has been well documented over the past 3 decades (Rose, Mallinson, & Walton-Moss, 2002). Family burden is multifaceted and includes, in part, the need to coordinate and provide care on an ongoing basis, respond to the actual symptoms of the illness, process personal emotional reactions brought about by the mental illness of a member, and endure the stigmatizing reactions of others (Crisp, Gelder, Rix, Meltzer, & Rowland, 2000; Doornbos, 2001a; Saunders, 2003; Saunders & Byrne, 2002). It seems apparent, then, that as families valiantly attempt to engage in caregiving for a loved one with a persistent mental illness in the face of a nonfunctional mental health care delivery system and enormous burdens, the health of their entire family system may be in jeopardy. For this reason, efforts to promote the health of these families are essential. The form and content of those efforts must be empirically based so as to provide appropriate, quality support that specifically addresses their needs.

The purpose of this chapter is to trace the development over time of an empirically tested middle range theory of family health in the families of adults with persistent mental illnesses. Family health theory (FHT) attempts to identify factors that predict family health. Such prediction will allow for the development of interventions that support and promote the health of these families as they engage in the critical work of caregiving.

THEORY DEVELOPMENT APPROACH

The theory development approach used for the FHT was primarily that of deduction. Deduction uses an established theory as the basis for a new theoretical effort. The original theory is typically broader and more comprehensive than the derived theory. The established theory is logically extended, often for the purpose of specifically addressing a particular population. It is anticipated that the derived theory would, however, be closely related to the established theory (Jacox, 1974).

Walker and Avant (1995) spoke of the theory-building process as iterative. Both inductive and deductive strategies may be employed sequentially until an adequate theoretical formulation is achieved. In so far as the empirical literature was consulted relative to the development of this middle range theory for the specific population of families with an adult member with a mental illness, there was an inductive element to the theory development strategy as well.

DESCRIPTION OF THE MIDDLE RANGE THEORY

Figure 3.1 summarizes the FHT. The FHT uses client, family, and professional factors in an attempt to explain the outcome of family health in the families of adults with persistent mental illnesses. Five specific variables

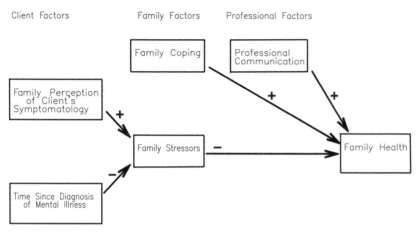

Figure 3.1. Family health theory in the families of adults with persistent mental illness. *Note.* "Predicting Family Health in Families of Young Adults With Severe Mental Illness," by M. M. Doornbos, 2002, *Journal of Family Nursing, 8,* p. 243. Copyright 2002 by Sage Publications, Inc. Reprinted with permission.

fall under these categories and each has either a direct or an indirect relationship with the outcome variable of family health. The FHT proposes a direct relationship between family coping and family health, between family stressors and family health, and between professional communication and family health. Family perception of the client's symptomatology and time since diagnosis of mental illness each have a direct relationship with family stressors. Table 3.1 shows the conceptual–theoretical–empirical indicator structure for the FHT in the families of the persistently mentally ill.

THEORY LINKAGES TO KING'S WORK

King's conceptual system proposes three dynamic and interacting systems—personal, interpersonal, and social. These systems pertain to individuals, groups, and society, respectively, and each is described in terms of relevant concepts (King, 1981, 1992, 1995).

King has suggested that although each of her concepts is placed in the context of either the personal, interpersonal, or social system, in fact the concepts can be used interchangeably between and among systems. Therefore, six of King's concepts were selected for use in the FHT: perception, time, coping, stressors, communication, and health. Each of these was adapted to address more specifically the families of those struggling

Table 3.1. Conceptual–Theoretical–Empirical Indicator Structure for Family Health Theory in the Families of Persistently Mentally Ill Clients

Conceptual System Concepts	Perception	Time	Coping	Stressors	Communication	Health
Theory concepts	Family perception of client symptomatology	Times since Dx	Family coping	Stressors	Professional	Family
Empirical indicators	IODB	No. months since informed of Dx	F-COPES	FILE	PSQ	Family APGAR

Dx = Diagnosis; IODB = Index of Disruptive Behavior; F-COPES = Family Crisis Oriented Personal Scales; FILE = Family Inventory of Life Events and Changes scale; PSQ = Professional Support Questionnaire.

with persistent mental illnesses and became (a) family perception of client symptomatology, (b) time since diagnosis of mental illness, (c) family coping, (d) family stressors, (e) professional communication, and (f) family health. Although these concepts are directly derived from King's conceptual system, the empirical literature base surrounding families of the mentally ill also influenced the concepts' labels and theoretical definitions. At this point, these concepts from King's system were arranged into new propositions that suggested relationships between five predictor factors and family health in the families of adults with persistent mental illnesses.

SELECTIVE LITERATURE REVIEW

Family Perception of Client Symptomatology

King (1983) was unequivocal about the fact that an understanding of the family's perception of a member's illness was critical. When speaking more generally about perception, she suggested that perception is subjective, personal, and selective—that is, one cannot assume that each person in a given situation perceives circumstances similarly (King, 1981). Thus, an important area of professional nursing activity involves verifying client (family) and nurse perceptions as they plan together to achieve specific goals (King, 1981).

This verification of perceptions is particularly necessary as it pertains to the family's perception of client symptomatology. For example, positive symptoms (an exaggeration or distortion of normal function) of schizophrenia cause difficulties for some families, whereas other families may take these symptoms in stride but have difficulty with the negative symptoms (a loss of normal function). In general, however, numerous studies have documented the significance of client symptoms to the family. The preponderance of the literature supports the notion that the perceived degree and frequency of symptomatology led to greater levels of family burden (Biegel, Milligan, Putnam, & Song, 1994; Doornbos, 1997; Jones 1996; Jungbauer, Wittmund, Dietrich, & Angermeyer, 2003; Ricard, Bonin, & Ezer, 1999; Song, Biegel, & Milligan, 1997; Tuck, duMont, Evans, & Schupe, 1997). Other authors have identified links between client symptoms and family functioning (Najarian, 1995; Saunders, 1999).

Time Since Diagnosis of Mental Illness

King (1983) asserted that time influenced behavior in family situations. Similarly, the variable of time in the families of persons with persistent mental illnesses has been recognized as significant. Researchers have suggested that parents of adult children with schizophrenia specifically demarcated time into before and after diagnosis categories (Tuck et al., 1997). A variety of findings have characterized the literature around this variable in that some found the burden of mental illness to increase over time (Miller, Dworkin, Ward, & Barone, 1990; Seymour & Dawson, 1986) and others have suggested that it actually decreases over time (Cook & Picket, 1988; Mays & Lund, 1999).

The variable of time has received increased attention recently. Rose et al. (2002) suggested that little is definitively known about the responses of families to mental illness over time and that our ability to assist these families has been hampered by a lack of understanding of their cumulative experience. In another study, the time-related development of subjective burden experienced by parents of persons with schizophrenia was categorized as constantly high, increased, reduced, shifting, or constantly low over a 12-month period (Jungbauer et al., 2003). Thus, time remains a central but insufficiently understood variable relative to the families of persons with mental illnesses.

Family Coping

King (1983) suggested that when a family is unable to cope with an event or health problem, they frequently seek the assistance of a health care professional. King (1981, 1990, 1992, 1994, 1995) was articulate about the fact that nursing should take an active role in assisting individuals and families to cope with events or stressors. She specifically suggested that nurses might be involved in supporting family coping efforts in the face of situational or maturational crises, conflict, rapid change, or the illness of a family member (King, 1983). Each of these circumstances may be applicable to the families of those with persistent mental illnesses.

Saunders (2003) suggested that effective family functioning in families with a member who has a persistent mental illness might be influenced by a variety of psychosocial factors. She cited coping as a central factor. The families of persons with persistent mental illnesses use an array of coping methods (Doornbos, 1996, 1997; Eakes, 1995; Ip & Mackenzie, 1998; Mays & Lund, 1999; Rose, 1998; Saunders, 1999; Yamashita, 1998) and, in fact, rely more on coping strategies than do normative families (Doornbos, 1996). These coping methods have been categorized in various ways: (a) as problem focused or behavioral (Saunders, 1999); (b) as psychological, physical, or social (Huang & Slevin, 1999); (c) as those methods that manage events, meanings and perceptions, or stress (Lundh, 1999); and (d) as encompassing various types of action (Hall, 2000).

Saunders (2003) concluded that the outcome of family coping might be either positive or negative—producing either additional burdens for an already overwhelmed family or serving as a method to make the situation more manageable for the entire family.

Family Stressors

King (1981) asserted that stressors are that which must be adjusted to maintain health. In addition, she suggested that "too many stressors in the family environment ... may precipitate a crisis"(King, 1983, p. 182), which presumably has the potential to affect adversely the health of the family. King (1981) was explicit that a central role of the nurse is to identify client and family stressors and intervene to mediate their effect. King (1981) suggested that there are pertinent nursing interventions that can be used to alleviate the impact of stressors.

It makes intuitive sense that families with a member who struggles with a persistent mental illness may have an array of stressors, some of which are common to all families and others that are specifically related to caring for the member with a mental illness. Doornbos (1996) found that these families did, indeed, have significantly more stressors than normative families. The specific types of stressors included intrafamily, marital, financial, employment, grief and loss, illness related, transition, legal, and mental health care system stressors (Doornbos, 1996, 1997, 2002a; Rose et al., 2002; Saunders & Byrne, 2002).

Professional Communication

King (1981) concisely stated that communication, understood as both verbal and nonverbal, is a vital concept to professional nursing. She explained this further by indicating that communication forms the basis for interactions with persons who may be experiencing unusual stress that leads them to seek professional intervention (King, 1981). King (1981) also suggests that communication between the nurse and individuals and families is essential for effective care and is the key in assisting others to achieve the health-related goals that they have set for themselves.

Families of persons with persistent mental illnesses have identified communication between themselves and health care professionals as their greatest need (Biegel, Song, & Milligan, 1995). By communication, they refer to attentiveness, listening, emotional support, affirmation, respect, and sharing of information (Dixon & Lehman, 1995; Doornbos, 2002a; Hall & Purdy, 2000; Ip & Mackenzie, 1998; Jungbauer et al., 2003; Rose, 1997, 1998; Winefield & Harvey, 1994). A recent comprehensive review of the literature indicated that educational interventions with these families led to a decrease in family burden, an increase in family functioning, enhanced coping strategies, and improved caregiver health (Biegel, Robinson, & Kennedy, 2000). Unfortunately, another recent study indicated that significant percentages of families engaged in caregiving for a mentally ill member did not receive critical information, advice, or encouragement from professionals (Doornbos, 2001b).

Family Health

Since her early writing about the conceptual system to the present, King (1971, 1981, 1983, 1990, 1995) has consistently identified health as the goal for nursing practice. Specifically, she stated, "The goal of nursing is to help individuals and groups attain, maintain, and restore health" (1971, p. 84). This goal was explicitly set forth relative to families as well (King, 1983).

Unfortunately, little of the literature pertaining to the families of persons with persistent mental illnesses to date has focused on the outcome of health. In a recent review of the past 30 years of literature regarding families living with severe mental illness, Saunders (2003) noted that only the more recent investigations have a focus on strengths and adaptive capabilities of families. She suggested a paradigm shift from stress responses to health behaviors for future studies.

METHODOLOGY

The FHT has been empirically tested twice (Doornbos, 2000, 2002b). A cross-sectional, predictive design was used in each instance. There has been an ongoing evolution of theoretical concepts, instrumentation, and conceptualizations of the FHT since its inception.

Evolving Theoretical Concepts

Tables 3.2 and 3.3 show the evolution of the theoretical concepts included in the FHT. Table 3.2 (Doornbos, 2000) shows the original five concepts along with their theoretical definitions, and Table 3.3 (Doornbos, 2002b) shows the six concepts included in the current conceptualization of the FHT. Several changes should be noted from the original conceptualization to the second empirical testing of the FHT.

First, the concept titled "family perception of client's level of health" was changed to "family perception of client's symptomatology." It should

Table 3.2. Theoretical Definitions of Family Health Theory Concepts—Initial Conceptualization and First Empirical Testing

Concept	Definition
Family stressors	Persons, objects, or events that have the potential to cause stress (King, 1981) for the family unit
Family coping	"The constantly changing cognitive and behavioral efforts to manage specific external and internal demands that are appraised as taxing or exceeding the resources" of the family (Lazarus & Folkman, 1984, p. 141)
Family perception of client's level of health	The family's sense of the client's ability to function and conduct business of living in terms of one's personal, social, and familial responsibilities
Time since diagnosis	The duration of the mental illness from the time of diagnosis to the present
Family health	The ability of the family to adjust to stressors and to function in their social roles (Frey, 1989)

Note. From "King's Systems Framework and Family Health: The Derivation and Testing of a Theory," by M. M. Doornbos, 2000, *Journal of Theory Construction and Testing, 4*, p. 20. Copyright 2000 by Tucker Publications, Inc. Reprinted with permission.

Table 3.3. Theoretical Definitions of Family Health Theory Concepts—Current Conceptualization

Concept	Definition
Family perception of client symptomatology	The family's sense of the frequency of client behaviors associated with the severe mental illness
Time since diagnosis of mental illness	The duration of the mental illness from the time of diagnosis to the present
Family coping	"The constantly changing cognitive and behavioral efforts to manage specific external and internal demands that are appraised as taxing or exceeding the resources" of the family (Lazarus & Folkman, 1984, p. 141)
Family stressors	Persons, objects, or events that have the potential to cause stress (King, 1981) for the family unit
Professional communication	The instrumental and affective support that is communicated by mental health care professionals to family caregivers
Family health	Perceived satisfaction with the functioning of the family

Note. From "Predicting Family Health in Families of Young Adults With Severe Mental Illness," by M. M. Doornbos, 2002, *Journal of Family Nursing, 8*, p. 243. Copyright 2002 by Sage Publications, Inc. Reprinted with permission.

be noted that the salient King concept of *perception* is consistent, but the focus of the families' perceptions has been shifted slightly. A careful reexamination of the current research, after the first testing of the theory, suggested that such a variable change was more consistent with the existing empirical support. Families of the mentally ill are stressed and burdened by the specific symptoms of the mental illness of their loved one. Although there may be some overlap, illness symptoms are distinctly different from the ability to function that characterizes health. King (1981) supported this contention by suggesting that health and illness are distinctly different concepts rather than part of a linear continuum. Thus, this change seemed a better reflection of the literature while maintaining consistency with King's concepts of perception, illness, and health.

Second, the theoretical definition of family health was altered from its original conceptualization. The definition changed from attempting to capture the families' ability to function to capturing the families' satisfaction with their functioning. Both the first and second conceptualizations are consistent with King's systems theory. King (1981) generally focused on function as an indicator of health and in fact spoke of health as "a functional state in the life cycle" (p. 5). She also suggested that health is needed to lead a "useful, satisfying, productive, and happy life" (p. 4). From these two statements, a definition that focuses on satisfaction with functioning seems warranted. Further, such a definition seems to suggest appropriately that family health is, in perhaps all but extreme cases, subjectively determined by those directly involved.

Finally, Table 3.3 shows the addition of the concept of professional communication. This concept was added as a logical extension of the FHT after the first empirical testing. On reflection, it seemed apparent that the first conceptualization of the FHT focused on client and family factors to the exclusion of salient nursing factors that might be used to protect the health of these families. From her earliest writing, King (1983) has spoken of the goal of nursing as helping "individuals (and families) maintain their health so they can function in their roles" (pp. 3–4). Thus, the complexity of families caring for a member with a persistent mental illness seems clearly to necessitate active nursing intervention to support the functioning of these families in their central roles. The concept itself was deemed appropriate given King's discussion of communication as the "vehicle by which human relations are developed and maintained" (p. 79). Such relationships are integral to the practice of nursing and thus to the care of families dealing with persistent mental illness. Further, King (1981) suggested that communication is the informational component of human interactions. The empirical literature emphasizes the critical role of dialogue between families caring for a mentally ill member and mental health providers as well as the necessity of information exchange.

Evolving Instrumentation

The general criteria used to select instruments to operationalize the concepts of the FHT were fit with the theoretical definition and psychometric adequacy. There were two instruments that performed well and thus were used in both studies. First, the Family Crisis Oriented Personal Scales (F-COPES; McCubbin, Olson, & Larson, 1996) was designed to identify problem-solving and behavioral strategies used by families in difficult situations. It was used to measure family coping. The F-COPES had evidence of construct validity, derived from factor analysis, and the Cronbach's alpha for the overall F-COPES, as found in previous studies, is .77. Second, the Family Inventory of Life Events and Changes scale (FILE; McCubbin, Patterson, & Wilson, 1996) functions as an index of family stress and seeks to evaluate the pileup of normative and nonnormative stressors. The FILE was used to measure family stressors. It also had evidence of construct validity, provided by factor analysis, and an overall reliability of .81 as calculated in previous studies. Time since diagnosis of mental illness was operationalized consistently in both studies as the number of months since the family was first told of a member's mental illness to the present. Finally, the Professional Support Questionnaire (PSQ; Reinhard, 1994) was the empirical measure of professional communication. The PSQ measured instrumental as well as affective support given by professionals to caregivers. There was evidence of content and concurrent validity, and the overall reliability of the scale is .74, as calculated in previous studies. It was used only in the second testing of the FHT because the variable was added at this point, but it performed well.

Changes in instrumentation occurred in several instances. First, the concept change from "family perception of client's level of health" to "family perception of client symptomatology" obviously necessitated a change in instrumentation. In the first empirical testing of the theory, the Progress Evaluation Scales (PES; Ihilevich, Gleser, Gritter, Kroman, & Watson, 1981) were used to capture the client's ability to function in terms of personal, social, and familial responsibilities. In previous studies, the PES had an interrater reliability of .65, and there was evidence of construct validity. The second study employed the Index of Disruptive Behaviors (IOBD; Horwitz & Reinhard, 1992) to capture the frequency of client behaviors associated with severe mental illness. The IOBD has been reviewed by an advisory group of family caregivers for content validity and the reliability coefficient for this scale was found to be .72 in previous studies (Reinhard, 1994).

Family health is one concept that has presented a challenge in terms of operationalization. First, as noted earlier, the definition of this concept has shifted slightly from the first to the second empirical testing of the FHT, and consequently the instrumentation has as well. Initially, the Family APGAR (Smilkstein, Ashworth, & Montano, 1982), the Family Adaptability and Cohesion Scale (FACES III; Olson, Portner, & Lavee, 1985), and the Family Environment Scale (FES)—Conflict subscale (Moos & Moos, 1994) were used to measure family health. The Family APGAR was used to assess the caregiver's satisfaction with the functioning of her or his family. It was found in previous studies to have construct validity as well as a reliability coefficient of .86. Relative to the FACES III, the scales were designed to measure the amount of cohesion that exists within a family unit as well as the family's ability to adjust to stressors. They have face, content, and construct validity. The internal consistency of the Cohesion Scale and the Adaptability Scale in previous studies were .77 and .62, respectively. Finally, the FES Conflict subscale was used to measure the family's ability to manage conflict. A body of research supports the construct, concurrent, and predictive validity of the total FES, and the internal consistency of the Conflict subscale was found to be .75 in previous studies (Moos, 1990; Moos & Moos, 1994).

There were difficulties with the FACES III in the initial empirical testing because it had items that did not fit the developmental stage of the families in the sample. For example, items regarding the discipline of children were not applicable to families with young adult or adult members who had a mental illness. Further, the FES Conflict subscale measures methods used within the family to manage the amount of aggression present. It was intended as an inverse measure of family health because it was assumed that significant amounts of openly expressed anger and conflict would be indicative of a lower level of family health. In reality, the fit between this instrument and each of the ensuing definitions of family health was poor. The initial focus on family functioning and the subsequent focus on satisfaction with family functioning were not captured by the FES Conflict subscale. Thus, at present only a single, brief measure is available for the concept of family health, which seems less than desirable.

Evolving Conceptualizations of the FHT

Figures 3.2 to 3.4 provide visual representations of how the FHT has evolved over time. Figure 3.2 (Doornbos, 1995) presents the original conceptualization in which family stressors, family coping, family perception of client's level of health, and time since diagnosis of mental illness were all hypothesized to affect directly the outcome variable of family health. As shown in Figure 3.3 (Doornbos, 1995), the empirical testing supported a direct relationship between family coping and family health as well as between family stressors and family health. In addition, family perception of client's level of health and time since diagnosis of mental illness had

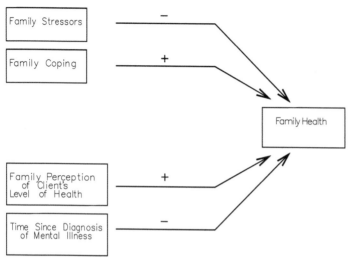

Figure 3.2. Originally proposed middle range theory of family health in the families of young adults with serious and persistent mental illness. *Note.* From "Using King's systems framework to explore family health in the families of the young chronically mentally ill," by M. M. Doornbos. In *Advancing King's Systems Framework and Theory of Nursing,* by M. A. Frey & C. L. Sieloff (Eds.), p. 196. Thousand Oaks, CA: Sage. Reprinted with permission.

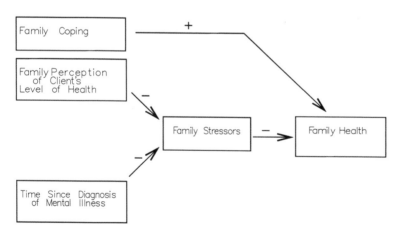

Figure 3.3. First revision of middle range theory of family health in the families of young adults with serious and persistent mental illness. *Note.* From "Using King's systems framework to explore family health in the families of the young chronically mentally ill," by M. M. Doornbos. In *Advancing King's Systems Framework and Theory of Nursing,* by M. A. Frey & C. L. Sieloff (Eds.), p. 200. Thousand Oaks, CA: Sage. Reprinted with permission.

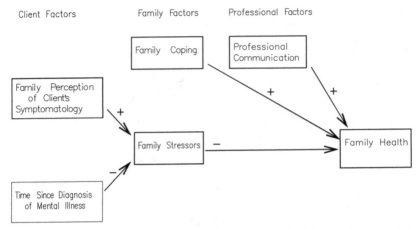

Figure 3.4. Current version of family health theory in the families of adults with persistent mental illness. *Note.* From "Predicting Family Health in Families of Young Adults With Severe Mental illness," by M. M. Doornbos, 2002, *Journal of Family Nursing, 8,* p. 243. Copyright 2002 by Sage Publications, Inc. Reprinted with permission.

direct relationships with family stressors. Finally, Figure 3.4 (Doornbos, 2002b) demonstrates that subsequent empirical testing of the FHT supported a direct relationship between family coping and family health, between family stressors and family health, and between professional communication and family health. In a manner similar to previous testing, the new variable, family perception of client's symptomatology, and the previously used variable, time since diagnosis of mental illness, had direct relationships with family stressors.

STRENGTHS AND LIMITATIONS

The FHT is unique in that it specifically addresses the health of the population of families caring for adult members with serious and persistent mental illnesses. In addition, it has been empirically tested twice with modifications made to the theory based on the results of those studies. The most recent version of the FHT explained 23% of the variance in family health, with professional communication, family stressors, and family coping functioning as significant predictors (Doornbos, 2002b). In addition, 15% of the variance in family stressors was explained by the family perception of the client symptomatology and time since diagnosis of mental illness (Doornbos, 2002b). Thus, the FHT offers the beginning of a theoretical base for provision of care to these families.

The FHT also has several limitations. First, a more representative sample in terms of the gender of family respondents, family socioeconomic status, and cultural diversity is needed. To date, the family respondents have been primarily women whereas the families themselves have been largely middle to upper-middle class and White. More diversity in the sample would allow for greater generalization and indicate whether the FHT, as is, is applicable to families challenged by a lack of financial resources or those that belong to other cultural groups.

A second limitation of the FHT pertains to instrumentation. A more comprehensive measure of family health than that provided by the Family APGAR alone is needed. Additional work will need to be done in terms of identifying an instrument that is consistent with the theoretical definition of family health and that has adequate psychometric data.

APPLICATION TO THE CLINICAL PROBLEM

The current conceptualization of the FHT provides specific direction in terms of nursing care that is designed for caregiving families with a member diagnosed with a persistent mental illness. For example, a family's perception of the client's symptomatology has a direct relationship with family stressors, and thus high-risk subgroups within this population can be identified. Families that perceive greater levels of client symptomatology will likely experience more stress, which, in turn, will adversely affect their experience of family health. Similarly, recognizing the role of the time since diagnosis of mental illness as it relates to family stressors can assist nurses in identifying families that are at particularly vulnerable points in the illness trajectory and in need of intervention. The nurse's efforts at partnering with a family around enhancing their repertoire of coping strategies is likely to have a direct effect on their experience of family health as well. Finally, nurses have long operated under the assumption that their communication and relationship skills and supportive presence were important to clients. The empirical testing of the FHT supports the validity of such an assumption with this specific population. Nurses can directly affect the families' experience of health by communicating instrumental and affective support to these burdened caregivers.

FUTURE RECOMMENDATIONS

As work on the FHT moves forward, there will likely be a focus on exploring linkages between family health and family caregiving efforts. Although it makes intuitive sense that these two concepts would be related, additional research is necessary to establish that link. Then, assuming a relationship between these concepts, the next logical step is to determine whether nurses can have a positive impact on the health of these family units by supporting their caregiving efforts. This complex and multifaceted caregiving role may negatively affect the family unit's health if it is not adequately supported. Thus, specific supportive interventions designed to sustain family health in these families needs to be planned and empirically tested.

SUMMARY

The FHT is an important initiative related to protecting the health of families challenged by the serious mental illness of a member. Derived from King's conceptual system, it has been empirically tested twice in an effort to provide a sound foundation for the design and implementation of quality nursing care for these families. An additional benefit is that a formulation such as the FHT, accompanied by empirical testing, can make a contribution to the ongoing development of the science of nursing.

REFERENCES

Biegel, D. E., Milligan, S. E., Putnam, P. L., & Song, L. (1994). Predictors of burden among lower socioeconomic status caregivers of persons with chronic mental illness. *Community Mental Health Journal, 30*, 473–494.

Biegel, D. E., Robinson, E. M., & Kennedy, M. (2000). A review of empirical studies of interventions for families of persons with mental illness. In J. Morrisey (Ed.), *Research in community mental health: Social factors in mental health and illness, Vol. 11.* Greenwich, CT: JAI Press.

Biegel, D. E., Song, L., & Milligan, S. E. (1995). A comparative analysis of family caregivers' perceived relationships with mental health professionals. *Psychiatric Services, 46*, 477–482.

Cook, J. A., & Pickett, S. (1988). Burden and criticalness among parents living with their chronically mentally ill offspring. *Journal of Applied Social Sciences, 12*, 79–107.

Crisp, A. H., Gelder, M., Rix, S., Meltzer, H. I., & Rowlands, O. J. (2000). Stigmatisation of people with mental illness. *British Journal of Psychiatry, 177*, 4–7.

Dixon, L. B., & Lehman, A. F. (1995). Family interventions for schizophrenia. *Schizophrenia Bulletin, 21*, 631–643.

Doornbos, M. M. (1995). Using King's systems framework to explore family health in the families of the young chronically mentally ill. In M. A. Frey & C. L. Sieloff (Eds.), *Advancing King's systems framework and theory of nursing* (pp. 192–203). Thousand Oaks, CA: Sage.

Doornbos, M. M. (1996). The strengths of families coping with serious mental illness. *Archives of Psychiatric Nursing, X,* 214–220.

Doornbos, M. M. (1997). The problems and coping methods of caregivers of young adults with mental illness. *Journal of Psychosocial Nursing, 35,* 22–26.

Doornbos, M. M. (2000). King's systems framework and family health: The derivation and testing of a theory. *Journal of Theory Construction and Testing, 4*(1), 20–26.

Doornbos, M. M. (2001a). The 24–7–52 job: Family caregiving for young adults with serious and persistent mental illness. *Journal of Family Nursing, 7,* 328–344.

Doornbos, M. M. (2001b). Professional support of family caregivers of people with serious and persistent mental illnesses. *Journal of Psychosocial Nursing, 39,* 38–45.

Doornbos, M. M. (2002a). Family caregivers and the mental health care system: Reality and dreams. *Archives of Psychiatric Nursing, XVI,* 39–46.

Doornbos, M. M. (2002b). Predicting family health in families of young adults with severe mental illness. *Journal of Family Nursing, 8,* 241–263.

Eakes, G. G. (1995). Chronic sorrow: The lived experience of parents of chronically mentally ill individuals. *Archives of Psychiatric Nursing, IX,* 77–84.

Frey, M. A. (1989). Social support and health: A theoretical formulation derived from King's conceptual framework. *Nursing Science Quarterly, 2,* 138–148.

Hall, M. (2000). Parent coping styles and schizophrenic patient behavior as predictors of expressed emotion. *Family Process, 39,* 435–445.

Hall, L. L., & Purdy, R. (2000). Recovery and serious brain disorders: The central role of families in nurturing roots and wings. *Community Mental Health Journal, 36,* 427–441.

Horwitz, A. V., & Reinhard, S. (1992). Family management of labeled mental illness in a deinstitutionalized era: An exploratory study. *Perspectives on Social Problems, 4,* 111–127.

Huang, M., & Slevin, E. (1999). The experiences of carers who live with someone who has schizophrenia: A review of the literature. *Mental Health Care, 31,* 89–93.

Ihilevich, D., Gleser, G. C., Gritter, G. W., Kroman, L. J., & Watson, A. S. (1981). Measuring program outcome: The progress evaluation scales. *Evaluation Review, 5,* 451–477.

Ip, G. S. H., & Mackenzie, A. E. (1998). Caring for relatives with serious mental illness at home: The experiences of family carers in Hong Kong. *Archives of Psychiatric Nursing, XII,* 288–294.

Jacox, A. (1974). Theory construction in nursing: An overview. *Nursing Research, 23,* 4–13.

Jones, S. L. (1996). The association between objective and subjective caregiver burden. *Archives of Psychiatric Nursing, X,* 77–84.

Jungbauer, J., Wittmund, B., Dietrich, S., & Angermeyer, M. C. (2003). Subjective burden over 12 months in parents of patients with schizophrenia. *Archives of Psychiatric Nursing, XVII,* 126–134.

King, I. (1971). *Toward a theory for nursing*. New York: Wiley.

King, I. (1981). *A theory for nursing: Systems, concepts, process*. New York: Wiley.

King, I. (1983). King's theory of nursing. In I. W. Clements & F. B. Roberts (Eds.), *Family health: A theoretical approach to nursing care* (pp. 87–99). New York: Wiley.

King, I. (1990). Health as the goal for nursing. *Nursing Science Quarterly, 3*, 123–128.

King, I. (1992). King's theory of goal attainment. *Nursing Science Quarterly, 5*, 19–26.

King, I. (1994). Quality of life and goal attainment. *Nursing Science Quarterly, 7*, 29–32.

King, I. (1995). A systems framework for nursing. In M. A. Frey & C. L. Sieloff (Eds.), *Advancing King's systems framework and theory of nursing* (pp. 14–21). Thousand Oaks, CA: Sage.

Lazarus, R., & Folkman, S. (1984). *Stress, appraisal, and coping*. New York: Springer Publishing Company.

Lundh, U. (1999). Family carers: Coping strategies among family carers in Sweden. *British Journal of Nursing, 8*, 735–740.

Mays, G. D., & Lund, C. H. (1999). Male caregivers of mentally ill relatives. *Perspectives in Psychiatric Care, 35*, 19–28.

McCubbin, H. I., Olson, D., & Larsen, A. (1996). Family Crisis Oriented Personal Scales (F-COPES). In H. I. McCubbin, A. I. Thompson, & M. A. McCubbin (Eds.), *Family assessment: Resiliency, coping and adaptation—Inventories for research and practice* (pp. 405–507). Madison: University of Wisconsin Press.

McCubbin, H. I., Patterson, J., & Wilson, L. (1996). Family Inventory of Life Events and Changes (FILE). In H. I. McCubbin, A. I. Thompson, & M. A. McCubbin (Eds.), *Family assessment: Resiliency, coping and adaptation—Inventories for research and practice* (pp. 103–178). Madison: University of Wisconsin Press.

Miller, F., Dworkin, J., Ward, M., & Barone, D. (1990). A preliminary study of unresolved grief in families of seriously mentally ill patients. *Hospital and Community Psychiatry, 41*, 1321–1325.

Moos, R. H. (1990). Conceptual and empirical approaches to developing family-based assessment procedures: Resolving the case of the Family Environment Scale. *Family Process, 29*, 199–208.

Moos, R. H., & Moos, B. S. (1994). *Family Environment Scale manual*. Palo Alto, CA: Consulting Psychologists Press.

Najarian, S. P. (1995). Family experience with positive clients' response to Clozapine. *Archives of Psychiatric Nursing, IX*, 11–21.

National Institute of Mental Health. (2001). *The numbers count: Mental disorders in America*. Retrieved June 2, 2004, from http://www.nimh.nih.gov/publicat/numbers.cfm

New Freedom Commission on Mental Health. (2003). *Achieving the promise: Transforming mental health care in America. Final Report* (DHHS Pub. No.

SMA-03-3832). Rockville, MD: U.S. Department of Health and Human Services.

Olson, D. H., Portner, J., & Lavee, Y. (1985). *Family Adaptability and Cohesion Scale (FACES III)*. St. Paul: University of Minnesota Press.

Reinhard, S. C. (1994). Living with mental illness: Effects of professional support and personal control on caregiver burden. *Research in Nursing and Health, 17*, 79–88.

Ricard, N., Bonin, J. P., & Ezer, H. (1999). Factors associated with burden in primary caregivers of mentally ill patients. *International Journal of Nursing Studies, 36*, 73–83.

Rose, L. E. (1997). Caring for caregivers: Perceptions of social support. *Journal of Psychosocial Nursing, 35*, 17–24.

Rose, L. E. (1998). Benefits and limitations of professional–family interactions: The family perspective. *Archives of Psychiatric Nursing, XII*, 140–147.

Rose, L., Mallinson, R. K., & Walton-Moss. (2002). A grounded theory of families responding to mental illness. *Western Journal of Nursing Research, 24*, 516–536.

Saunders, J. C. (1999). Family functioning in families providing care for a family member with schizophrenia. *Issues in Mental Health Nursing, 20*, 95–113.

Saunders, J. C. (2003). Families living with severe mental illness: A literature review. *Issues in Mental Health Nursing, 24*, 175–198.

Saunders, J. C., & Byrne, M. M. (2002). A thematic analysis of families living with schizophrenia. *Archives of Psychiatric Nursing, XVI*, 217–223.

Seymour, R., & Dawson, N. (1986). The schizophrenic at home. *Journal of Psychosocial Nursing, 26*, 28–30.

Smilkstein, G., Ashworth, C., & Montano, D. (1982). Validity and reliability of the Family APGAR as a test of family function. *Journal of Family Practice, 15*, 303–311.

Song, L., Biegel, D. E., & Milligan, S. E. (1997). Predictors of depressive symptomatology among lower social class caregivers of persons with chronic mental illness. *Community Mental Health Journal, 33*, 269–286.

Tuck I., du Mont, P., Evans, G., & Shupe, J. (1997). The experience of caring for an adult child with schizophrenia. *Archives of Psychiatric Nursing, XI*, 188–125.

Walker, L. O., & Avant, K. C. (1995). *Strategies for theory construction in nursing*. Norwalk, CT: Appleton and Lange.

Winefield, H. R., & Harvey, E. J. (1994). Needs of family caregivers in chronic schizophrenia. *Schizophrenia Bulletin, 20*, 557–566.

Yamashita, M. (1998). Family coping with mental illness: A comparative study. *Journal of Psychiatric and Mental Health Nursing, 5*, 515–523.

CHAPTER FOUR

A Theory of Asynchronous Development

A Midlevel Theory Derived From a Synthesis of King and Peplau

Phyllis du Mont

Across cultures and independent of race, socioeconomic class, or early school achievement, girls who experience early menarche (at less than 12 years old) are at risk for depression, early coital debut, drug and alcohol abuse, smoking, and low educational/occupational attainment (du Mont, 1998; Johansson & Ritzen, 2005; Kaltiala-Heino, Kosunen, & Rimpela, 2003; Lanza & Collins, 2002; Stattin & Magnusson, 1990; Waylen & Wolke, 2004). Much of the work that has been done to investigate the antecedents of risky behaviors in this population has been atheoretical.

This chapter illustrates the value of using nursing theory to guide empirical investigation of a puzzling clinical phenomenon. To be truly useful, the explanatory model should be consistent with existing empirical data and should also direct the researcher in the identification of important factors that can be empirically explored to advance the science. Specifically, this analysis of the phenomenon of early menarche led to the development and testing of a midlevel nursing theory derived from the synthesis of works by Imogene King and Hildegard Peplau.

Girls who experience menarche earlier than their peers exhibit high rates of participation in health risk behaviors. Several mechanisms that might influence this observed increase in health risk behaviors have been

50

proposed and studied, but they do not have consistent empirical support. These include low self-esteem (Bolden & Williams, 1995; Connor, Poyrazli, Ferrer-Wreder, Grahame, & Maraj, 2004; Shrier, Harris, Sternberg, & Beardslee, 2001; Wild, Flisher, Bhana, & Lombard, 2004) and excessive stress (Aseltine & Gore, 2000; Tschann et al., 1994). Hormonal factors play a role, but in humans, hormones exert limited direct control over behavior (Masten, 2004). Several authors (Cairns & Cairns, 1994; Johansson & Ritzen, 2005; Paul, Fitzjohn, Herbison, & Dickson, 2000; Stattin & Magnusson, 1990) confirmed an association between socializing with an older, deviant peer group and an increase in health risk behaviors but offered no explanation for this observation. Not all girls who experience early menarche suffer unfortunate outcomes. Explanations invoking both protective and predisposing factors that might account for this variation in outcomes have been proposed and evaluated. Factors that have been explored and that have not adequately explained the phenomenon include direct hormonal effects, self-esteem, and problem-solving ability. Behaviors commonly exhibited in adolescence (interest in sex, striving for autonomy) show modest correlations with hormonal peaks (Halpern, Udry, & Suchindran, 1997); however, the influence of social context is much greater (Masten, 2004). Although body mass index (BMI), early menarche, and lower self-esteem seem interrelated (Rierdan & Koff, 1997), research to date has not demonstrated a clear link between low self-esteem and risk-taking behaviors (Connelly, 1998; Connor et al., 2004; Stevenson, Maton, & Teti, 1999). South African researchers (Wild et al., 2004) devised and tested an interesting variant of the hypothesis that self-esteem is inversely correlated with participation in health risk behaviors. They concluded that the mixed results obtained in previous studies resulted from a failure to recognize that self-esteem varies across various domains. Accordingly, they identified six domains or subscales for self-esteem: peers, school, family, sports and athletics, body image, and global self-worth. They found that participation in health risk behaviors was associated with high levels of self-esteem in the peer domain and low self-esteem in family and school domains.

Empirical data are mixed on the relation between problem-solving abilities and responsible health-related behavior. Recent studies have not confirmed the hypothesis that superior problem-solving ability results in decreased participation in health risk behaviors (Ellickson, Tucker, Klein, & Saner, 2004; Koniak-Griffin, Lesser, Uman, & Nyamathi, 2003; Sutton, McVey, & Glanz, 1999). Research has established that high levels of ego development seem to be an important protective factor against participation in risky behaviors and depression. Adolescent girls who correctly used contraceptives demonstrated higher levels of ego development than all other categories of adolescents studied, including those who abstained from intercourse (Hart & Hilton, 1988; Resnick & Blum, 1985). Rierdan (1998) found that among sixth-grade girls who had reached menarche, those with low levels of ego development had high rates of depressive symptoms, whereas girls who had high levels of ego development did not. There has been comparatively little recent research investigation into the relationship between level of ego development and risk behaviors, and this lack of research is apparently related to a relative lack of enthusiasm among researchers for stage theories of maturation. A recent meta-analysis (Cohn, Westenberg, & Cohn, 2004) found that the Washington University Sentence Completion Test, a popular measure of ego development used in more than 300 published studies (Cohn, 1998), appears to quantify a distinct construct and that there is a significant body of empirical evidence to support that ego development increases incrementally over an individual's course of development.

Although this body of work has helped nurses identify an at-risk subgroup of early adolescents, no satisfying theoretical explanation had empirical support. Although some of the discrepant findings in the literature might be attributed to methodological issues (i.e., underpowered or poorly designed research), the existing research did not suggest an obvious direction for future research. Without a cogent theoretical explanation, no specific remedy could be proposed.

In choosing a nursing framework to guide this research, the goal was to select a perspective that would allow specific aspects of the person in the environment to be considered while continuously relating those to the unified whole in interaction with the world. Viewing the early-maturing girl as a complex whole integrated in the environment of a social context avoids the reductionist error of examining parts to infer the qualities of the whole. However, the whole does have parts and particulars, and in the assessment and or treatment of individuals, it is often the variation of accidental qualities of the person that are of interest or concern to nurses.

According to Fawcett and Downs (1992), it is critical to specify the linkages between the empirical indicators of a proposed research project, the theoretical constructs they are meant to represent, and the conceptual model that frames the domain of interest. This is perhaps best visualized as a process that begins with an explicit acknowledgment of the conceptual model, a clear exposition of how the theory is anchored in that framework, and a careful consideration of the ways in which the empirical indicators can be said to capture the concepts outlined by the theory.

The conceptual model developed by Imogene King (1981) allows integration of context, person, and interaction within a cogent framework. In her general systems framework, King described several characteristics of the individual or personal system that have clear relevance for the study of adolescent developmental processes. However, it is evident that King assumed these ideas to be part of the established nursing knowledge base and therefore did not amplify or expand on them. Perhaps most critically, clarification of the concepts of the self and of growth and development was frustratingly absent. In short, King alluded to a theory of human growth and development but did not explicate it.

Hildegard Peplau (1952) developed a theory of interpersonal relations for nursing. Although best known for her formulation of the stages of the nurse–patient relationship, she also provided a nursing interpretation of the interpersonal psychology theories of Harry Stack Sullivan (1953). This aspect of Peplau's work, which evolved from a psychological perspective, focused on the concepts of growth and development of the individual. She called the psychological structure of the individual the *self-system* (recall that King defined the self as a personal system). Peplau specified a role for feelings, especially anxiety, in motivating action. King saw goal setting as the outcome of having perceived the features of a situation and thus becoming "motivated to exert some control over events to achieve goals" (1976, p. 54). Peplau elaborated on the mechanism of motivation when she identified the relationship between language, thought, actions and feelings that occur in response to a particular situation. She went on to state that if an individual experiences a wish, desire, or goal and cannot achieve it, anxiety will result. However, that anxiety will be unconsciously converted into a "relief behavior." Acting out the relief behavior dissipates the energy generated by anxiety. Peplau's specific elaboration of the person is a compatible and useful extension of the personal system as King outlined it. Embedding the self-system as described by Peplau within King's framework anchors King's theory in the larger environment of social systems and explicates the details of the development of the self. This synthesis supports the development of a middle range theory of asynchronous development, intended to explain why individuals who face a developmental challenge prematurely are at risk for poor outcomes.

KING'S CONCEPTUAL SYSTEM

Imogene King (1990) used a system theory approach to achieve a comprehensive view of the person as a manifestation of three interacting and dynamic systems. She called these interacting systems the personal system (the individual), the interpersonal system (dyads, triads, and small groups), and the social system (institutions and organizations). She stated that the goal for nursing is health, which she defined as "the dynamic life experiences of a human being, which implies continuous adjustment to stressors in the internal and external environment through optimum use of one's resources to achieve maximum potential for daily living" (1990, p. 76).

King described the individual as a personal system interacting through perception with the environment. It is via perception that one comes to "know self, to know other persons, and to know objects in the environment" (King, 1980, p. 19). She identified growth and development as an important concept needed to help understand individuals. The focus of her framework was on the interaction of individuals with others in diverse social systems, but knowledge of the individual was explicitly identified as relevant to nursing care.

The concept of growth and development, as described by King (1981), is the result of the interaction of genetic potential with the environment. Influenced by the stage theorists (Gesell, Freud, Erikson, Piaget, and Havighurst are cited in her 1981 work), she conceptualized growth and development as an orderly process with predictable patterns and manifestations subject to individual variation. The environment could be—or not be—conducive to helping individuals move toward maturity. "Patterns develop in people that are predictable but vary because of individual differences. The manner in which a person grows and develops is influenced positively and negatively by other people and objects in the environment" (King, 1981, p. 31).

The concept of the self is key to an understanding of the personal system. King's discussion of the self is abstract. She described the person as a unified whole. "A personal system is a unified, complex whole, self who perceives, thinks, desires, imagines, decides, identifies goals and selects means to achieve them" (1981, p. 27).

An important component of the self (as described by King) is the concept of body image. Body image is defined as a dynamic characteristic that is shaped by growth and developmental changes and the person's awareness of the ways in which others react to these changes (King, 1981). It is an internalized mental representation of the body intimately connected to the idea of self.

Body image, growth and development, and the self are all interacting components of an indivisible whole. "Body image may be viewed as an integral component of growth and development, which in turn influences a concept of self" (King, 1981, p. 31). She also stated that "body image is a part of each stage of growth and development" (p. 32). King identified knowledge about growth and development as important for nurses as they assess patients. She stated that the nurse should be aware that for patients the "stage of their developmental tasks...may be influenced by the stages that they have successfully achieved" (1981, p. 31). This statement substantiates the claim that King accepted Peplau's premise that to respond appropriately to developmental tasks, a person must have successfully achieved the tasks of the preceding developmental level. Thus, King implied the existence of an orderly progression of developmental stages and associated tasks without specifying what this would look like.

Peplau explicated an orderly progression of life stages and ego development tasks. I will demonstrate that both King and Peplau endorsed a concept of development as occurring along a continuum and as a sequential series of tasks to be achieved. This connection strengthens the validity of the argument for the proposed embedding of Peplau's developmental theory of the self within King's personal system and the larger conceptual framework.

PEPLAU'S THEORY

Peplau has defined the goal of nursing as "moving the personality forward in the direction of constructive, productive, personal and community living" (1952, p. 15). She stated, "The central feature of nursing is the nurse–patient interaction" (1992, p. 13). She further stated:

> "The interaction of the nurse-with-patient occurs as a joint enterprise in which data about a person's problems are described by the patient. They are then observed by the nurse, brought into the open, discussed, clarified, identified and formulated. . . . Options for the solution of the problems by the patient are also an outcome of this effort." (1992, p. 14)

She defined *clients* as "patient-persons [who] have problems for which expert nursing services are needed or sought" (p. 14).

Peplau described the self-system as "an organizing structure through which experiences, events, and people are perceived and known, accepted or rejected" (1992, p. 296). The contents of the self-system include self-view, attitudes, opinions, and goals. Self-worth is a part of the self-system, said to develop in late childhood as the result of acceptance and affirmations by same-sex friends (generally age 9 through 12).

Forchuk (1991) reported, based on personal communication with Peplau, that the concept of pattern integration, an interpersonal process whereby the patterns of one person are used to interact with the patterns of another person, is a process which may be an " intrapersonal, interpersonal and systems phenomena" (p. 56). This statement again illustrates the underlying consistency of Peplau's theory with King's conceptual framework (1991). King described nursing as occurring in a framework of dynamically interacting systems that, as noted earlier, she called the personal system, the interpersonal system and the social system. There is parallelism and congruity between these ideas.

Takahashi (1992) wrote an account of a nursing forum during which Peplau drew a parallel between goal attainment and her own idea of beneficial outcomes and King explicitly acknowledged Peplau's influence on her work. Analysis of the two theories reveals other similarities and compatibilities. Peplau's theory can be thought of as a detailed description of the personal system and the nurse–client relationship. King, whose work is explicitly inclusive of the personal, interpersonal, and social systems, focused her attention at the interpersonal level (and, to a lesser degree, at the systems level), in essence implying that the details of the personal system were a given.

The theory of human development as elaborated by Peplau and the conceptual framework of Imogene King are fundamentally compatible. Each body of work grants the nurse a different but complementary view of the person. A synthesis of these two explanatory systems allows the researcher to focus on the developmental aspects of personality in a more holistic and meaningful way than could be achieved using either alone. King's conceptual framework provides a context for Peplau's elaboration of individual growth and development.

Peplau defined the goal of nursing as health and defined health as "a word symbol that implies the forward movement of personality and other on-going human processes in the direction of creative, constructive, personal and community living" (1952, p. 12). She specifically directed nurses to study personality development (1964). She described this process as a series of steps with predictable "tasks" to be achieved using newly acquired "tools" (O'Toole & Welt, 1989). This suggests that each individual should have congruency between "his chronological age and his present accomplishments" (1964, p. 39).

Peplau proposed a theory of personality development composed of stages. Of interest here are conceptualizations of the juvenile, preadolescent, and adolescent phases of personality development. The juvenile phase is roughly equivalent to the grammar school period. The child has language and the ability to communicate and to engage in interpersonal interactions. Peplau proposed that to move successfully from a childhood phase of egotistic preoccupation with one's self, the juvenile has to learn to compete and compromise with his or her peers. Toward the end of this phase and in ushering in the preadolescent phase, the child must come to identify with a same-age, same-sex friend and come to see the world from this other person's perspective. This ability to see the world from the perspective of another is a tool needed to form successful intimate interpersonal relationships. This phase ends with the onset of puberty.

Puberty is marked physiologically by the development of secondary sex changes and psychologically by the need to find appropriate objects for the emerging lust dynamic (O'Toole & Welt, 1989; Sullivan, 1953). As adulthood approaches, adolescents need to develop a successful pattern of interpersonal behavior that allows them to fulfill both intimacy and sexual needs. Adolescence is a time of heightened vulnerability because the growing adolescent assumes increasing responsibility for making important decisions including those regarding life goals, sexual activity, smoking, and the use of alcohol, tobacco, and illicit drugs.

Both Sullivan and Peplau regarded the beginning of each developmental phase as a time of potential for change, either good or bad.

> The self-system...is much more subject to influence through new experience, either fortunate or unfortunate, at each of the developmental thresholds.... And it is this capacity for distinct change in the self-system which begins to be almost fantastically important in preadolescence. (Sullivan, 1953, p. 247)

Although there has not been a satisfying theoretical explanation of the observed relationship between early menarche and participation in high-risk behaviors, some ideas are supported. There is ample evidence to support the claim that girls who mature earlier than their peers are at increased risk for participation in health-damaging behaviors. There are discrepant results regarding the predictive value of levels of self-esteem, hormonal changes, intention to abstain, or stress in identifying which of these girls will suffer deleterious outcomes. It appears that level of ego development and certain subsets of self-esteem (as conceptualized by King and others) may serve as protective factors at this vulnerable time. In addition, several studies have confirmed that early life stress and genetic factors seem to promote early menarche. Some data support association with a deviant older peer group fosters participation in health risk behaviors among these girls. Thus, the literature confirms that there is a relationship between early maturation and risk behaviors but provides few answers as to what factors mediate this relationship.

Peplau's theory of personality development as described in her "Tools and Tasks Outline" (O'Toole & Welt, 1989) offers a framework for examining this phenomenon. She stated that at each stage or era of personality development, the individual is equipped with certain tools and faced with certain predictable tasks. She defined a task as "a learning experience that arises at or about a certain period in the life of an individual, as a result of biological maturation, cultural pressures, and level of aspiration. *Each task that is learned becomes a tool for the next era*" (O'Toole & Welt, 1989, p. 32, emphasis added). Therefore, it is proposed that a child who is in the juvenile era and suddenly faced with the out-of-sequence task of adjusting to the biological and interpersonal changes associated with puberty does not yet possess the tools needed for successful resolution of these tasks. This hypothesis formed the basis of the current research.

SYNTHESIS OF A THEORY OF ASYNCHRONOUS DEVELOPMENT

There were no convincing empirical data to support with certainty any of the proposed mechanisms mediating the observed relationship between early puberty and participation in health risk behaviors. The purpose of this study was to determine whether level of ego development, as described by Hildegard Peplau, could serve as a framework to explain the observed association of early pubertal timing and health risk behaviors. Early puberty is an example of a situation in which there exists a high likelihood of asynchrony of personality development and physiological maturity. Specifically, it was proposed that reliance on the psychological tools belonging to the juvenile era (which proceeds the adolescent era) results in an increased risk of early coital debut and other deviant behaviors with significant health consequences. The tools acquired in late childhood include the ability to share experiences with a same-sex friend, the ability to project oneself into the situation of another, the ability to accept the body as it changes, and a beginning interest in satisfying intimacy needs in interpersonal relationships. It is during this time that, through interaction with same-sex friends, a sense of self-worth develops (Peplau, 1952, p. 308).

If a person is regarded as a personal system, composed of the self, containing a body image (King, 1981) and an evolving self-worth (O'Toole & Welt, 1989), in forward movement in the direction of constructive, productive, personal, and community living (Peplau, 1954), and if successful completion of a learning experience (an event that arises at or near a certain period in the life of an individual) is dependent on the availability of tools developed in preceding developmental eras (King, 1981; Peplau, 1954), then it was proposed a girl who reaches physical maturity before she has accomplished the tasks of late childhood will exhibit difficulties adjusting to puberty. Thus, the researcher proposes a special case of a theory of asynchronous development as the mechanism to explain the observed associations of early menarche and deleterious health outcomes.

Briefly stated, it can be posited that biological factors (physical maturation), social context (peer group age and behaviors), and intrapersonal factors (level of personality development) all interact to raise or lower the likelihood that a young girl will exhibit risk behaviors or depression. It is critical that there be tight linkages among these abstract concepts and the empirical indicators chosen to measure them (see Figure 4.1).

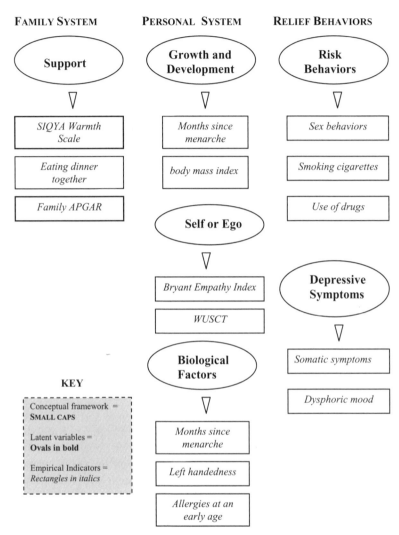

Figure 4.1. Substruction. WUSCT = Washington University Sentence Completion Test. SIQYA = Self Image Questionnaire for Young Adolescents.

Theoretical Definitions

Personality development is the predictable progression from each stage of personality to the next. It is dependent on biological maturation and cultural pressures (Peplau, 1954). *Personality development level* is indicated by the tools available for use by the individual to deal with the developmental tasks facing the individual. These tools are acquired sequentially, through personal experience. The process of developing these tools involves the interaction of physiological development, intrapersonal characteristics, and interpersonal experience in relationships (Peplau, 1954).

An era is a period in time distinguished by certain criteria of a physiological or psychological nature. Peplau, following Sullivan, delineated several predictable, developmental eras (O'Toole & Welt, 1989). *The juvenile era* is that age roughly equivalent with grammar school years during which the child uses symbolic communication and faces the task of defining herself through cooperation and competition with peers. As this era ends, the child enters the *preadolescent era* (O'Toole & Welt, 1989). The preadolescent era extends roughly from age 10 until puberty. In this era, the hallmark task is the need to establish close same-sex friends and to gradually develop the capacity to see the world from their perspective (empathy). This new tool lays the foundation for the development of intimate interpersonal relationships (O'Toole & Welt, 1989).

Empathy can be described as a vicarious emotional response to the perceived emotional experience of another. It is not simply the correct recognition of cues to the present emotional state of others but also encompasses the ability of the empathetic person to understand the situation of another person. This ability to project oneself into the situation of another and to identify with that person's needs and desires is central to the concept of empathy as described by Peplau. This is more than just an affective response that undergirds altruism or sympathetic feelings; it is also a tool that allows one to read accurately the motivations and intent of others.

Adolescence is the era wherein the task is to learn to form a durable and mutually satisfying relationship with a selected individual to fulfill the needs for personal and physical intimacy. The onset of puberty with the emergence of biologically based drives for satisfaction (or sublimation) of sexual urges propels the individual into adolescence (O'Toole & Welt, 1989). The behavior that results from the interaction of these factors is largely shaped by the interpersonal and cultural environment.

For females, *puberty* can be conceptualized as a gradual process, the outcome of which is signaled by the menarche. The process begins with the onset of hypothalamic activity at approximately 8 years of age and is completed with the attainment of ovulatory cycles, signaling full reproductive capacity. The development of secondary sex characteristics accompanies this process (Stevens-Simon, 1993).

Age at coital debut is the age at which a girl first has heterosexual intercourse. For the purposes of this project, coital debut was assumed to have been consensual. In reality, the issue of consent is complex, especially when one contemplates the fact that among unwed teenage mothers fully half report that the father is an adult.

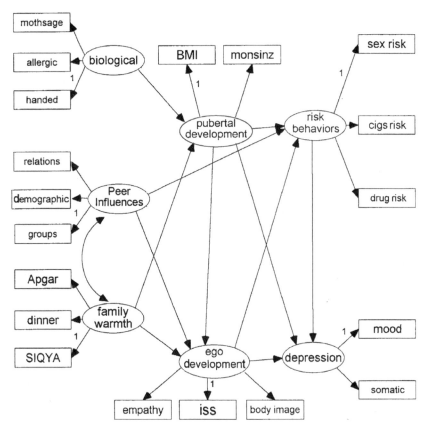

Figure 4.2. Originally proposed model. BMI = body mass index; SIQYA = Self Image Questionnaire for Young Adolescents.

The Model

Model and causal pathways were developed based on the midlevel theory of asynchronous development. The initial model (see Figure 4.2) incorporated three exogenous latent variables (predictor variables) and four endogenous variables (two mediators and two outcomes). In this model, the exogenous variables *biological factors* and *family warmth* and *family conflict* influence the endogenous variable *level of pubertal development*. The model predicted that family conflict would accelerate the rate of pubertal development, whereas family warmth would foster ego development. When these variables proved to be multicollinear, the model was modified by dropping the family conflict predictor and pathway. The latent exogenous variable *family warmth* directly influences the endogenous latent variable *level of ego development*. The *level of pubertal development* was hypothesized to influence *participation in risk behaviors* through its effects on the *level of ego development*. In the model, *level of ego development* directly influences the likelihood of participation in *health risk behaviors*. Furthermore, the *level of pubertal development* has indirect effects on the likelihood of *depressive symptoms* mediated via the *health risk behaviors* latent variable.

Manifest variables (empirical indicators)

The tools chosen to capture the concepts of interest were selected on both their psychometric properties (when applicable) and their ability to establish a meaningful conceptual link to the proposed theory within the framework of this research. A structural equation model requires that multiple empirical indicators represent each of the latent variables in the model. In this case, the challenge was to choose measurement instruments capable of accurately measuring ego development and empathy in a way that would be consistent with the theoretical constructs. The diagram in Figure 4.1 illustrates the relationship or linkages between the framework concepts of family system, personal system, and relief behaviors, and the latent variables (family warmth is linked to family system; ego or self, growth and development, and biological factors are linked to the personal system; and risk behaviors and depression are linked to relief behaviors). The empirical indicators (operationalized variables) are also shown linked to the corresponding latent variables they represent indicators to represent them.

Family system

The literature is replete with support for the idea that commitment and appreciation (Stinnet & Frain, 1985) are qualities of family life that aid the forward development of the child's personality. King described the family as "a social system" with the purpose of influencing "individuals as they grow, develop, and move from dependency in childhood to interdependence in adulthood" (1983, p. 180). Peplau (1952) has described the person as a "self-system" in the environment of a family. She considered the quality of the interpersonal relations within the family to make a key contribution to the growth and development of the individual. Each individual needs human connection and is motivated to act so as to reduce the anxiety of separateness or abandonment. If anxiety is not allayed by the presence of and connection with significant others, then learning and growth and development will be inhibited (Peplau, 1952). Thus, within this framework, the affiliative nature of family relations is critical to foster forward movement of the personality, and by extension, health.

The level of family warmth was operationalized as the score on the Family Warmth subscale of the Self Image Questionnaire for Young Adolescents (Petersen, Schulenburg, Abramovitch, Offer, & Jarcho, 1984). A second empirical indicator of the latent variable family warmth was the score on the Family APGAR (Smilkstein, 1976). In addition to these indicators, a third empirical indicator, the number of times per week that the family sits down to dinner as a unit, was used as a marker of family cohesiveness and warmth.

Personal system

The level of ego development was assessed using the Washington University Sentence Completion Test (WUSCT; Hy & Loevinger, 1996; Loevinger, 1998; Loevinger & Wessler, 1970). The concept of ego development, as measured by this instrument, is the individual's evolving framework of meaning that is imposed on his or her perceptions, inner experience, and perceptions of people and events (Hauser & Sayfer, 1994). This framework assumes that the dimensions of ego development evolve along a continuum. Therefore, the level of ego development represents a continuous variable and can be used in structural equation modeling.

Loevinger derived her theory of personality and ego development from the perspective of an interpersonal framework based in part on the work of Sullivan (who influenced Peplau) and also the field theory of Kurt Lewin (who influenced King). It is logical to conclude that her work is likely to be congruent with that of Peplau and King because they share conceptual and philosophical foundations.

As measured by the WUSCT, the early stage of ego development is characterized by a sense of control by external forces, an egocentric view of the environment, and a limited ability to relate to others. Loevinger termed this the *preconformist* level, and it is indicated by an E-level score of 3 or below (Hauser & Sayfer, 1994). In this study, it was proposed that this is analogous to Peplau's childhood phase, which she described as "The period of living that begins with communication and ends with a beginning need for association with compeers, when the child begins to form relationships with people of his own level" (O'Toole & Welt, p. 35). Peplau also stated that the child responds to "external events" during this phase.

The next stage of ego development, as measured by this instrument, is called the *conformist* level or E-4 (Hauser & Sayfer, 1994). This level is characterized by social concerns, the need for approval, and an understanding of some sort of mutuality in relationships, although this is still limited in terms of understanding motives. This stage ends with a transition marked by self-awareness and a greater understanding of the emotions of others. It is proposed that this is analogous to Peplau's preadolescent phase: "The period of living that begins with the capacity to love and ends with the first evidence of puberty" (O'Toole & Welt, 1989, p. 39). She defines the capacity to love as the tool that enables the individual to express himself freely and naturally. Tolerance, sympathy, generosity, and optimism are described as flowing out of this ability to love.

In the next level of ego development (E-5) as measured by the WUSCT, the individual exhibits increased awareness of the complexity of relationships and less reliance on stereotypes, with relationships being understood as a series of connections and interrelated feelings. This is called the *conscientious* stage (Hauser & Sayfer, 1994). It is proposed that this level is analogous to Peplau's early adolescent stage. According to Peplau, it is during this period that there is "further realization of oneself as an individual in relation to other individuals" (O'Toole & Welt, p. 40). There is also an intense evaluation of authority, ideals, attitudes, and beliefs.

The next stages of ego development as measured by the WUSCT are the autonomous stage (E-6) and the integrated stage (E-7). Collectively, these are termed the *postconformist level* (Hauser & Sayfer, 1994). These levels are characterized by increasing individuality, increased inner awareness, and increased respect for others. It is proposed that the late adolescent phase as described by Peplau is analogous to Loevinger's postconformist stage. In the late adolescent phase, the individual becomes "economically, intellectually, and emotionally self-sufficient" (O'Toole & Welt, p. 41). In this phase of development, there is a newfound focus on the reciprocality of relationships.

Scoring gives both an ordinal-level option and a total score option (treated as interval-level data). It has been used extensively with more than 300 published analyses (Cohn, 1998). A recent review of the reliability and validity of the tool (Gilmore & Durkin, 2001) found extensive empirical evidence supporting the construct, predictive, and discriminant validity of the WUSCT. Use of the manual and adherence to recommended methods of interpretation produce high interrater reliability (Hy & Loevinger, 1996, Loevinger, 1998). Loevinger reported a high level of structural unity for the WUSCT with a principal component analysis demonstrating one major component with an eigen value of 8.8. This high internal unity was created by the constant refinement of the scoring manual toward the end that all items reflect the same underlying variable or total protocol rating (Loevinger, 1998). In this sample, an alpha of .88 was obtained, and the values were normally distributed.

Index of empathy for children and adolescents

If the task of a preadolescent child is to learn to relate to a same-age, same-sex friend and to come to see the world from this other person's perspective, it is proposed that an important tool developed during this era is a capacity for empathy. This ability to see the world from the perspective of another will develop into the beginning of the ability to form intimate interpersonal relationships (O'Toole & Welt, 1989). Through the use of a hermeneutical analysis of King's work, Alligood and May (2000) concluded that the theory of interacting systems implicitly contains several theoretical propositions related to empathy. Here, the two of most relevant include their finding that "empathy facilitates awareness of self and others... (and) facilitates understanding of individuals within a social context" (p. 245).

Because empathy is a concept that has been interpreted in different ways by different theorists (Walker & Alligood, 2001), it is important to chose an instrument that is congruent with the intended definition and that is suitable for use with children and adolescents. Bryant (1982) developed the Index of Empathy for Children and Adolescents (IECA; 1982) based on a widely used adult index of empathy, the Meharabian and Epstein (1972) empathy index. Meharabian and Epstein defined empathy as a vicarious emotional response to the perceived emotional experience of another. This contrasts with definitions of empathy which emphasize correct recognition of the cues to the emotional states of others, in that it encompasses a responsive, shared feeling tone. It also encompasses a sense that the person can understand the situation of the other. The ability to project oneself into the situation of another and identify with their needs and desires (as described by Peplau) has a logical correspondence with this definition of empathy.

Because empathy, in this context, is conceptualized as a trait rather than a state, it was particularly important for the measure to exhibit stability in test–retest scores. Test–retest scores on the IECA for seventh-grade students showed an adequate level of stability at a 2-week interval ($r = .85$). Convergent validity was satisfactory (Bryant, 1982) using an existing empathy measure, the Feshbach and Roe (1968) childhood measure of empathy. Tests of discriminant validity and controls for social desirability responses were acceptable. Thus, the IECA is a valid and reliable, age-appropriate measure of empathy suitable for use in this context.

In the initial development of a model to explain why early-maturing girls participate in high-risk behaviors at higher rates than their peers, King's work suggested that body image would be an important component of ego development, especially at this age. Body image was defined by King (1981) as a dynamic characteristic that is shaped by growth and developmental changes and the person's awareness of the ways in which others react to these changes. It is an internalized mental representation of the body intimately connected to the idea of self. Peplau (O'Toole & Welt, 1989) described one of the tasks of the preadolescent phase as the acceptance of the changing body. It was proposed that children who have a higher degree of personality development would exhibit higher scores on a measure of body image satisfaction. The inability to use this variable in the model is an example of how ensuring tight correspondence between an empirical indicator and a theoretical definition will not ensure that model analysis will go forward without problems. Entry of the data for variables tapping into the concept of body image caused our model to "crash" (i.e., to have no solution). Analysis of the modification indices in AMOS software (1997, version 3.61) seemed to indicate a tendency for this factor to load on other factors (e. g., body mass index, pubertal development, and other single empirical indicators). Given the focal nature of body changes for this age group and the fact that bodily sensations are a preoccupation of individuals at the preconformist or E-3 level of ego development (E-3 was the modal score for level of ego development in this sample), this is not a surprising finding. It may be useful to think of body image as so overwhelmingly focal for early adolescent girls that it is almost a ground rather than a useful predictor variable.

Relief behaviors

Peplau spoke of relief behaviors as patient responses to frustration that can be observed, described, and understood. Relief behaviors are pattern interactions that are essential to the functioning of the whole person and that tend to become automatic. These behaviors dissipate the energy that frustration or anxiety engender. In this model, it is proposed that risk-taking behaviors (smoking, drug use, sexual activity) are one form of relief behaviors. Standard survey instruments based on the CDC Youth Risk Surveillance survey can adequately quantify these behaviors. Peplau viewed maladaptive affective responses as alternative relief behaviors. Beeber, Canuso, and Emory (2004) recently updated the role of relief behaviors (which they call *security operations*) in the development of depression. They propose that depressive symptoms represent one form of transient relief behaviors that can become repetitive patterns resulting in persistent depression. In this model, it is proposed that these two types of relief behaviors should be inversely related. That is, risk-taking behaviors should dissipate the energy that might otherwise result in depression. Depressive symptoms can be captured by measures of somatic symptoms and dysphoric mood.

TESTING THE MODEL

Using the graphical interface in AMOS 3.61, the path model was created to reflect the proposed structural relations of the model. Two competing models were developed to explain the dynamics of family warmth, ego development, and pubertal development and their possible interactions and to explain how these variables affect the outcomes of depressive symptoms and risk-taking behaviors. The only difference between these models was the existence of a path from the latent variable risk behaviors to the latent variable depression. The path weight on this path was in the expected direction but did not reach statistical significance. As with all structural equation programs, AMOS tests to determine whether the parameters specified in the model produce an implied covariance matrix that closely resembles the covariance matrix of the observed variables.

If the specified models are alike in all ways except for the number of restraints placed on parameters, the models can be said to be hierarchically nested and direct comparisons of their relative goodness of fit can be made. The chi-square of the weaker model can be subtracted from the chi-square of the stronger model. The difference here is $117.96 - 117.24 = .72$; for degrees of freedom, it is $80 - 79 = 1$. For 1 degree of freedom, chi-squares greater than 3.84 are significant at the .05 level. Based on this test, we should accept Model B (see Figure 4.3).

The full model has a chi-square of 117.24 with 79 degrees of freedom. The CFI, Bentler's comparative fit index, should be .9 or higher to accept a model. Here, the CFI is .90. The adjusted goodness of fit is an often-reported fit index, and here it is .94, which is also quite acceptable. Other fit indices are the root mean square error of approximation (RMSEA), which is used to compensate for the effects of model complexity. Browne and Cudek (1993) recommend a value of .05 or less on the RMSEA as an indication of a good fit for the model, taking the degrees of freedom into account. They suggested an upper limit of .08 and felt that a value any higher invalidated a model. Here, this index suggests that the model can be accepted because the RMSEA is .04.

The model had an acceptable fit, the standardized path coefficients were interpretable, and the critical ratios of the path weights were acceptable. The squared multiple correlations option in AMOS provides estimations of the amount of variance accounted for by the model. These are printed on the path diagram in Figure 4.3.

DISCUSSION

Careful analysis of the conceptual framework developed by King and the theory of development implied by Peplau in her "Tools and Tasks Outline" resulted in their synthesis to form a middle range theory of asynchronous development. The special case of the child experiencing early menarche was examined and a testable hypothesis was developed. This hypothesis stated that if a person is regarded as a personal system, composed of the self (King, 1981) and an evolving self-worth (O'Toole & Welt, 1989),

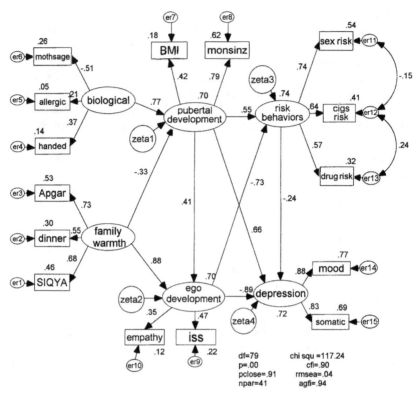

Figure 4.3. Full model with standardized coefficient, using asymptotically distribution free estimate. BMI = body mass index; RMSEA = root mean square error of approximation.

in forward movement (Peplau, 1954); and if successful completion of a learning experience (an event that arises at or near a certain period in the life of an individual) is dependent on the availability of tools developed in preceding developmental eras (King, 1981; Peplau, 1954), a girl who reaches physical maturity before she has accomplished the tasks of late childhood will exhibit difficulties adjusting to puberty. The tools that are acquired in late childhood include the ability to share experiences with a same-sex friend, the ability to project oneself into another's situation, the ability to accept the body as it changes, and a beginning awareness of an emerging need for physical intimacy.

Evidence in Support of the Theory

The theory states that a girl who reaches physical maturity before she has accomplished the tasks of late childhood will exhibit difficulties adjusting to puberty. Two latent variables, participation in health risk behaviors and reports of depressive symptoms, were identified from the literature as meaningful problem areas for girls who experience menarche earlier than their peers. The theory also proposed that the level of ego development was an important aspect of human development and a tool for coping with the tasks of adolescence. Ego development is posited to be fostered by warm and supportive interpersonal relations within the family system. The biological aspects of being human (embodied) are, by the principle of isomorphy, also subject to influence by interpersonal relations within the family system. In this case, it is posited that family conflict (the polar opposite of family warmth and support) would tend to decrease age at menarche. It is proposed that the level of pubertal development predicts the likelihood of participation in risky behaviors as well as the likelihood of manifesting depressive symptoms; however, this is seen as the result of attempting to cope with the tasks of the adolescent era without the benefit of the tools that should have been developed in the juvenile era. Level of ego development, encompassing both empathy and general ego development, opposes the influence of early pubertal development, offering a buffering effect against the influence of early menarche and decreasing the asynchrony.

The model specifying these relationships was developed and tested for the described variables and sample (see Figure 4.3). In this context, the model offers strong support of the theory, explaining approximately 70% of the variance of the dependent variables.

Limitations

Although the method used is generally held to be robust, the failure to demonstrate multivariate normality and the need to use an alternate model estimation is a common problem in the social sciences, fields in which many variables of interest are liable to be not multivariate normal. The difficulty making reasonable determinations regarding sample size, number of variables that should be permitted in the model, which goodness of fit indices to use, and how to gauge the trustworthiness of the path weights have been areas of change within the field of structural equation modeling.

There is almost always the possibility that an important variable has not been specified in the model. Theories of interpersonal development, including Peplau and King, suggest that peer interaction ought to be increasingly focal as the child moves away from family influence. In this case, it is not possible to evaluate whether a theoretically appealing peer interaction variable would have altered the way the model ran.

Another potential difficulty has to do with the ability of the instruments to capture the latent constructs. Although good linkages through theory can greatly increase the likelihood that testing will capture the variables of interest, problems can still occur. Survey data of youth and children under the conditions that are common at school can increase the amount of random error that any instrument captures.

Implications for Future Research

The implications for future research can be divided into two broad categories: measurement issues and theoretical issues. Measurement issues include problems with the validity and reliability of empirical indicators and steps to improve existing measures or develop new tools. There is also the issue of replication with other samples. If the failure to develop meaningful friendships with same-sex friends is the root cause of poor judgment regarding interpersonal relations, then it holds that the corrective experience would be to encourage the development of meaningful friendships. It is possible to speculate that many social conventions of mid- to late adolescence provide opportunities for this to happen (teams, roommates, group experiences of many sorts). For adolescent girls who become alienated from their peer group, interventions might be designed to target this need for affiliation and shared experiences in safe, supervised environments. Theoretical issues include consideration of ways to explore further the special case of developmental asynchrony represented by the girl experiencing early menarche but also consideration of other developmental eras and challenges when asynchrony is likely.

CONCLUSION

In nursing science, there has been a disturbing trend toward regarding the linkage between theory and research as optional, or even as an artificial distraction. Yet it is clear that our most powerful research tools, such as structural equation modeling, only retain their power when used as confirmatory procedures. This means that one must have predicted an outcome before one can look for it. Furthermore, the amount of information captured by any empirical indicator is directly related to the strength of its relationship to the actual phenomenon of interest. Without these two conditions, each of which implies that careful consideration has been given to theoretical issues of concept development, instrument evaluation for the specific application, and the theory based relationships between variables, it is unlikely that a research project can accurately develop and test explanatory models. This is not to suggest that there is any real value to retrospectively "tacking on" a nursing theory to a project that was conceived atheoretically.

In this instance, review of the existing literature revealed that many researchers had, from an atheoretical stance, examined a multitude of factors as possible influential antecedents to the observed vulnerabilities among early-maturing girls. No satisfying explanatory model had substantive empirical support. In an effort to reconceptualize the approach to this problem, a review of nursing theories was undertaken to discover which theory might best address the key issues of early maturity. From this work, a midlevel theory of asynchronous development evolved. The resulting analysis and synthesis of King's interacting systems framework with Peplau's theory of interpersonal relationships directed attention to the possible role of ego development and empathy as mediating factors. A model incorporating these ideas was developed and tested. The results support both the midlevel theory and the value of theory-driven research.

REFERENCES

Alligood, M. R., & May, B. (2000). A nursing theory of personal system empathy: Interpreting a conceptualization of empathy in King's interacting systems. *Nursing Science Quarterly, 13*, 243–247.

Arbuckle, J. L. (1997). *AMOS User's guide.* Version 3.61. Chicago, IL: Salt Waters Corporation.

Aseltine, R. H., & Gore, S. L. (2000). The variable effects of stress on alcohol use from adolescence to early adulthood. *Substance Use and Misuse, 35*, 643–668.

Beeber, L. S., Canuso, R., & Emory, S. (2004). Instrumental inputs: Moving the interpersonal theory of nursing into practice. *Advances in Nursing Science, 27*, 275–286.

Bolden, L., & Williams, B. G. (1995). A measurement of self-esteem in pregnant teenagers. *Clinical Nursing Research, 4*, 223–231.

Browne, M. W., & Cudeck, R. (1993). Alternative ways of assessing model fit. In K. A. Bollen & J. S. Long (Eds.), *Testing structural equation models* (pp. 136–162). Newbury Park, CA: Sage.

Bryant, B. K. (1982). An index of empathy for children and adolescents. *Child Development, 53*, 413–425.

Cairns, R. B., & Cairns, B. D. (1994). *Lifelines and risks.* Cambridge, England: Cambridge University Press.

Cohn, L. D. (1998). Age trends in personality development: A quantitative review. In P. M. Westenberg, A. Blasi, & L. D. Cohn (Eds.), *Personality development: Theoretical, empirical, and clinical investigations of Loevinger's conception of ego development* (pp. 133–144). Mahwah, NJ: Erlbaum.

Cohn, L. D., Westenberg, P. M., & Cohn, L. D. (2004). Intelligence and maturity: Meta-analytic evidence for the incremental and discriminant validity of Loevinger's measure of ego development. *Journal of Personality and Social Psychology, 86*, 760–772.

Connelly, C. D. (1998). Hopefulness, self-esteem, and perceived social support among pregnant and nonpregnant adolescents. *Western Journal of Nursing Research, 20,* 195–209.

Connor, J. M., Poyrazli, J., Ferrer-Wreder, S., Grahame, L., & Maraj, K. (2004). The relation of age, gender, ethnicity, and risk behaviors to self-esteem among students in non-mainstream schools. *Adolescence, 39,* 457–473.

Ellickson, P. L., Tucker, J. S., Klein, D. J., & Saner, H. (2004). Antecedents and outcomes of marijuana use initiation during adolescence. *Preventive Medicine, 39,* 976–984.

Fawcett, J., & Downs, F. (1992). *The relationship of theory and research.* Philadelphia: Davis.

Feshbach, N. D., & Roe, K. (1968). Empathy in six- and seven-year-olds. *Child Development, 39,* 133–145.

Forchuk, C. (1991). Peplau's theory: Concepts and their relations. *Nursing Science Quarterly, 4*(2), 54–60.

Gilmore, J. M., & Durkin, K. (2001). Critical review of the validity of ego development theory and its measurement. *Journal of Personality Assessment, 77,* 541–567.

Halpern, C. T., Udry, J. R., & Suchindran, C. (1997). Monthly measures of salivary testosterone predict sexual activity in adolescent males. *Archives of Sexual Behavior, 27,* 445–465.

Hauser, S. T., & Sayfer, A. W. (1994). Ego development and adolescent emotions. *Journal of Research on Adolescence, 4,* 487–502.

Hy, L. X., & Loevinger, J. (1996). *Measuring ego development* (2nd ed.). Hillsdale, NJ: Erlbaum.

Johansson, T., & Ritzen, E. M. (2005). Very long-term follow-up of girls with early and late menarche. *Endocrine Development, 8,* 126–36.

King, I. M. (1971). *Toward a theory for nursing: General concepts of human behavior.* New York: Wiley.

King, I. M. (1981). *A theory for nursing: Systems, concepts, process.* New York: Wiley.

King, I. M. (1983). King's theory of nursing. In I. W. Clements & F. B. Roberts (Eds.), *Family health: A theoretical approach to nursing care* (pp. 177–188). New York: Wiley.

King, I. M. (1987). King's theory of goal attainment. In R. R. Parse (Ed.), *Nursing science: Major paradigms, theories and critiques* (pp. 107–114). Philadelphia: Saunders.

King, I. M. (1990). King's conceptual framework and theory of goal attainment. In M. E. Parker (Ed.), *Nursing theories in practice* (pp. 73–84). New York: National League for Nursing.

Koniak-Griffin, D., Lesser, J., Uman, G., & Nyamathi, A. (2003). Teen pregnancy, motherhood, and unprotected sexual activity. *Research in Nursing and Health, 26,* 4–19.

Lanza, S. T., & Collins, L. M. (2003). Pubertal timing and the onset of substance abuse in females during early adolescence. *Prevention Science, 3,* 369–382.

Loevinger, J. (1998). History of the Sentence Completion Test (SCT) for ego development. In J. Loevinger (Ed.), *Technical foundations for measuring ego development: The Washington University Sentence Completion Test.* Mahwah, NJ: Lawrence Erlbaum Associates.

Loevinger, J., & Wessler, R. (1970). *Measuring ego development: 1. Construction and use of a sentence completion test.* San Francisco: Jossey-Bass.

Masten, A. S. (2004). Regulatory processes, risk, and resilience in adolescent development. *Annals of the New York Academy of Sciences, 1021,* 310–319.

Meharabian, A., & Epstein, N. (1972). A measure of emotional empathy. *Journal of Personality, 40,* 525–543.

O'Toole, A. W., & Welt, S. R. (1989). *Interpersonal theory in nursing practice: Selected works of Hildegard E. Peplau.* New York: Springer Publishing Company.

Paul, C., Fitzjohn, J., Herbison, P., & Dickson, N. (2000). The determinants of sexual intercourse before age 16. *Journal of Adolescent Health, 27,* 136–147.

Peplau, H. E. (1952). *Interpersonal relations in nursing.* New York: Putnam.

Peplau, H. E. (1964). Psychiatric nursing skills and the general hospital patient. *Nursing Forum, 16,* 28–37.

Peplau, H. E. (1992). Interpersonal relations: A theoretical framework for application in nursing practice. *Nursing Science Quarterly, 5,* 13–18.

Resnick, M. D., & Blum, R. W. (1985). Developmental and personalogical correlates of adolescent sexual behavior and outcome. *International Journal of Adolescent Medicine and Health, 1,* 293–313.

Rierdan, J. (1998). Ego development, pubertal development, and depressive symptoms in adolescent girls. In P. M. Westenberg, A. Blasi, & L. D. Cohn (Eds.), *Personality development: Theoretical, empirical, and clinical investigations of Loevinger's conception of ego development* (pp. 253–269). Mahwah, NJ: Erlbaum.

Rierdan, J., & Koff, E. (1997). Weight, weight-related aspects of body image, and depression in early adolescent girls. *Adolescence, 32,* 615–624.

Shrier, L. A., Harris, S. K., Sternberg, M., & Beardslee, W. R. (2001). Associations of depression, self-esteem, and substance use with sexual risk among adolescents. *Prevention Medicine, 33,* 179–189.

Smilkstein, G. (1978). The family APGAR: A proposal for a family function test and its use by physicians. *Journal of Family Practice, 6*(6), 1231–1239.

Stattin, H., & Magnusson, D. (1990). *Pubertal maturation in female development.* Hillsdale, NJ: Erlbaum.

Stevenson, W., Maston, K. I., & Teti, D. M. (1999). Social support, relationship quality, and well-being among pregnant adolescents. *Journal of Adolescence, 22,* 109–121.

Sullivan, H. S. (1953). *The interpersonal theory of psychiatry.* New York: Norton.

Sutton, S., McVey, D., & Glanz, A. (1999). A comparative test of the theory of reasoned action and the theory of planned behavior in the prediction of condom use intentions in a national sample of English young people. *Health Psychology, 18,* 72–81.

Takahashi, T. (1992). Perspectives on nursing knowledge. *Nursing Science Quarterly, 5,* 86–91.

Tschann, J. M., Adler, N., Irwin, C. E., Millstein, S. G., Turner, R. A., & Kegeles, S. M. (1994). Initiation of substance use in early adolescence: The roles of pubertal timing and emotional distress. *Health Psychology, 4,* 326–333.

Walker, K. M., & Alligood, M. R. (2001). Empathy from a nursing perspective: Moving beyond borrowed theory. *Archives of Psychiatric Nursing, 15,* 140–147.

Waylen, A., & Wolke, D. (2004). Sex 'n' drugs 'n' rock 'n' roll: The meaning and social consequences of pubertal timing. *European Journal of Endocrinology, 161*(Suppl. 3), U151–U159.

Wild, L. G., Flisher, A. J., Bhana, A., & Lombard, C. (2004). Associations among adolescent risk behaviours and self-esteem in six domains. *Journal of Child Psychology, 45,* 1454–1467.

CHAPTER FIVE

Testing a Theory of Decision Making Derived From King's Systems Framework in Women Eligible for a Cancer Clinical Trial

Heidi E. Ehrenberger, Martha Raile Alligood, Sandra P. Thomas, Debra C. Wallace, and Cynthia M. Licavoli

The purpose of this study was to test an explanatory theory of decision making in women eligible for a cancer clinical trial. The theory derived from King's framework proposed that the concepts of uncertainty, role functioning, and social support relate to emotional health (hope and mood state), which in turn relates to the treatment decision. A correlational study design was used to test the theory in a sample af 40 women. Findings provided empirical evidence of the adequacy of King's framework and supported, in part, theorized relationships among the critical factors. However, these factors did not illuminate the treatment decision.

Optimal cancer treatments can only be devised through patient enrollment in cancer clinical trials. Yet less than 3% of all persons with cancer enroll in clinical trials (Ho, 1994; National Cancer Institute, 2000; Tejeda et al., 1996). There remains a critical need to increase the number of

Authors' Note: Research support for this work was provided by a doctoral scholarship (FO05) from the Oncology Nursing Society Foundation (Thomas Jordan Doctoral Scholarship, Bristol-Myers Squibb Oncology Division).

persons with cancer who participate in clinical trials. Because women have been grossly underrepresented in multiple therapeutic areas of investigations (Thomas, 1997), it is vital to understand their unique approach to decision making regarding clinical trial enrollment. Despite efforts by social scientists and physicians to study the phenomenon of cancer clinical trial enrollment, the problem of low and slow enrollment persists (Gotay, 1991). The inadequate specification of the personal and psychological factors of patient refusal, as well as the complexity of the response regarding entry into the clinical trial, are no doubt responsible, to a great extent, for the lack of progress. Clearly, there is an expedient need to improve understanding of the patient factors surrounding the enrollment process (Huizinga, Sleijfer, van de Wiel, & van der Graaf, 1999; Schain, 1994).

Recently, nurse researchers have begun to investigate the psychosocial aspects of the cancer clinical trial enrollment process (Cox & Avis, 1996; Crago, Schaefer, & Gyaunch, 1997; Yoder, O'Rourke, Etnyre, Spears, & Brown, 1997). Previous findings from Dwyer's (1993) research on decision making maintained that the cancer patient's decision relies primarily on human emotion and less on the cognition of decision analysis, expected utility theory, or judgment heuristics. Additionally, Dwyer (1993) found that the actual decision is dependent on how the patient sees the self as able to pursue and psychologically manage a given treatment. Dwyer not only emphasized the role of human emotions but also the role of emotional wellness or health in the decision-making process. These findings by Dwyer are congruent with the theoretical perspective offered by King (1981). Both King and Dwyer emphasized the individual's perception of the situation and the nature of subjectivity in the decision-making process. To date, studies that examine the psychosocial influences on women's emotional health in relation to the treatment decision have been absent from the literature. This chapter describes the testing of a theory of decision making in women eligible for a cancer clinical trial.

BACKGROUND

Identifying barriers to optimal clinical trial accrual and subsequently developing strategies to overcome them are of critical importance (Gotay, 1991). Despite the urgent need for effective strategies, there are only a few systematic studies of patients in cancer clinical trials, and the findings rarely go beyond demographics and exclusion criteria (Gotay, 1991; Swanson & Ward, 1995). Patient demographic characteristics such as age and sociodemographic status are fairly well understood in the enrollment process; however, they are not readily changeable or amenable to interventions to increase accrual (Morrow, Hickock, & Burish, 1994). Additionally, these characteristics are inadequate by themselves in explaining the patient's emotional health. Gotay (1991) recommended that additional research should focus on the perspectives of patients who accept and decline trial participation and on subsequent interventions designed to affect enrollment. Yet rarely have the perspectives of patients been assessed. Given the complexity of the patient's response regarding entry into or avoidance of a clinical trial, Schain (1994) maintained that researchers must try and isolate a few of the major variables to learn more about this phenomenon. Cox and Avis (1996) and Yoder et al. (1997) clearly identified the significance of hope in the enrollment process, whereas Crago et al. (1997) identified the significance of uncertainty and social support. Therefore, the present nursing study extends the previous patient-focused research on demographics and exclusion criteria. It builds on the previous studies by Cox and Avis (1996), Crago et al. (1997), Dwyer (1993), and Yoder et al. (1997), but goes beyond those studies by assessing the indicators of emotional health and the relationship between emotional health and enrollment. This research was designed to begin addressing the critical issues raised by Dwyer (1993), Gotay (1991), and Schain (1994).

PURPOSE OF THE STUDY

The purpose of this study was to test an explanatory theory of decision making derived from King's (1981) framework in women who had been given the option to enroll in a cancer treatment trial. The theory proposes that concepts of uncertainty, role functioning, and social support relate to emotional health (hope and mood state), which in turn relate to the treatment decision. The primary research questions formulated to test the proposed theory were: (a) What is the extent of the relationship among personal, interpersonal, and social systems' concepts (uncertainty, role functioning, social support) and emotional health (hope and mood state)? and (b) What is the extent of the relationship between emotional health (hope and mood state) and the treatment decision?

CONCEPTUAL FRAMEWORK AND THEORY

King's (1981) framework provides a reference for the domain of nursing. It is based on the overall assumption that the focus of nursing is human beings interacting with their environment leading to a state of health for individuals (King, 1981). This framework consists of three interacting systems: the personal system, the interpersonal system, and the social

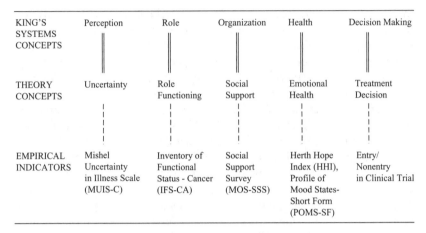

KING'S SYSTEMS CONCEPTS	Perception	Role	Organization	Health	Decision Making
THEORY CONCEPTS	Uncertainty	Role Functioning	Social Support	Emotional Health	Treatment Decision
EMPIRICAL INDICATORS	Mishel Uncertainty in Illness Scale (MUIS-C)	Inventory of Functional Status - Cancer (IFS-CA)	Social Support Survey (MOS-SSS)	Herth Hope Index (HHI), Profile of Mood States-Short Form (POMS-SF)	Entry/ Nonentry in Clinical Trial

Figure 5.1. Conceptual–Theoretical–Empirical Structure.

system. The boundaries of each system are open, such that each system influences the others. In each system there are interrelated concepts such as perception, role, and organization. King (1995) asserted, "This framework differs from other conceptual schema in that it is concerned not with fragmenting human beings and the environment but with human transactions in different types of environments" (p. 21). The theory derived from King's (1981) framework proposes relationships between the variable of emotional health and several systems concepts: (a) the woman's uncertainty about the illness situation, (b) her ability to function in her roles, and (c) her social support network. A relationship between emotional health and the treatment decision is also proposed. The concepts are linked to King's systems as indicated in Figure 5.1. These linkages, also supported with the literature pertaining to cancer nursing and cancer clinical trials, are further described here.

King's (1981) personal system contained several key concepts, including perception. According to Mishel (1983), uncertainty is a perceptual variable. When a physician presents a clinical trial as a treatment option to an individual, it introduces into the illness situation the fact that the best answer for treating the illness remains unknown. Stetz (1993) stated that little is known about how patients manage uncertainty with respect to making the decision to enter a clinical trial. Uncertainty occurs when the decision maker (the woman eligible for a cancer clinical trial) is unable to assign definite values to objects and events, is unable to accurately predict outcomes, or both (Mishel, 1988). Moreover, perceptions of uncertainty can lead to problems in psychosocial adjustment and a pessimistic view of the future (Mishel, 1983).

King's (1981) description of the interpersonal system contained the concept of role. According to King, several elements give meaning to the concept of role, including the "relationship with one or more individuals interacting in specific situations for a purpose" (p. 93). Whereas the ability or inability to function in roles is certainly related to health, it is not the overall definition of health (Winker, 1995). Role function in the tested theory is clearly viewed as influencing health or more precisely, emotional health. Accordingly, "role functioning refers to the degree to which an individual performs or has the capacity to perform activities typical for a specified age and social responsibility" (Sherbourne, Stewart, & Wells, 1992, p. 205). Unfortunately, the important roles held by women have often not been assessed in the context of role functioning (Sherbourne et al., 1992). During the treatment decision-making process, the person with cancer must rebalance his or her roles within the family and society while attempting to regain and maintain a state of physical and emotional well-being (Dwyer, 1993). Women may have a more difficult time rebalancing the roles because of role multiplicity, which in turn may create distress.

King (1981) characterized social systems as the family, religious systems, work systems, educational systems, and peer groups. She identified the organization as a major concept of the social system, noting an "organization as a system exhibits patterns of individual and group behavior, patterns of communication and patterns of interaction" (p. 121). Thus, an organization can represent a social support system. Family support can be a significant factor in the patient's decision making process as members provide emotional support throughout the process (Johansen, Mayer, & Hoover, 1991). Conversely, the absence of informal and formal networks can pose major problems to patients with cancer who are seeking care (Guidry et al., 1996). Morrow et al. (1994) went so far as to say that "support groups may improve the likelihood of study entry of patients with inadequate social networks" (p. 2681). The presence or absence of an adequate social support system or network may influence how the individual emotionally pursues the decision to participate in a complex clinical trial.

King (1971) stated that health "encompasses the whole man physical, emotional, and social . . . within the cultural pattern in which he was born and to which he attempts to conform" (p. 67). King (1981) also stated that the goal of nursing "is to help individuals maintain their health so they can function in their roles" (pp. 3–4). In examining King's (1971, 1981) various definitions of health, Winker (1995) noted, "Limiting the definition of health to role function does not comprehend the interaction of people and the universe and the teleological nature of humanity" (p. 42). Therefore, a new definition of health was created by Winker

(1995), who stated that "health is the ability of the individual to create meaningful symbols based on either biological or human values within his or her cultural and individual-value systems" (p. 42). Furthermore, Dwyer (1993) believed that there is a relationship between the process of making the treatment decision and emotional well-being. In the proposed theory, health is viewed as emotional health that takes into account King's (1971) and Winker's (1995) definitions of health. A state of emotional health is desired prior to engaging in an active course of cancer therapy, although it is not always present in optimal form due to factors such as grief or denial (Dwyer, 1993). Within the theory, the indicators of emotional health are hope and mood state.

King (1981) stated, "Decisions are individual, personal, and subjective" (p. 132). Dwyer (1993) contended that for the person with cancer, the treatment decision stems from human emotion, which the proposed theory conceptualizes as emotional health. The action of decision making manifests itself in the treatment decision. Therefore, the treatment decision is consenting to enter or not to enter the clinical trial.

METHODOLOGY

Design

A descriptive, correlational study design was used. The primary measurements of all variables were made at entry into this study using self-report, paper-and-pencil scales that were conceptually linked with empirical indicators of the concepts in the theory (see Figure 5.1). This approach yielded reports about emotional health in close relation to the precise day of finalizing the treatment decision. The design avoided placing high demands on the participant, which could lead to refusal to participate in the proposed nursing study (Hinds, Quargnenti, & Madison, 1995).

Sample and Setting

A sample of women newly diagnosed with cancer was drawn from four cancer care facilities. A woman was eligible for participation if she (a) was at least 18 years old, (b) could communicate in English verbally and in writing, (c) had a cancer diagnosis ≤ 6 months, (d) had a Karnofsky Performance Status (KPS) score of ≥ 60, (e) had no history of psychiatric illness, (f) had been given the option to enroll in a treatment trial by her physician, and (g) reported the personal treatment decision had been made 28 days prior. The sample was one of convenience according to the availability of participants. Power analysis using SamplePower 1.0 software indicated that with a sample size of 40 and alpha set at .05, the study would have a power of 0.92.

Instruments

The Mishel Uncertainty in Illness Scale—Community Form (MUIS-C) is used to measure the uncertainty perceived in illness by those persons who are not hospitalized (Mishel, 1997). The MUIS-C is a 23-item scale with a 5-point Likert-format response set ranging from *strongly disagree* to *strongly agree*. The verb tense has been modified in three items in consultation with the author (M. Mishel, personal communication, September 17, 1997). A score is obtained for the total scale, which represents the one-factor. To calculate the one-factor/total score, all items are summed. The total uncertainty score ranges from 23 to 115. Higher scores indicate more uncertainty. The MUIS-C has been used in samples of participants with breast cancer and other illnesses (Mishel, 1997). The reliabilities for the MUIS-C were reported to be in the moderate-to-high range (alpha = .74 to .92). Evidence of content and construct validity has also been provided (Mishel, 1997).

The Inventory of Functional Status-Cancer (IFS-CA) measures functional status in women who have cancer. Functional status is defined "as a multidimensional concept that encompasses continuation of usual household and family, social and community, personal care, and occupational activities following diagnosis of cancer" (Tulman, Fawcett, & McEvoy, 1991, p. 254). The IFS-CA is conceptually based on the Roy adaptation model role function response mode, which reflects activities associated with a person's primary, secondary, and tertiary roles (Fawcett & Tulman, 1996). The IFS-CA, a 39-item questionnaire, measures the extent to which the woman continues her usual activities. All items use a 4-point rating scale ranging from 1 (*not at all*) to 4 (*fully*) for household, family, social, and community activities, and 1 (*never*) to 4 (*all of the time*) for personal care and occupational activities. The total IFS-CA score is computed such that the possible range of scores is 1 to 4; the higher the score, the greater the total functional status. The IFS-CA has been used in women diagnosed with different types of cancer (Tulman & Fawcett, 1996; Tulman et al., 1991). Content validity was established at 98.5%. Test–retest reliability coefficient for the total IFS-CA has been reported at .91 (Tulman et al., 1991).

The Medical Outcomes Study—Social Support Survey (MOS-SSS) is used to assess the perceived availability, if needed, of various components of functional support in an adult patient population (Sherbourne &

Stewart, 1991). The MOS-SSS is a 19-item survey that assesses emotional–informational support, tangible support, affectionate support, and positive social interaction. All items use a 5-point Likert response format with choices ranging from 1 (*none of the time*) to 5 (*all of the time*). The observed scores range from 1 to 5 for the overall support index. The scores can be transformed to 0 to 100. Higher scores indicate more frequent availability of different types of support, as needed. The transformed score for the overall support index was used in the present study. This tool has been used in various patient populations, including chronically ill women. The reported alpha reliability for the total support index is .97. Evidence of validity testing with multitrait scaling has also been reported (Sherbourne & Stewart, 1991).

The Herth Hope Index (HHI) is used to assess hope in adult patients within the clinical setting. Hope is defined as a multidimensional dynamic life force characterized by a confident yet uncertain expectation of achieving good, which to the hoping person is realistically possible and personally significant (Herth, 1992). The HHI is a 12-item instrument adapted from the Herth Hope Scale (HHS); it was designed specifically for clinical application and research. The HHI uses a Likert-type response set ranging from 1 (*strongly disagree*) to 4 (*strongly agree*), with a total range of scores from 12 to 48. The higher the total scale score, the higher the level of hope. This tool has been used in adult men and women diagnosed with various types of cancer (Herth, 1989, 1992). Alpha coefficient is reported to be .97 with a 2-week test–retest reliability of 0.91; correlation with the parent HHS is 0.92 (Herth, 1992).

The Profile of Mood States—Short Form (POMS-SF) is used to identify and assess transient, fluctuating affective states. According to McNair, Lorr, and Droppleman (1992), "The understanding of the psychology of emotion requires not only the inclusion of physiological and behavioral data but also the subjective data of feeling, affect and mood" (p. 1). The POMS-SF is a 30-item measure that uses a 5-point adjective rating scale ranging from 0 (*not at all*) to 4 (*extremely*) for assessing identifiable mood or affective states: tension–anxiety, depression–dejection, anger–hostility, vigor–activity, fatigue–inertia, and confusion–bewilderment. From the POMS-SF, a Total Mood Disturbance (TMD) score is calculated that provides an overall measure of adjustment. The score ranges from −20 to 100; the higher the score, the greater the mood disturbance. The POMS has been used in numerous studies of female cancer patients (McNair et al., 1992). Alpha reliabilities reported for the POMS-SF in a female sample range from .75 to .90 (McNair et al., 1992).

Participants also completed a 10-item demographic data form that ascertained the following: date, approximate date of the treatment decision, actual treatment decision, type and stage of cancer, age, ethnic group, marital status, educational level, number of children, employment status, and financial concern.

Procedures

The appropriate human participants review committees at each of the four cancer care facilities approved the study. Designated clinical trial nurses (CTNs) at each facility were oriented to study procedures. The actual data collection procedure was imbedded in the regular process of clinical trial consideration. The CTN typically saw the patient after the physician discussed treatment options and provided details of the treatment trial. When the patient met the criteria for the present study, the potential participant was given a brief explanation of the nursing study by the CTN at the closure of the initial meeting with the CTN. The patient usually made the enrollment decision within 2 weeks after the physician recommendation. At the point of informing the physician or CTN of the therapy decision, the patient was again given an explanation of the nursing study by the CTN. If the patient was interested in participating, the informed consent statement attached to the questionnaire was given in conjunction with verbal instruction for completion. Completion of the questionnaire required approximately 15 to 20 minutes. Data from the questionnaires were analyzed using SPSS 7.5 statistical software.

RESULTS

Sample

A convenience sample of 40 women newly diagnosed with cancer and eligible for a treatment trial participated. Select characteristics are presented in Table 5.1. The average age of the participants was 55.32 years (range = 23–76, $SD = 12.35$). The average number of years of education completed by the participants was 13.45 (range = 7–17, $SD = 2.12$). All participants completed the questionnaire within 28 days of making their self-reported treatment decision. The mean time to completion was 6.02 days (range = 0 to 28, $SD = 7.87$). Of the participants, 27 (67.5%) decided to enroll in a treatment trial, whereas 13 (32.5%) decided not to enroll. Efforts were made to obtain a more evenly distributed sample; however, each data collection site reported challenges in securing participants who had decided not to enroll in a treatment trial. Hence, the decision was made to use the present sample because it was sufficient for the analysis.

Table 5.1. Distribution of Categorical
Sociodemographic Variables ($N = 40$)

Variable	n	%
Ethnic group		
Caucasian	37	92.5
African American	3	7.5
Marital status		
Married	23	57.5
Widowed	7	17.5
Never married	5	12.5
Other	5	12.5
Children		
Yes	33	82.5
No	7	17.5
Employment status		
Not employed	22	55.0
Employed full time	15	37.5
Employed part time	3	7.5
Diagnosis		
Breast	30	75.0
Colorectal	5	12.5
Other	5	12.5
Stage		
I/II	30	75.0
III/IV	9	22.5
Not reported	1	2.5
Enrollment		
Yes	27	67.5
No	13	32.5

Main Study Variables

Preliminary data analysis involved examination of the main study variables (uncertainty, role functioning, social support, hope, and mood state) using descriptive statistics and comparisons to the means reported for various samples in the literature. Table 5.2 includes the means, standard deviations, and ranges of scores for these continuous variables. The level of statistical significance was set at alpha $\leq .05$. Tests for normal distribution were performed on the data. Distributions from the HHI, the POMS-SF, and the MOS-SSS were all negatively skewed. Because the sample did not meet the criteria for normal distribution, nonparametric statistics were used to perform data analysis.

Data analysis to answer the first research question involved examination of the Spearman rank-order correlation coefficients among the main study variables (see Table 5.3). The initial part of this question

Table 5.2. Means, Standard Deviations, and Ranges of Main Variables for Sample ($N = 40$)

Variable	M	SD	Range
Uncertainty (MUIS-C)	47.92	14.06	26 to 100
Role functioning (IFS-CA)	3.09	0.47	1.77 to 3.94
Social support (MOS-SSS)	87.36	18.77	32 to 100
Hope (HHI)	43.07	4.97	31 to 48
Mood state (POMS-SF)	15.55	20.0	−14 to 58

Note. MUIS-C = Mishel Uncertainty in Illness Scale—Community; IFS-CA = Inventory of Functional Status–Cancer: MOS-SSS = Medical Outcomes Study—Social Support Survey; HHI = Herth Hope Index; POMS-SF = Profile of Mood States—Short Form.

Table 5.3. Correlation Matrix for Main Variables

Variable	MUIS-C	IFS-CA	MOS-SSS	HHI	POMS-SF
Uncertainty (MUIS-C)	—				
Role functioning (IFS-CA)	−.476*	—			
Social support (MOS-SSS)	−.303*	.007	—		
Hope (HHI)	−.557*	.451*	−.434*	—	
Mood state (POMS-SF)	−.501*	−.448*	−.170	−.598*	—

Note. MUIS-C = Mishel Uncertainty in Illness Scale—Community; IFS-CA = Inventory of Functional Status–Cancer; MOS-SSS = Medical Outcomes Study—Social Support Survey; HHI = Herth Hope Index; and POMS-SF = Profile of Mood States—Short Form.
*Spearman rank-order correlation is significant at the .01 level (two-tailed).

sought to examine the relationship of hope to the three variables of uncertainty, role functioning, and social support. All three variables had a statistically significant relationship with the variable of hope. Uncertainty was negatively correlated with hope ($r_s = -.557, p = .0001$), whereas role functioning and social support were positively correlated with hope ($r_s = .451, p = .004; r_s = .434, p = .005$). The second part of this question sought to examine the relationship of mood state to the three variables of uncertainty, role functioning, and social support. Two of the three variables had a statistically significant relationship to the variable of mood state. Uncertainty was positively correlated with mood disturbance ($r_s = .501, p = .001.$), whereas role functioning was negatively correlated with mood disturbance ($r_s = -.448, p = .004$). There was no statistically significant relationship between social support and mood state ($r_s = -.170, p = .294$).

For the second research question, a point biserial correlation was to be undertaken to examine the strength of the association between emotional health (hope and mood state) and the treatment decision. However, the critical assumptions for the statistic could not be met. Thus, the

Mann–Whitney U Test was used to examine hope and mood state among women who enrolled in a treatment trial and those who did not. There was no significant difference in the level of hope among women who enrolled in a treatment trial and those who did not ($z = -.102$, $p = .919$). There was also no significant difference in the level of mood disturbance among women who enrolled in the trial and those who did not ($z = -.766$, $p = .444$).

DISCUSSION

Systems Concepts and Emotional Health

The first research question examined the extent of the relationships among personal, interpersonal, and social systems concepts and emotional health. Uncertainty, role functioning, and social support were all significantly correlated with hope, whereas uncertainty and role functioning were also significantly correlated with mood state. The magnitude of all of these associations was either interpreted as moderate or strong. Surprisingly, there was no statistically significant relationship between social support and mood state. In terms of the theory, these findings suggest sufficient empirical evidence for how select concepts from the personal, interpersonal, and social systems relate to emotional health, an aspect of health as a whole, reflecting an organismic view of the individual. King (1995) maintained that the goal of her nursing system, as a whole, is health for individuals. Nonetheless, the specific finding that social support was not significantly related to mood state was not as the theory predicted. Because social support was significantly related to hope, it raises questions about the relationship between social support and the indicators of emotional health. It may be that hope is a mediating variable and that mood state is the outcome variable. It may also be that the two indicators of emotional health interact differently with the systems variable of social support. Path analytic research is indicated to answer this question.

In nursing practice CTNs are frequently involved in alleviating uncertainty in the illness situation, assisting women with role-functioninig issues, and providing professional support. Clinical trial nurses engaging in these professional activities may have an effect on emotional health among women eligible for a cancer clinical trial. In mediating uncertainty, Ruckdeschel, Albrecht, Blanchard, and Hemmick (1996) suggested that nurses and physicians need to frame the accrual process as a prime opportunity for meeting patient information needs and, importantly, for providing an explanation of complex, ambiguous elements of the disease and disease experience. Furthermore, CTNs should be more keenly aware of the support they provide to women either eligible for a cancer clinical trial during the decision making process or already enrolled in a clinical trial. A recent study by Skrutkowska and Weijer (1997) found that women with breast cancer enrolled in clinical trials had more phone interactions with nursing staff ($p = .003$) and received teaching ($p = <.001$) and reassurance ($p = .005$) from nursing staff more often than women not enrolled in clinical trials.

Emotional Health and the Treatment Decision

The second question sought to examine the relationship between emotional health and the treatment decision. There was no significant difference in the presentation of emotional health between the two groups of women. Although this finding was unexpected, the sample was not as evenly distributed as desired between women who chose to enroll and those who did not.

An additional explanation for the lack of significant findings may be related to the instruments themselves and their reference to time. The HHI is a trait-like instrument that asks the participant to respond based on how much they agree with the statement right now. In contrast, the POMS-SF is a transient-like instrument that asks participants to respond based on how they have been feeling during the past week. From a theoretical stance, King (1981) identified the concept of time as a significant concept that helps nurses understand persons as personal systems. King (1981) defined time "as the duration between the occurrence of one event and the occurrence of another event. It is a change from one state to another state" (p. 44). In the present study, participants were asked to respond to the HHI based on "right now" and to the POMS-SF based on "during the past week." King (1981) stated, "Either lengthening or shortening the order and duration of time determines how one perceives the succession of events in the environment" (p. 43). Perhaps the response to the questions on these two instruments by the participant would have been different than reported had they been similarly oriented to time.

Conceivably, the issue of timing is more significant than one would have expected. Hinds (P. Hinds, personal communication, August 17, 1998) noted in an ongoing study of decision making examining the process parents, patients, and physicians experience when making end-of-life decisions that the highest rate of refusal was within the first 72 hours, when individuals were highly emotional. Agreement to participate in a study about their decision making was notably higher 4 to 6 weeks after making the actual end-of-life decision. These initial findings suggest the significant influence of time on the decision-making process (P. Hinds, personal communication, August 17, 1998).

Whereas all participants completed the questionnaire within 28 days of making their self-reported treatment decision, it may very well be that differences would have been seen in the responses had the duration of time been significantly less. This would have captured the woman's perception of the treatment decision even closer to the actual time of decision making. Surely, the timing of the administration of the questionnaire factors into the present study results, although only through additional studies could one confirm this. Unfortunately, most other studies that have been done in the area have extended the time to questionnaire or interview completion (3–6 months) by the participant instead of shortening it, thus making it difficult to compare findings.

It was proposed in this study that the treatment decision stems from human emotion, conceptualized as emotional health, with the action of decision making manifesting itself in the treatment decision. Evidently, most of the women reported hope without significant differences in mood disturbance in spite of the two different decisions (to enter or not to enter a clinical trial). The exact reason for this finding remains unclear, and additional theoretical and design limitations may exist, necessitating theory revision. Finally, whereas the findings from this research question are probably related to the decision-making process as a whole, factors differentiating those women who did enter a clinical trial and those who did not were not captured by the present study.

CONCLUSION

King (1981) clearly stated that the focus of nursing is the care of human beings with the premise that human beings are open systems interacting with the environment. The conceptual framework represents personal, interpersonal, and social systems as the domain of nursing. In the present study, findings provided empirical evidence of the adequacy of King's systems framework and supported, in part, theorized relationships among the critical factors. However, these factors did not illuminate the treatment decision.

This study expanded nursing science as it relates to women eligible for a cancer clinical trial by providing a clearer perspective of the inter-relationships among systems concepts and emotional health. As Fawcett and Whall (1995) stated. "The credibility of the general systems framework requires continuous investigation by means of systematic tests of conceptual–theoretical–empirical structures derived from the framework" (pp. 332–333). Although the tested theory advances King's (1981) systems framework, future research should focus on theory revision. It is only with further understanding of the theoretical concepts underlying enrollment that the appropriate interventions can be systematically developed, tested, and incorporated into nursing practice.

REFERENCES

Cox, K., & Avis, M. (1996). Psychosocial aspects of participation in early anticancer drug trials. *Cancer Nursing, 19*(3), 177–186.

Crago, E., Schaefer, K., & Gyaunch, L. (1997). Backing and forthing: Process of decision making by women considering clinical trials. *Oncology Nursing Forum, 24*(2), 299.

Dwyer, M. (1993). The oncology patient's experience in making a treatment decision (Doctoral dissertation, Catholic University of America, 1993). *Dissertation Abstracts International, 54*, 03B.

Fawcett, J., & Tulman, L. (1996). Assessment of function. In R. McCorkle, M. Grant, M. Frank-Stromberg, & S. Baird (Eds.), *Cancer nursing* (pp. 66–73). Philadelphia: Saunders.

Fawcett, J., & Whall, A. (1995). State of the science and future directions. In M. A. Frey & C. L. Sieloff (Eds.), *Advancing King's systems framework and theory of nursing* (pp. 327–334). Thousand Oaks, CA: Sage.

Gotay, C. (1991). Accrual to cancer clinical trials: Directions from the research literature. *Social Science and Medicine, 33*, 569–577.

Guidry, J., Greisinger, A., Aday, L., Winn, R., Vernon, S., & Throckmorton, T. (1996). Barriers to cancer treatment. *Oncology Nursing Forum, 23*, 1393–1398.

Herth, K. (1989). Relationship of hope, coping styles, concurrent losses, and setting to grief resolution in the elderly widow(er). *Research in Nursing & Health, 13*, 109–117.

Herth, K. (1992). Abbreviated instrument to measure hope: Development and psychometric evaluation. *Journal of Advanced Nursing, 17*, 1251–1259.

Hinds, P., Quargnenti, A., & Madison, J. (1995). Refusal to participate in clinical nursing research. *Western Journal of Nursing Research, 17*, 232–236.

Ho, R. (1994). The future direction of clinical trials. *Cancer, 74*, 2739–2744.

Huizinga, G., Sleijfer, D., van de Wiel, H., & van der Graaf, W. (1999). Decision making process in patients before entering phase III cancer clinical trials: A pilot study. *Cancer Nursing, 22*, 119–125.

Johansen, M., Mayer, D., & Hoover, H. (1991). Obstacles to implementing cancer clinical trials. *Seminars in Oncology Nursing, 7*, 260–267.

King, I. M. (1971). *Toward a theory for nursing: General concept of human behavior.* New York: Wiley.

King, I. M. (1981). *A theory for nursing.* Albany, NY: Delmar.

King, I. M. (1995). A systems framework for nursing. In M. A. Frey & C. L. Sieloff (Eds.), *Advancing King's systems framework and theory of nursing* (pp. 14–22). Thousand Oaks, CA: Sage.

McNair, D., Lorr, M., & Droppleman, L. (1992). *EdITS manual for the profile of mood states*. San Diego, CA: EdITS/Educational and Industrial Testing Service.

Mishel, M. (1983). Adjusting the fit: Development of uncertainty scales for specific clinical populations. *Western Journal of Nursing Research, 5*, 355–370.

Mishel, M. (1988). Uncertainty in illness. *Image: Journal of Nursing Scholarship, 20*, 225–231.

Mishel, M. (1997). *Uncertainty in illness scales manual*. Chapel Hill: University of North Carolina.

Morrow, G., Hickock, J., & Burish, T. (1994). Behavioral aspects of clinical trials. *Cancer, 74*, 2676–2682.

National Cancer Institute. (2000). *Facts and figures about cancer clinical trials*. Retrieved December 4, 2001, from http://cancertrials.nci.nih.gov/understanding/basics/facts/1200.html

Ruckdeschel, J., Albrecht, T., Blanchard, C., & Hemmick, R. (1996). Communication, accrual to clinical trials, and the physician-patient relationship: Implications for training programs. *Journal of Cancer Education, 11*, 73–79.

Schain, W. (1994). Barriers to clinical trials part II: Knowledge and attitudes of potential participants. *Cancer, 74*, 2666–2671.

Sherbourne, C., & Stewart, A. (1991). The MOS social support survey. *Social Science and Medicine, 32*, 705–714.

Sherbourne, C., Stewart, A., & Wells, K. (1992). Role functioning measures. In A. L. Stewart & J. E. Ware (Eds.), *Measuring functioning and well-being: The medical outcomes study approach* (pp. 204–219). Durham, NC: Duke University Press.

Skrutkowska, M., & Weijer, C. (1997). Do patients with breast cancer participating in clinical trials receive better nursing care? *Oncology Nursing Forum, 24*, 1411–1416.

Stetz, K. M. (1993). Survival work: The experience of the patient and the spouse involved in the experimental treatment for cancer. *Seminars in Oncology Nursing, 9*, 121–126.

Swanson, G. M., & Ward, A. J. (1995). Recruiting minorities into clinical trials: Toward a participant-friendly system. *Journal of the National Cancer Institute, 87*, 1747–1759.

Tejeda, H., Green, S., Trimble, E., Ford, L., High, J., Ungerleider, R., et al. (1996). Representation of African Americans, Hispanics, and Whites in National Cancer Institute cancer treatment trials. *Journal of the National Cancer Institute, 88*, 812–816.

Thomas, S. P. (1997). Distressing aspects of women's roles, vicarious stress, and health consequences. *Issues in Mental Health Nursing, 18*, 539–557.

Tulman, L., & Fawcett, J. (1996). Lessons learned from a pilot study of biobehavioral correlates of functional status in women with breast cancer. *Nursing Research, 45*, 365–358.

Tulman, L., Fawcett, J., & McEvoy, M. (1991). Development of the inventory of functional status – cancer. *Cancer Nursing, 14*, 254–260.

Winker, C. (1995). A systems view of health. In M. A. Frey & C. L. Sieloff (Eds.), *Advancing King's systems framework and theory of nursing* (pp. 35–45). Thousand Oaks, CA: Sage.

Yoder, L., O'Rourke, T., Etnyre, A., Spears, D., & Brown, T. (1997). Expectations and experiences of patients with cancer participating in phase I clinical trials. *Oncology Nursing Forum, 24,* 891–896.

CHAPTER SIX

Social Support and Health of Older Adults

Janice E. Fries Reed

It is well known that the U. S. population is aging. It has been estimated that by 2020, every fourth American will be 65 years of age or older. This aging is a success for our culture as well as a challenge in terms of how to maintain and promote the health of the increasing numbers of elderly. In this chapter, I present the findings from a descriptive correlation study that focused on the health and social support of older adults living independently in their communities. A primary purpose of this study was to develop a reciprocal measure of social support that accounted for the types of social support older adults provided to their network members in addition to what support they received from their network members. The reciprocal measure of social support was then used to investigate the relationship that social support has with the health of older adults.

Social support has been shown to have beneficial effects on morbidity and mortality (House, Landis, & Umberson, 1988). Evidence indicates that individuals with strong social support have a decreased risk of death from such diverse conditions as heart disease, cancer, cerebrovascular disease (House, Robbins, & Metzner, 1982), and rheumatoid arthritis (Lambert, Lambert, Klipple, & Mewshaw, 1989).

It is commonly accepted that families provide the majority of informal social support that older adults need to maintain their health and to continue living independently. However, changing family dynamics are taxing this tradition. Families have fewer children, and the children frequently live farther away from aging parents than they used to. In addition, increased numbers of women are in the workforce, making them less available to care for aging parents. At the same time, older adults are more vulnerable to losses within their social networks from retirement, relocation, or death. Exactly how the composition of social networks and the interactions among network members affects the social support and health of older adults is not clear. Perhaps friends and neighbors are assuming a greater role in the exchange of social support as families are increasingly taxed to provide for elderly members. There may be an increasing dependence on formal sources of support within the community.

The focus of this study is in the informal social support exchanged between family members and between friends and neighbors rather than the formal support provided by professionals. Formal support, provided by professionals, lacks the element of reciprocity. Lenrow and Burch (1981) and Pearlin (1985) advocated that social support only occurs in interactions between layperson networks and not between professionals and laypersons because exchange of support is missing from the latter. Few researchers measure the reciprocal aspect of social support. Instead, they measure the types, sources, and frequency of support provided to individuals. A reciprocal measure of social support would more accurately reflect the theoretical definition of social support, which embodies the concept of reciprocity.

The Norbeck Social Support Questionnaire (NSSQ) was selected to measure social support of older adults because of its conciseness and suitability for modification to reflect reciprocity of social support. The questionnaire also has established evidence of reliability and validity. J. S. Norbeck (personal communication, June 15, 1996) agreed to modification of questions to reflect reciprocity on her instrument, acknowledging that reciprocity is an important component of social support. Measures of reciprocal support were subsequently used to investigate whether social support was a predictor of health for older adults.

The research question was: Is there a difference in social support (emotional and tangible) that older adults receive from their social networks and social support they provide to their social networks of family members and friends and neighbors? A hypothesis of the study was: Health (activities of daily living [ADLs] and instrumental ADLs [IADLs], and self-perception of health) of older adults will be predicted by the social support received from and provided to family members and friends and neighbors.

THEORY DEVELOPMENT APPROACH

King's conceptual system for nursing provided the theoretical perspective for this study. King (1971, 1981) focused on three interacting systems: the personal system made up of the individual, the interpersonal system of individuals interacting with one another, and the larger social system. For this study, older adults comprise the individual systems that are seen as interacting with their network members of family and friends and neighbors (forming interpersonal systems), all within the larger social system of their communities. King stated that human interactions are goal oriented toward health and that they are reciprocal.

King (1981) described health as "the dynamic life experiences of a human being, which implies continuous adjustment to stressors in the internal and external environment through optimum use of one's resources to achieve maximum potential for daily living (p. 5)." She stated that individual health is achieved through interaction goals accomplished within the larger environment of society (King, 1993). *Interaction* is the key word in this definition of health because social support in this study was defined as interactions. Kahn and Antonucci (1980) identified that interactions of social support involve affect, affirmation, and tangible aid. Norbeck (1981) used these elements to develop her social support questionnaire. It follows, then, that if social support is an interaction and if health is achieved through interaction, then social support must have an effect on one's health.

Dulock and Holzemer (1991) developed substruction of theory to show the congruence between the theoretical and operational aspects of the research study design. In Figure 6.1, substruction of this study's theoretical perspective is diagrammed from the highest to lowest levels of abstraction. By linking the concepts of health and social support to the theoretical constructs of King's conceptual system and to empirical indicators, one is able to provide support for King's conceptual system.

At the highest level of abstraction, at the top of Figure 6.1, are the three theoretical constructs of the dynamic interacting systems derived from King's conceptual system: the personal system, the interpersonal system, and the social system. Arrows linking all three of these constructs indicate the interaction that goes on between all three systems.

Within the construct of the personal system, the concept of adult health was identified. Similarly, Frey (1989) developed the concept of health for children and adolescents with Type I diabetes and their families within the personal system. Specific for this study, the concept of health was further divided into two subconcepts specific to older adults: functional health and perception of health. Functional health was operationalized by measuring ADLs and IADLs on a Likert scale of 1 to 5. Perception of health was operationalized by using a self-rating of health status.

Similarly, the concept of social support was substructed from King's construct of the interpersonal system. The subconcepts of social support pertinent for this study were identified as the reciprocal social support between older adults and (a) their family members and (b) their friends

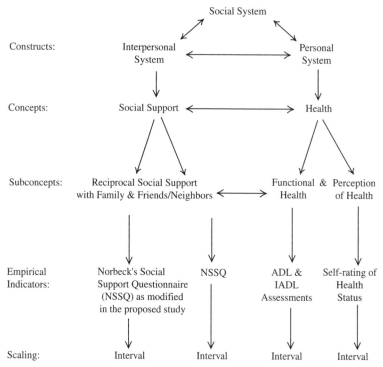

Figure 6.1. Theory substruction of social support and health as derived from King's (1981) conceptual system.

and neighbors. These subconcepts of reciprocal social support with family and with friends and neighbors were then operationalized using the NSSQ (Norbeck, 1995) as modified in this study to measure reciprocity of support.

LITERATURE REVIEW

Several investigators have looked at social support and social networks of older adults. In 1987, Antonucci and Akiyama (1987) examined the structure and function of social networks among 718 older adults aged 50 to 95 years. Six types of social support were measured: (a) confiding about things that are important; (b) being reassured when feeling uncertain; (c) being respected; (d) being cared for when ill; (e) talking with someone when upset, nervous, or depressed; and (f) talking with someone about one's health. The participants reported receiving similar numbers of the six types of support. It is of interest that they reported providing more types of support than they received from their networks of family, friends, and neighbors, although the reciprocity was approximately balanced. In 1992, however, Ingersoll-Dayton and Talbot, in a qualitative study to assess equity in exchanges of social support, found that the elderly 75 years and older maximized the support they provided to others and minimized the support they received. Morgan, Schuster, and Butler (1991) also found that, even for adults 85 years and older, the mean for giving social support was greater than the mean for receiving support.

Krause and Markides (1990) looked at whether older adults were satisfied with the reciprocity of their social support. They found that 90% of respondents indicated they were most satisfied with the amount of tangible support they received, and only 59% said they were satisfied with the reciprocity of their social support; 39% wished they could provide more support. Wolfson, Handfield-Jones, Glass, McClaran, and Keyserlingk (1993) found that adult children feel a strong moral obligation that they should provide high levels of care for elderly parents. In general, researchers have focused on describing the numbers and types of social support that older adults receive without regard to the quality or amount of social support exchanged with specific persons.

Pertinent to this study about the perception of health, La Rue, Bank, Jarvik, and Hetland (1979) found that physicians' ratings on physical health were significantly correlated with the self-perception of health by older adults. Mossey and Shapiro (1982) further found that irrespective of objective health, age, gender, income, or life satisfaction, self-perceived health was a strong predictor of mortality that was stable over time for noninstitutionalized elderly 65 years and older.

METHODS

Participants

The sample population included 140 older adults living either in their own homes or in housing for senior citizens. A community-based, convenience sample was selected from senior citizen centers, churches, and senior citizen retirement housing. Individuals were also referred to the study by colleagues and network sampling was employed to reach prospective older participants out in the community. Criteria for taking part in the study were that the participants be (a) aged at least 70 years, (b) living independently within the community, and (c) able to speak English. The mean age of the sample was 79 years with an SD of 6.51. Ages ranged from 70 to 100 years. There were 109 women and 31 men in the sample. Most (125) were Caucasian; 15 were African American.

Instruments

Health

Indicators of health were perception of health status and activities of daily living. Perception of health was measured by a single-item rating scale described by Maddox and Douglas (1973). Participants were asked the following question: "Generally speaking, how do you rate your health at the present time?" Responses were scored as: Excellent = 8, Excellent for my age = 7, Good = 6, Good for my age = 5, Fair = 4, Fair for my age = 3, Poor = 2, Poor for my age = 1. Magnani (1990) reported a correlation of .74 over a 2-week period using a test–retest method to establish reliability of a self-rating of health among independently functioning older adults.

ADLs were measured using the traditional ADL items (dressing, feeding, bathing, toileting, and grooming) on the scale developed by Katz, Ford, Moskowitz, Jackson and Jaffe (1963). Instrumental activities of daily living were measured using the IADL (Lawton & Brody, 1969). These activities included telephoning, walking upstairs, grocery shopping, meal preparation, repairing or cleaning, doing laundry, and money management. Participants received 2 points if they could perform the activity without help and 1 point if they needed any help. Higher numerical values of performance indicated greater independence.

Social support

The NSSQ (Norbeck, Lindsey, & Carrieri, 1981, 1983) was chosen to measure social support in this study because of the theoretical congruence between Norbeck's conceptualization of social support and the conceptualization used in this study. Three main properties of social support are measured by the NSSQ: total functional support (emotional and tangible), total network support, and total loss of support. Descriptive data can be calculated for total support in all of these areas or for specific subscales and variables.

Participants were first asked to list their family members and their friends and neighbors who were important to them. Then they were asked to rate the total functional support (emotional and tangible) they exchanged with each network member using a Likert scale of 0 (*no support at all*) to 4 (*a great deal of support*). Participants were asked to respond to 12 questions about their exchange of social support. The first 6 questions asked about the amount of emotional and tangible support received from each network member whom they had identified as important in their social network. These questions came directly from the NSSQ. The next 6 questions were modifications of the first 6 questions that had been reworded to reflect the reciprocity aspect of social support. They asked about the amount of emotional and tangible support the older adult provided to each network member using the same Likert scale.

Mean scores were calculated for support (emotional and tangible) from family members and friends and neighbors and provided to family members and friends and neighbors. Data were also collapsed to form eight support variables: emotional support received from family members, emotional support received from friends and neighbors, tangible support received from family members, tangible support received from friends and neighbors, emotional support provided to family members, emotional support provided to friends and neighbors, tangible support provided to family members, and tangible support provided to friends and neighbors. Differences between these two sets of scores, those that represented support received from the network and those that represented support provided to the network, were used as the measure of reciprocity of social support.

The NSSQ has demonstrated high test–retest reliability of equal to or greater than .80 in previous studies (Norbeck et al., 1981). Internal consistency measures were reported to be from .69 to .97. Content and concurrent validity have been reported, and the instrument appears to be free from the social desirability response bias. For this study, Cronbach's alpha ranged from .90 to .98 for all subscales and scale totals.

RESULTS

Descriptive Analysis

There were two dependent variables of health: self-perceived health status and ADLs and IADLs. The mean for perception of health status was 5.6 (SD 1.64) Thirty-three percent perceived their health as "excellent for my age." The mean score of the ADLs and IADLs was 23 (SD 1.69) indicating that this population of older adults rated themselves very high for independence with ADLs.

Older adults in this study identified a mean number of 9 people in their social networks. The range was 1–24 people. The mean number of family members was 5 (SD 3.31) and the mean number of friends and neighbors was 4 (SD 2.83). Mean scores for the calculated subscales and scale totals are shown in Table 6.1. The Hotelling's trace test showed no significant differences between either the emotional or tangible support that older adults exchanged between their network of family members or friends and neighbors (F = 1.95, p = .11).

Table **6.1.** Descriptive Statistics for Support Subscales and Scale Totals

| | Emotional | | Tangible | |
Source	Mean	SD	Mean	SD
Received From				
Family	13.32	3.49	5.28	2.36
Friends and Neighbors	10.64	4.49	4.12	2.47
Total	23.96	5.84	9.40	4.04
Provided to				
Family	13.17	3.28	5.44	2.41
Friends and Neighbors	10.44	4.49	4.42	2.51
Total	23.61	5.82	9.85	4.36

Multiple Regression Analysis

Initially, the two indicators of health (ADLs and IADLs and self-perception of health) were to be regressed onto the eight subscales of social support. However, when multicolinearity of the eight independent variables was identified, a principle component factor analysis with varimax rotation was performed. The factor analysis resulted in a two-factor solution, which accounted for 81.1% of the variance in social support. The four social support subscales relating to exchange of social support with friends and neighbors loaded on the first factor and accounted for 50.5% of the variance. The other four social support subscales relating to exchange of social support with family members loaded on the second factor and accounted for 30.6% of the variance. As a result, the subscales were further reduced to two: social support exchanged with family members and social support exchanged with friends and neighbors. Each of these subscales included the exchange of both emotional and tangible social support.

Results for the regression of self-perception of health on social support controlling for demographic variables are shown in Tables 6.2 and 6.3. This model only explained 5% of the variance in health status. Emotional and tangible social support that older adults exchanged with their network members did not account for a significant amount of variance in perception of health.

The regression analysis was repeated with ADLs and IADLs as the dependent variable (Tables 6.4 and 6.5). This model accounted for 12% of the variance in ADLs and IADLs. However, the only individually significant variable was age. Thus, the main hypothesis of this study was not supported. Social support did not predict the health of older adults.

Table 6.2. Coefficients for the Regression of Self-Perception of Health on Social Support

Variables	Standardized Beta	t	Significance
Control			
Age	.146	1.653	.101
Gender	−.028	−.282	.778
Education	−.032	−.280	.780
Income	.152	1.295	.198
Ethnicity	.066	.714	.477
Social Support			
Family Social Support	.037	.399	.691
Friends and Neighbors Social Support	.098	1.067	.288

Alpha = .05

Table 6.3. Summary of Simultaneous Regression of Self-Perception of Health on Social Support

Variables	R	R Square	R Square Change	F Change	Sig F Change
Step 1					
Age, Gender, Education, Income Ethnicity	.206	.042	.042	1.175	.325
Step 2					
Social Support Exchanged with Family					
	.232	.054	.012	.797	.453
Social Support Exchanged with Friends and Neighbors					

Alpha = .05

Table 6.4. Coefficients for the Regression of ADLs and IADLs on Social Support

Variables	Standardized Beta	t	Significance
Control			
Age	−.248	−2.913	.004*
Gender	.042	.431	.667
Education	.128	1.161	.248
Income	.059	.520	.604
Ethnicity	.042	.463	.644
Social Support			
Family Social Support	.004	.040	.968
Friends and Neighbors Social Support	.059	.660	.510

Alpha = .05 * = Level of significance truly significant at the alpha level.

Table 6.5. Summary of Simultaneous Regression of ADLs and IADLs on Social Support

Variables	R	R Square	R Square Change	F Change	Sig F Change
Step 1					
Age, Gender Education, Income Ethnicity	.336	.113	.113	3.378	.007*
Step 2					
Social Support Exchanged with Family					
	.340	.116	.003	.239	.788
Social Support Exchanged with Friends and Neighbors					

Alpha = .05 * = Level of significance truly significant at the alpha level.

DISCUSSION

The aims of this study were to measure the reciprocal nature of social support from family and nonfamily members, compare the amount of support received from family and nonfamily members, and to determine if social support was a predictor of health in older adults living in the community. Societal changes in families have created opportunity for friends and neighbors to take an increasingly active role in the informal social support of older adults and this had not been systematically investigated to date. The theoretical formulation was derived from King's (1981) conceptual system related to the concepts of social support and health. It was hypothesized that social support would be a predictor of health for this population.

As modified, the NSSQ showed high reliability as a measure of reciprocal support from family and nonfamily members. Previous studies showed that older adults have increasingly identified friends as important members of their social networks (Antonucci & Akiyama, 1987; Morgan et al., 1991). This study also supported that trend, in that, approximately 50% of the participants' social network were family and friends. In addition, there was a close balance of the emotional and tangible support that they exchanged with their family members and with their friends and neighbors. Finding little difference in the amounts of social support that older adults exchange with family and friends and neighbors was contrary to anticipated findings. It was anticipated that older adults might receive more tangible aid than they would be able to give because of physical restrictions or limited financial funds. However, this may have been due to the nature of the sample and may not generalize to other populations of older adults.

Prediction of Health Related to Reciprocity of Informal Social Support

The primary hypothesis of this study, that health (ADLs and IADLs and self-perception of health) would be predicted by the social support exchanged with family members and friends and neighbors, was not supported. This may have been because of the significant skewness of the scores for ADLs and IADLs. Not surprisingly, the older adults in this study rated their abilities to perform ADLs and IADLs very high. Again, this may have been due to sampling bias. Contrary to expectations, the development of a reciprocal measurement of social support did not improve the prediction of the health variables in this study. The reciprocity of scores for social support were so evenly balanced that any anticipated improvement to predict health was negated.

Summary

The findings of this study do not provide direct support for the credibility of King's conceptual system. However, this is most likely due to the limited number of variables in the model as tested. For example, there could be many other interactions between and among systems that influence health as well as other factors that mediate or moderate the effect of social support on health for this population. Knowledge about the health of individuals and factors that influence the health of individuals is critical to the discipline of nursing. This study and King's conceptual system provide a foundation for increasing knowledge about the health of older individuals.

REFERENCES

Antonucci, T. C., & Akiyama, H. (1987). Social networks in adult life and a preliminary examination of the convoy model. *Journal of Gerontology, 42,* 519–527.

Dulock, H. L., & Holzemer, W. L. (1991). Substruction: Improving the linkage from theory to method. *Nursing Science Quarterly, 4,* 83–87.

Frey, M. A. (1989). Social support and health: Theoretical formulation derived from King's conceptual framework. *Nursing Science Quarterly, 2,* 138–148.

House, J. S., Landis, K. R., & Umberson, D. (1988). Social relationships and health. *Science, 241,* 540–545.

House, J. S., Robbins, C., & Metzner, H. C. (1982). The association of social relationships and activities with mortality: Prospective evidence from the Tecumseh community health study. *American Journal of Epidemiology, 116,* 123–140.

Ingersoll-Dayton, B., & Talbott, M. M. (1992). Assessments of social support exchanges: Cognitions of the old-old. *American Journal of Epidemiology, 115,* 684–694.

Kahn, R. L., & Antonucci, T. C. (1980). Convoys over the life course: Attachment, roles, and social support. In P. B. Baltes & O. G. Brim (Eds.), *Life-span development and behavior* (pp. 253–386). New York: Academic Press.

Katz, S., Ford, A. S., Moskowitz, R. W., Jackson, B. A., & Jaffe, M. W. (1963). Studies of illness in the aged. The index of ADL: A standardized measure of biological and psychosocial function. *Journal of the American Medical Association, 185,* 914–919.

King, I. (1971). *Toward a theory for nursing: General concepts of human behavior.* New York: Wiley.

King, I. (1981). *A theory for nursing: Systems, concepts, process.* New York: Wiley.

King, I. (1993). Quality of life and goal attainment. *Nursing Science Quarterly, 7,* 29–32.

Krause, N., & Markides, K. (1990). Measuring social support among older adults. *International Journal on Aging and Human Development, 30,* 37–53.

LaRue, A., Bank, L., Jarvik, L., & Hetland, M. (1979). Health in old age: How do physicians' ratings and self-ratings compare? *Journal of Gerontology, 34,* 687–691.

Lambert, V. A., Lambert, C. E., Klipple, G. L., & Mewshaw, E. A. (1989). Social support, hardiness and psychological well-being in women with arthritis. *Image: Journal of Nursing Scholarship, 21,* 128–131.

Lawton, M. P., & Brody, E. M. (1969). Assessment of older people: Self-maintaining and instrumental activities of daily living. *The Gerontologist, 9,* 179–186.

Lenrow, P. B., & Burch, R. W. (1981). Mutual aid and professional services: Opposing or complementary? In B. H. Gottlieb (Ed.), *Social networks and social support* (pp. 233–257). Beverly Hills, CA: Sage.

Maddox, G. L., & Douglas, E. B. (1973). Self-assessment of health: A longitudinal study of elderly subjects. *Journal of Health and Social Behavior, 4,* 87–93.

Magnani, L. E. (1990). Hardiness, self-perceived health, and activity among independently functioning older adults. *Scholarly Inquiry for Nursing Practice: An International Journal, 4,* 171–184.

Morgan, D. L., Schuster, T. L., & Butler, E. W. (1991). Role reversals in the exchange of social support. *Journal of Gerontology: Social Sciences, 46,* S278–287.

Mossey, J. M., & Shapiro, E. (1982). Self-rated health: A predictor of mortality among the elderly. *American Journal of Public Health, 72,* 800–808.

Norbeck, J. S. (1981). Social support: A model for clinical research and application. *Advances In Nursing Science, 3,* 43–59.

Norbeck, J. S. (1995). *Scoring instructions for the Norbeck Social Support Questionnaire (NSSQ)*. San Francisco: University of California.

Norbeck, J. S., Lindsey, A. M., & Carrieri, V. L. (1981). The development of an instrument to measure social support. *Nursing Research, 30*, 264–269.

Norbeck, J. S., Lindsey, A. M., & Carrieri, V. L. (1983). The development of the Norbeck Social Support Questionnaire: Normative data and validity testing. *Nursing Research, 32*, 4–10.

Pearlin, L. (1985). Social structure and processes of social support. In S. Cohen & S. L. Syme (Eds.), *Social support and health* (pp. 43–60). Orlando, FL: Academic Press.

Wolfson, C., Handfield-Jones, R. H., Glass, K. C., McClaran, J., & Keyserlingk, E. (1993). Adult children's perceptions of their responsibility to provide care for dependent elderly parents. *The Gerontologist, 33*, 315–323.

The Theory of Integration

Congruency With King's Conceptual System

Cheri Ann Hernandez

Liehr and Smith (1999) identified five approaches to the development of middle range theory, one of which was by induction through research and practice. The theory of integration is a middle range theory that was developed using grounded theory research, an inductive research method. This chapter (a) outlines the development of the theory of integration, (b) describes the theory and relevant research, (c) demonstrates the congruency of its major constructs with those of Imogene King's conceptual system (KCS), and (d) suggests one method of further explicating a major construct of integration theory—collaborative alliance relationship—using some of the concepts identified in KCS.

DEVELOPMENT OF THE THEORY OF INTEGRATION

The theory of integration emerged during a study of Type 1 diabetes (Hernandez, 1991) using the grounded theory research method (Glaser & Strauss, 1967). According to Glaser (1992), "the grounded theory approach is a general methodology of analysis linked with data collection that uses a systematically applied set of methods to generate an inductive theory about a substantive area" (p. 16). The grounded theory method and the way in which grounded theory was used to develop the theory of integration, a middle range theory that is applied to a specific population (diabetes), is described in this section.

Grounded Theory Method

Grounded theory generates a theory that accounts for behavior that is relevant and problematic for those involved (Glaser, 1978). In the grounded theory method, data collection, data analysis, theory write-up, and theoretical sampling continue simultaneously. Research participants are selected on the basis of emerging theory needs, a process called theoretical sampling. The constant comparative method of analysis is the functional pivot of the grounded theory method and involves "continually checking out concepts and producing properties of categories and theoretical codes to relate them" (Glaser, 1992, p. 76). During the analysis process, two types of codes are identified: substantive codes and theoretical codes. Initially, the researcher begins with *open coding* (concepts or categories that represent lines or chunks of data), but once the core category is found, *selective coding* (coding of only those concepts and categories that relate to the core category) is done.

The identification of the core category is through emergence, as the researcher constantly compares each chunk of data to every other chunk of data and continually asks two questions of the data: (a) What is the main concern or problem of these adults with diabetes, and what accounts for most of the variation in processing this problem or concern? (b) What category or property of category does this incident indicate (Glaser, 1992, p. 4)? These concepts and categories developed so far are known as the substantive codes. Finally, these substantive codes are related to each other through *theoretical coding,* that is, the conceptual model of the relationship of the core category to its properties and other categories is determined.

Throughout this data collection and analysis process, the researcher is memoing. Memos are "the theorizing write-up of ideas as they emerge while coding for categories, their properties and their theoretical codes. They are written up as they strike the analyst while constantly comparing, coding and analyzing" (Glaser, 1992, p. 108). For example, the researcher might memo about his or her reflections on the development or formulation of the theory, where to go next in terms of choice of participants based on the theory as it is emerging, hunches or theoretical ideas that need to be captured for later use, and so on. The result of the grounded theory research method is a substantive theory, consisting of the identification and explanation of a core category and its related properties, as well as categories of lesser importance (Glaser, 1992). This final substantive theory explains the major problem or concern of research participants and how this problem is being resolved.

Development of the Theory

Initial development of the theory of integration occurred when four young adults with Type 1 diabetes were interviewed over a 2-year period. In addition to the interviews, participants completed two writing tasks: a diabetes paper and a diabetes journal. No specific format guidelines were given for the diabetes paper; instead, participants were asked to tell the researcher what was important for her to know to understand diabetes from their perspective—it was a story about their particular diabetes. The journal was essentially a diary of thoughts and activities over a 3- to 5-day period. Participants were asked to write down what they were thinking related to diabetes throughout the day, including both unusual and mundane incidents, the individuals involved, the internal dialogue, personal reactions and actions taken, as well as their reflection on these actions or experiences.

An initial meeting was held with each participant to provide an opportunity for them to become familiar with the researcher and ask questions about the research protocol. The subsequent interviews were conducted in the privacy of participants' homes and were audiotaped and transcribed verbatim.

During the analysis process, the researcher listened to the interviews and reviewed the transcripts on a line-by-line basis, identifying relevant substantive codes as she went along. As the data were coded, the coded concepts (categories) were written into the margins of the transcripts beside the data they depicted. Coding of the diabetes papers and journals proceeded in a similar manner. An important aspect of this open coding process was comparison of each piece of data with every other piece of data, that is, comparing incidents within a transcript, comparing incidents between transcripts, and comparing transcript incidents with those in the diabetes papers and journals. From this constant comparison process emerged the core category of integration (originally termed "the becoming diabetic process"). The theoretical model through which the substantive codes were found to link together was a three-phase process of integration, a process described in detail in the next section.

In later studies, ongoing theoretical sampling was done to compare the experiences of Type 1 participants from a different geographic location (Bradish, 1994), older adults, health professionals, and those who had longer duration of diabetes (Hernandez, 1996), and First Nations (aboriginal) persons with Type 2 diabetes (Hernandez, Antone, & Cornelius, 1999). Within a typical grounded theory study, once the core category is found, selective coding can begin. However, this theoretical sampling took place through separate studies, and therefore the researcher intentionally used the emergent fit mode (Glaser, 1978) of grounded theory—that is, the theory of integration was used as a starting point for the data analysis process, but the researcher continually tried to remain unbiased by the theory and, instead, allowed the data to speak and revised the theory based on the data. For this reason, the researcher continued using the open coding method throughout the research process as a means of remaining "open" to the data rather than limiting herself to a particular theoretical framework (integration). In addition to the research participants, countless others have talked to the researcher at professional meetings or in everyday life and have verified that their diabetes experiences fit the integration framework. In addition, clients with other chronic illnesses and nurses with specialties in other chronic illnesses have indicated that they believe the theory of integration might actually be appropriate in areas such as Crohn's disease, cancer, weight loss, and others.

DESCRIPTION OF THE THEORY OF INTEGRATION

The findings of the studies described in the previous section point to a three-phase process of integration, that is, the basic problem of individuals with Type 1 and Type 2 diabetes is how to resolve the problem of having a new and intrusive diagnosis, diabetes. This problem is resolved through integration of the *personal* and *diabetic* selves, through a three-phase process of integration. According to the middle range theory of integration, the experience of living with diabetes can be seen as a three-phase process of integration: (a) having diabetes, (b) the turning point, and (c) the science of one phase. *Integration* is defined as

> an ongoing process by which the two selves (diabetic and personal) more fully merge to create an individual who is healthy, both mentally and physically. This unification of the selves is manifested in the person's ways of thinking, being and acting (including verbalization). (Hernandez, 1995a, p. 19)

The *personal self* refers to the person as she or he existed prior to the diagnosis of diabetes, and the *diabetic self* refers to the new entity that emerged and had to be contended with upon diabetes diagnosis (Hernandez, 1996). Characteristics of the three phases of integration are summarized in Table 7.1. Integration is minimal in the first phase but increases as the person progresses throughout the remaining two phases; this initial phase lasts for 3 years or more, but some individuals remain in this phase for more than 50 years, perhaps throughout their lives. It is not known how long the other phases can last; however, one individual remained in the *turning point* phase for 1 year before reverting back to the *having diabetes* phase.

Table 7.1. Characteristics of the Three Phases of Integration

Characteristic	Phase 1: Having diabetes	Phase 2: The turning point	Phase 3: Science of one
Beginning event	Diagnosis of diabetes	Single or multiple significant life events	Gradual shift beyond the turning point
Focus	Personal self-focus on living as one did before diabetes diagnosis	Diabetic self-focus on the diabetes	Focus on both the diabetic and personal selves
Knowledge	Minimal diabetes knowledge or piecemeal bits of knowledge	More diabetes knowledge; interest in learning more about diabetes	Diabetes knowledge plus knowledge of one's own body with diabetes
Lifeways used	Denying Normalizing Minimizing		Tuning in exercise Constant thinking Spirituality Balancing– rebalancing
Degree of integration	Minimal integration	More integration	Higher levels of integration plus ongoing increase in integration
Glycemic control (hemoglobin A1c)	Poor control	Unknown	Good control

Several lifeways, defined as the "characteristic patterns of thought or action used without conscious knowledge" (Hernandez, 1991, p. 99) were found that either inhibited or facilitated this integration of the diabetic and personal selves. There were also metaphors that characterized the lives of these individuals; each of these metaphors for living served as an overarching lifeway, pervading the individual's life and either inhibiting or facilitating integration. Passive metaphors worked to prevent change, that is, to prevent the integration of the personal and diabetic selves, whereas active metaphors facilitated change toward more integration of the personal and diabetic selves.

The *having diabetes* phase begins with the diagnosis of diabetes. During this phase the focus is on the personal self, trying to be as normal as possible and to live as one did prior to diabetes diagnosis. Those in the *having diabetes* phase tended to have poor glycemic control and lacked useful knowledge about diabetes. This lack of knowledge ranged from minimal knowledge to factual knowledge about diabetes, but this knowledge remained piecemeal, therefore did not involve a deep knowledge useful to living with diabetes. Three common lifeways kept the person in this first phase, therefore served to prevent integration of the personal and diabetic selves: denying, normalizing, and minimizing (Hernandez, Bradish, Rodger, & Rybansky, 1999). *Denying* involves denying that one has diabetes and is reflected in activities such as missing insulin injections or oral hypoglycemic agents. Another form of denying is seen in the "to tell or not to tell" tension that begins in this first phase. Often the decision is made not to tell others, even close friends or family members, about their diabetes. *Minimizing* is shown by a downplaying of the impact of diabetes on how one thinks and feels and on the usual way in which one lives. Examples of minimizing include statements that one does not think about diabetes at all or that one is not affected or bothered by diabetes. *Normalizing* involves asserting that one continues to live as one did before the diagnosis of diabetes or that one is living as normal. The word *normal* is frequently used to refer to various aspects of the diabetes regimen. In addition, individuals had an overarching lifeway, consisting of passive metaphors that characterized their speech and living style or patterns of living. These passive metaphors also prevented movement to the *turning point* phase. Examples of these passive metaphors were things such as "going along with" (Hernandez, 1996) and "carrying on" (Hernandez et al., 1999).

The second phase of integration is the *turning point*, a label borrowed from one of the participants. The *turning point* occurs when one or more physical or psychosocial life events affect the individual in such a major way that the decision is made that diabetes has to be contended with; no longer can it be normalized, denied, or minimized. In this phase, the focus changes from a focus on living as a normal individual (the personal self) to a focus on the diabetes (the diabetic self). During this phase, information about diabetes is actively sought, and there is increased involvement in diabetes care activities. Some individuals remain in the turning point for a year or more and then return to the having diabetes phase, whereas others go on to the third phase (Hernandez, 1996).

The *science of one* is a gradual progression out of the *turning point*. This phase was named the *science of one* because "It involves the ongoing, incremental process of building a unique, personalized, and exact science of living with diabetes" (Hernandez, 1996, p. 46). The focus in this phase is on living (personal self) but not to the detriment of the diabetes (diabetic self). Type 1 participants in this phase were in good glycemic control (Bradish, 1994; Hernandez, 1991, 1995b, 1996). In this phase, the individual tunes in to his or her own body and develops self-awareness knowledge that is used to make appropriate decisions related to diabetes. This tuning-in process is only one of several physical, emotional, and cognitive lifeways that promote the integration of the personal and diabetic selves. Exercise, constant thinking, and spirituality are other examples. Metaphors of integration (active, overarching lifeways that promoted integration) were used in this phase. Examples are "diabetes as work" (Hernandez, 1996) and "taking care" (Hernandez et al., 1999). Participants in this phase recognize that they have the expertise related to their own diabetes and expressed the desire to work in collaborative alliance relationships with their health care professionals.

RESEARCH RELATED TO THE THEORY OF INTEGRATION

Research related to the theory of integration is ongoing, by both the author and other colleagues (researchers and students). This section includes examples of three types of research that have been conducted.

Development of the Diabetes Questionnaire

The Diabetes Questionnaire (TDQ) is a 15-item questionnaire that was developed through focus group methodology and pilot tested on 224 clients with Type 1 and Type 2 diabetes (Hernandez, 1995a). Each item is scored on a 6-point Likert response format ranging from 1 (*strongly agree*) to 6 (*strongly disagree*). The results of the pilot test of the questionnaire indicated that the questionnaire was valid (content and construct validity) and reliable (test–retest reliability and internal consistency). Test–retest reliability was Pearson's $r = .75$ with a period of 7 to 10 days between test administration times. Internal consistency was Cronbach's alpha .84 for the total scale and .77 and .80 for the Psychoemotional Adjustment and Somatic Sensitivity subscales, respectively. The author has given permission for many students and other nurse researchers to use the TDQ in their research; however, most have not provided the author with reliability data from their studies. When researchers have used the TDQ, internal consistency estimates have ranged from Cronbach's alpha .80 to .92 for the total scale (Craig, 2002; Hernandez, Hume, & Rodger, 2003; Whittemore, Chase, Mandle, & Roy, 2001; Whittemore, Sullivan, Melkus, & Grey, 2004), and .86 for Psychoemotional Adjustment and .89 for Somatic Sensitivity (Craig, 2002). Whittemore, Melkus, and Grey (2005) found a significant negative correlation ($r = - .54, p < .01$) between the TDQ and the PAID scale (instrument that measures problems related to diabetes), which provides further support for the construct validity of the TDQ. The TDQ has also shown sensitivity to change in intervention studies in Type 1 diabetes (Hernandez et al., 2003) and Type 2 diabetes (Whittemore et al., 2001, 2004). Other nurse researchers have proposed revising the TDQ for use with other chronic illnesses such as mental health and chronic pain. It is possible that such revisions could be done specific to each chronic illness, or perhaps a more general revision would allow this instrument to be used in multiple chronic illnesses.

Research Using the Theory of Integration as Theoretical Framework

In diabetes, the theory of integration has been used as the theoretical framework in several intervention studies designed to increase self-awareness in subjects with Type 1 diabetes. Studies have included a 1-hour intervention with adolescents and young adults (Hernandez & Williamson, 2004), six 5-hour sessions with Type 1 adults (Hernandez, Laschinger, Rodger, Bradish, & Rybansky, 2004), and eight 3-hour sessions with adults with Type 1 diabetes and hypoglycemia unawareness (Hernandez et al., 2003). The theory of integration has also been used in an emergent fit mode grounded theory study of women with Crohn's disease (Compton, 2002).

Research Using the TDQ

Craig (2002) studied 41 employed mothers who had diabetes. She found a moderate correlation between mothers' time to manage competing life demands (work, family, and diabetes) and mothers' integration, as well as between family health work and mothers' integration.

Whittemore et al. (2001) evaluated the content, integrity, and efficacy of an 8-week nurse coaching intervention in nine female participants with Type 2 diabetes. Participants demonstrated increased psychosocial adaptation (integration) and enhanced physiologic adaptation (lower fasting blood glucose, increase in health-promoting behaviors).

Whittemore et al. (2004) used the TDQ in a pilot study to determine the efficacy of a 6-month nurse coaching intervention (educational, behavioral, and affective strategies) that was provided after diabetes education for women with Type 2 diabetes. Women in the treatment group demonstrated significantly better diet self-management ($p = .02$), less diabetes-related stress ($p = .01$), and better integration ($p = .03$).

CONGRUENCY OF THE THEORY OF INTEGRATION WITH KING'S CONCEPTUAL SYSTEM

The previous section demonstrated the usefulness of the theory of integration. In addition to being used as a framework to guide research, the

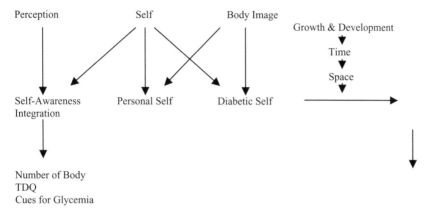

Figure 7.1. Theory of integration within King's personal system.

theory of integration can be used in clinical practice, as a way of obtaining a deeper understanding of the ongoing impact of the diagnosis of diabetes. The use of this theory within a broader conceptual framework such as King's conceptual system (KCS) may broaden its potential for a positive impact on clinical practice. The theory of integration is a middle range theory that can be used within KCS because of the congruency of its major constructs with those of the KCS. In this section, central concepts of the KCS are mapped onto the three major constructs of the theory of integration to demonstrate the congruency with the KCS. The constructs are defined and the congruency argument is then demonstrated. The first two constructs, integration and self-awareness, fit within the personal system of the KCS (refer to Figure 7.1). The final construct, collaborative alliance, reflects concepts from the personal, interpersonal, and social systems of the KCS.

Integration

Integration is defined as

> an ongoing process by which the two selves (diabetic and personal) more fully merge to create an individual who is healthy, both men- tally and physically. This unification of the selves is manifested in the person's ways of thinking, being and acting (including verbalization). (Hernandez, 1995a, p. 19)

The *personal self* refers to the person as she or he existed before the di- agnosis of diabetes, and the *diabetic self* refers to the new entity that emerged and had to be contended with upon diabetes diagnosis. Key ele- ments within the definition and description of integration are congruent with the King's personal system concepts of perception, self, body image, growth, and development. These areas of congruence are demonstrated here through comparison of the description of integration with the descriptions of these concepts. King (1981) expressed the belief that the diagnosis of a chronic disease such as diabetes results in a threat to the person's perception of self and body image (p. 33).

Perception is the major concept in King's personal system; King (1981) defined it as "a process of organizing, interpreting, and transforming information from sense data and memory" (p. 24), "a process of human transactions with environment" (p. 24), "each person's representation of reality" (p. 146), and "an awareness of persons, objects, and events" (p. 146). King's assertion that perception is a transaction with the environment that will affect a person's identity is reflected in the integration process of the personal and diabetic selves.

During the integration process, it is the client's view of his or her identity or *self* that is being organized, interpreted, and transformed as he or she interacts with others and with the newly developed diabetes (diabetic self). This developmental view of self as depicted in integration theory is consistent with King's characteristics of *self* as a dynamic, open system that is goal-oriented and with the description of the self as

> the way I define *me* to myself and to others. Self is all that I am. I am a whole person. Self is what I think of me and what I am capable of being and doing. Self is subjective in that it is what I think I should be or would like to be. (p. 26)

Within integration theory, there is the notion of the two selves, the personal and the diabetic, that need to integrate to become a whole person who retains the essential essence of the prior (personal) self but also includes the characteristics and demands of the new (diabetic) self.

A critical component of integration is related to body image. *Body image* "is defined as a person's perceptions of his own body, others' reactions to his appearance, and is a result of others' reaction to self" (King, 1981, p. 33). During the integration process, body image must be reconstructed to include the diabetic self. During the first phase of integration, the diabetic self is denied, minimized, and normalized so as not to become part of one's body image, but as integration proceeds, diabetes becomes an integral part of the body image. However, most individuals do not wish to be defined by their diabetes, that is, diabetes is not their essential characteristic but rather is merely an important aspect of who they are. It is the concern about body image, in particular, the worry about other's reactions to the new self, that provokes the "to tell or not to tell" controversy and often keeps individuals from telling others about their diabetes.

Ongoing integration is a process of *growth and development* in the behavioral sense, and this is a process that occurs over *time* as the individual moderates and negotiates personal *space*. "Growth and development describe the processes that take place in people's lives that help them move from potential capacity for achievement to self-actualization" (King, 1981, p. 31). The definition of integration describes the ongoing process by which the unification of the selves results in an individual who is healthy both mentally and physically, which can be viewed as a fundamental characteristic of the actualized self. This ongoing process indicates the passage of *time*, that integration is developed over time, and that certain issues such as "to tell or not to tell" may be resolved over time. *Space*, in terms of personal space, is also relevant in integration. Personal space is "that invisible territory in which individuals place themselves" (King, p. 35) and "is related to time, distance, area, volume, perception, and communication" (King, p. 38). In the having diabetes phase, the person distances himself or herself from the diabetic self through denial, minimizing, or normalizing, frequently relegating diabetes to a small corner of life. This distancing is resolved over time through integration of the personal and diabetic selves. In the "to tell or not to tell" dilemma, the person creates privacy space between the self and others and manages this space in different ways with different individuals over time.

Integration is the major construct in the middle range theory of integration. In this section, integration has been shown to be consistent with each of the six concepts in the personal system of KCS, including perception, the major concept of the KCS (refer to Figure 7.1).

Self-Awareness

Self-awareness is a characteristic that is essential for the occurrence of integration. The definition and description that follow demonstrate its congruence with King's (1981) personal systems' concepts of perception, self, body image, space, time, and growth and development. Self-awareness in diabetes involves a deep awareness of one's body and how it reacts to various circumstances. Self-awareness includes the following aspects: (a) being constantly sensitive to body cues and sensations—listening to one's body; (b) knowing the body's particular cues and signals that result from low, normal, and high blood glucose; (c) understanding the circumstances that might precipitate these cues; and (d) knowing the body's norms for different times of the day, days of the month, perhaps even seasons of the year (Hernandez & Bradish, 1996). Four types of self-awareness work in Type 1 diabetes were identified in focus-group research (Hernandez, Bradish, Laschinger, Rodger, & Rybansky, 1997): body listening (noticing, constant awareness), body knowing (differentiating, pattern seeking, reasoning), body balancing (monitoring, decision making, precautionary and anticipatory planning), and engaging others (knowledge checking and swapping, collaborative alliance). The congruency of the self-awareness concept with the personal systems concepts are articulated in the following paragraphs.

The concept of *perception* is critical to understanding self-awareness. Self-awareness can readily be seen as a continuous and heightened mode of *perception,* that is, "a process of organizing, interpreting, and transforming information from sense data and memory" (King, 1981, p. 24). Being constantly sensitive to body cues and sensations involves a conscious openness to sensory data from which one derives useful self-awareness knowledge. Knowing the body's particular cues for the various levels of glycemia, understanding the circumstances that precipitate the various body cues, and knowing the body's norms are all activities that involve organizing, interpreting, and transformation of information as well as the use of one's memory. According to King, *perception* is "an awareness of persons, objects, and events" (p. 146), and self-awareness is an in-depth awareness of self that may involve an awareness of how one's body will respond during certain events, in relation to particular objects such as food, or even in relation to others. Self-awareness knowledge can be viewed as a depth and breadth of perceptual knowledge that is continuously being derived and organized into usable information for present and future decision making. Therefore, self-awareness is consistent with King's assertion that "Human beings are in a continuous state of active participation in a perceptual milieu" (p. 23).

The *self* of self-awareness is consistent with King's (1981) characteristics of *self* as a dynamic, open system that is goal-oriented and as a whole person (p. 26) but is incongruent with the notion of self as subjective: "*Self* is subjective in that it is what I think I should be or would like to be" (p. 26). In self-awareness, the person must tap into the objective self—the somatic and emotional cues that are being experienced, not what he or she wishes were so. Accuracy in self-awareness is critical to appropriate decision making and treatment measures taken, as well as to good health.

Body image is defined as "the picture one has of one's own body bound in space, which constitutes one aspect of the idea of I" (King, 1981, p. 31). In self-awareness, the person with diabetes has a conceptual image of how one's body responds in *space,* and over *time,* in situations of hypoglycemia, hyperglycemia, and even euglycemia. Personal space is "that invisible territory in which individuals place themselves" (King, p. 35). The aspect of *personal space* that is relevant in self-awareness includes glycemic cues that relate to positioning of the muscles or other body parts as a result of low or high blood glucose. King defined time as "the duration between the occurrence of one event and the occurrence of another event" (p. 44) and as "a sequence of events moving onward to the future and influenced by the past" (p. 45). This conveys the essence of time in self-awareness and is reflected in examples such as the person expecting that hypoglycemia may be more likely to occur during peak action times of one's insulin or in knowing how quickly one's body cues will subside once hypoglycemia is treated, for example.

Development of a self-awareness ability is an example of behavioral *growth and development* but is also based on cellular changes over time. "Growth and development describe the processes that take place in people's lives that help them move from potential capacity for achievement to self-actualization" (King, 1981, p. 31). Without self-awareness ability, the person is unable to achieve the goal of glycemic control, with the subsequent inability to prevent the microvascular and macrovascular complications that occur due to prolonged hyperglycemia resulting from inadequate diabetes control.

The concept of self-awareness has been shown to be congruent with each of the six concepts of the personal system of the KCS (King, 1981; refer to Figure 7.1). Only one inconsistency was found in that what is essential and relevant in self-awareness is the objective self rather than subjective self.

Collaborative Alliance

The collaborative alliance is a relationship between the person with diabetes and the educator in which the interaction is characterized by mutual trust and respect and reciprocity in the areas of participation, power, and acknowledgment of expertise (Hernandez, 1991). This definition is shown here to be congruent with the KCS by comparing major aspects of the definition with eight of the key KCS concepts (King, 1981).

The *collaborative alliance relationship* can be considered a specific type of interaction. *Interaction* between the client and the nurse is specifically stated in the definition of collaborative alliance and is consistent with the person-to-person type of interaction described by King (1981). Interaction is "defined as a process of perception and communication between person and environment and between person and person represented by verbal and nonverbal behaviors that are goal-directed" (King, p. 145). Furthermore, King described the interaction between two individuals as such that they "collaborate to achieve a common goal" (p. 85), which further demonstrates the consistency of these two theoretical frameworks. The characteristics of this special form of interaction are now described, along with the concepts in the KCS to which they correspond.

The atmosphere of *mutual trust, respect,* and *reciprocity* that is characteristic of the collaborative alliance relationship can only be experienced by the client and nurse through the internal process of perception and external process of communication as delineated by King. *Perception* is an awareness of persons, objects, and events that is each person's representation of reality, his or her subjective world of experience (King, 1981, p. 146). *Communication* is "defined as a process whereby information is given from one person to another either directly in face-to-face meetings or indirectly through telephone, television or the written word" (King, p. 146). Communication is the vehicle by which the mutuality between the nurse and client is established and "is the means by which information is given in specific nursing situations to identify concerns and/or problems, to share information that assists individuals in making decisions that lead to goal attainment in the environment" (King, p. 146).

According to King (1981), *status* "is defined as the position of an individual in a group or a group in relation to other groups in an organization" and "is related to who you are, what you do, who you know, and what you have achieved" (pp. 129–130). In the collaborative alliance, the nurse and client collaborate (equality of status) rather than cooperate, and there is reciprocity in the areas of participation, power, and acknowledgment of expertise. This reciprocity does not mean that client and nurse have the exact same position or the exact same knowledge, but rather the status of each is such that they complement each other and there is equality of influence and proportion (not of type).

The definition of collaborative alliance depicts the role of both client and nurse as "reciprocity in the areas of participation, power, and acknowledgment of expertise" (Hernandez, 1991). According to King (1981), *role*

> is defined as a set of behaviors expected of persons occupying a position in a social system; rules that define rights and obligations in a position; a relationship with one or more individuals interacting in specific situation for a purpose. (p. 147)

King identified the functional role of the nurse as assessment of clients, using the assessment information to plan for goal setting, implementing the means to achieve the goal, and evaluating whether the goal is attained. Application of collaborative alliance relationships to this process would mean that there is client–nurse reciprocity in participation, power, and acknowledgment of expertise throughout the assessing, planning, implementing, and evaluating phases.

The *participation* characteristic of the role of the client and nurse is partially reflected through King's (1981) concept of *decision making,* "a dynamic and systematic process by which goal-directed choice of perceived alternatives is made and acted upon by individuals or groups to answer a question and attain a goal" (p. 132). Two of King's assumptions about nurse–client interactions are that clients have (a) a right to participate in decisions that influence their life, health, and community services and (b) a right to accept or reject health care (p. 143). In addition, the participation characteristic of collaborative alliance involves active participation in choosing, modifying, regulating, and performing activities of the diabetes regimen.

The *power* characteristic of the role of client and nurse in the collaborative alliance is consistent with the way King (1981) characterized *power* as situational rather than a personal attribute and with two of her seven premises of power, that is, power as a function of human interactions and decision making (p. 127).

The final characteristic of the collaborative alliance, reciprocity in acknowledgment of *expertise,* is reflected through King's (1981) concept of *authority.* "Authority is a transactional process characterized by active, reciprocal relations in which members' values, background, and perception play a role in defining, validating, and accepting the authority of individuals within an organization" (p. 124). Gulich (as cited in King, 1981, p. 122) believed authority came from those with expert knowledge and that one view of the authority of professionals is that it resides in them because of their knowledge and expertise (King, 1981, p. 123). Clients have the knowledge related to how their bodies react to diabetes in different situations and at different times, whereas nurses have a more generalized "science of diabetes" knowledge. Both types of knowledge are essential; therefore both client and nurse have—and recognize each other's—authority by virtue of their particular knowledge and expertise.

The collaborative alliance relationship construct is congruent with KCS. This congruence has been demonstrated through comparison of major components of the collaborative alliance definition with key concepts from the KCS: perception from the personal system; role, interaction, and communication from the interpersonal system; and power, authority, status, and decision making from the social system.

FURTHER EXPLICATION OF COLLABORATIVE ALLIANCE RELATIONSHIP USING KCS

Hernandez (1991, 1994) defined the collaborative alliance and suggested its use as a practice model for diabetes education but an in-depth description of what this type of relationship would look like in practice and

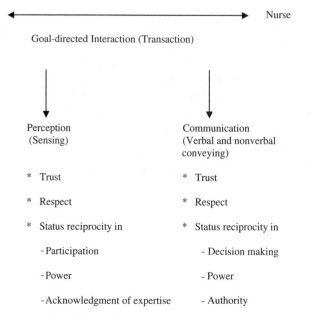

Figure 7.2. Model of the collaborative alliance conceptual components.

studies investigating collaborative alliance have not yet been completed. The decision was made to further explicate the collaborative alliance by using selected concepts within KCS to develop an operational definition of the collaborative alliance. The development of an operational definition of collaborative alliance was considered essential to its use in nursing practice and research.

The concepts used in the operational definition of collaborative alliance are depicted in Figure 7.2. The broad, overarching concept for the operational definition was *interaction*, which contains the two major subconcepts of *perception* and *communication*; these two subconcepts are further divided into other concepts. Perception includes the concepts of *status* and reciprocity of participation, *power*, and acknowledgment of expertise. Communication includes the concepts of *status*, *decision-making, power*, and *authority*. This depiction is consistent with King's (1981) definition of interaction as "a process of perception and communication between person and environment and between person and person represented by verbal and nonverbal behaviors that are goal-directed" (p. 145) with one exception: goal-directed. The theoretical definition of collaborative alliance does not contain a reference regarding goal-direction. However, it describes the relationship between the educator and the nurse and therefore is presumed to be health related (i.e., goal orientation) rather than merely social. To incorporate this goal orientation, it was necessary to add the concept *transaction,* which is a "process of interaction in which human beings communicate with environment to achieve goals that are valued" (King, 1981, p. 82). Therefore, transactions are goal-directed interactions.

The operational definition of a collaborative alliance is goal-directed interaction between a client and nurse consisting of perceptions and communications of a specific type. The interaction between clients and nurses is such that each perceives the other trusts and respects them; there is status reciprocity in participation, power, and acknowledgment of expertise; and there is recognition that these are shared perceptions. Verbal and nonverbal communications convey trust and respect for the other and status reciprocity in decision-making, power, and authority.

Additional theoretical work is necessary—and planned—to develop a paper-and-pencil instrument to measure collaborative alliance relationships. Potential questionnaire items will be derived from King's writings about the concepts specified in the model, as well as from Hernandez et al.'s (1997) delineation of the "engaging others" work that is necessary in diabetes self-awareness. Such an instrument would be useful in clinical practice and in teaching students about therapeutic relationships, and it would allow researchers to develop a body of knowledge about collaborative alliances between nurses and clients with diabetes.

CONCLUSION

The original development and refinement of the middle range theory of integration was through grounded theory research. The congruency of the theory of integration with King's (1981) conceptual system was demonstrated in this chapter. Current and future theoretical development of *collaborative alliance,* one of the major constructs in the theory of integration, is through using concept definitions and descriptions of KCS. This theoretical development is expected to have a positive impact on nursing clinical and educational practice as well as in further knowledge gains through research. As more is known about collaborative alliances and how to develop them, these types of relationships can be developed with clients and taught to nursing students and other nurses. The development of an instrument to measure collaborative alliance will allow it to be used in research, which will then further nursing knowledge related to the impact of such relationships on the health and well-being of clients.

REFERENCES

Bradish, G. I. (1994). *The lived experience of Type 1 diabetes: A replication study of the implications for diabetes education.* Unpublished master's thesis, University of Western Ontario, London, Canada.

Compton, L. (2002). *Women living with Crohn's disease.* Unpublished master's thesis, University of Windsor, Windsor, Canada.

Craig, L. A. (2002). *Time for managing competing life demands, health work, and integration of illness in families of mothers with diabetes mellitus.* Unpublished master's thesis, University of Western Ontario, London, Canada.

Glaser, B. G. (1978). *Theoretical sensitivity.* Mill Valley, CA: Sociology Press.

Glaser, B. G. (1992). *Basics of grounded theory analysis: Emergence vs. forcing.* Mill Valley, CA: Sociology Press.

Glaser, B. G., & Strauss, A. L. (1967). *The discovery of grounded theory.* New York: Aldine.

Hernandez, C. A. (1991). *The lived experience of Type 1 diabetes: Implications for diabetes education.* Unpublished doctoral dissertation, University of Toronto, Toronto, Canada.

Hernandez, C. A. (1994). Collaborative alliance: A practice model whose time has come. *Canadian Journal of Diabetes Care, 18*(4), 6–7.

Hernandez, C. A. (1995a). The development and testing of an instrument to measure integration in adults with diabetes mellitus. *Canadian Journal of Diabetes Care, 19*(3), 18–26.

Hernandez, C. A. (1995b). The experience of living with insulin-dependent diabetes: Lessons for the diabetes educator. *The Diabetes Educator, 21,* 33–37.

Hernandez, C. A. (1996). Integration: The experience of living with insulin dependent (Type 1) diabetes mellitus. *Canadian Journal of Nursing Research, 28*(4), 37–56.

Hernandez, C. A., Antone, I., & Cornelius, I. (1999). A grounded theory study of the experience of Type 2 diabetes mellitus in First Nations adults in Canada. *Journal of Transcultural Nursing, 10,* 220–228.

Hernandez, C. A., & Bradish, G. I. (1996). *Becoming self-aware: Cuing up to body listening.* London, Canada: University of Western Ontario.

Hernandez, C. A., Bradish, G. I., Laschinger, H. K. S., Rodger, N. W., & Rybansky, S. I. (1997). Self-awareness work in Type 1 diabetes: Traversing experience and negotiating collaboration. *Canadian Journal of Diabetes Care, 21*(4), 21–27.

Hernandez, C. A., Bradish, G. I., Rodger, N. W., & Rybansky, S. I. (1999). Self-awareness in diabetes: Using body cues, circumstances, and strategies. *The Diabetes Educator, 25,* 576–584.

Hernandez, C. A., Hume, M., & Rodger, N. W. (2003). Six month evaluation of a diabetes self-awareness intervention. *Outcomes Management, 7,* 148–156.

Hernandez, C. A., Laschinger, H. K. S., Rodger, N. W., Bradish, G. I., & Rybansky, S. I. (2004). Evaluation of a self-awareness intervention for adults with Type 1 diabetes. *Guidance & Counselling, 19*(1), 28–36.

Hernandez, C. A., & Williamson, K. M. (2004). Evaluation of a self-awareness education session for youth with Type 1 diabetes. *Pediatric Nursing, 30*, 459–464.

King, I. M. (1981). *A theory for nursing.* New York: Wiley.

Liehr, P., & Smith, M. J. (1999). Middle range theory: Spinning research and practice to create knowledge for the new millennium. *Advances in Nursing Science, 21*, 81–91.

Whittemore, R., Chase, S., Mandle, C. L., & Roy, C., Sr. (2001). The content, integrity and efficacy of a nurse coaching intervention in Type 2 diabetes. *The Diabetes Educator, 27*, 887–898.

Whittemore, R., Melkus, G. D., & Grey, M. (2005). Metabolic control, self-management and psychosocial adjustment in women with Type 2 diabetes. *Journal of Clinical Nursing, 14*, 195–203.

Whittemore, R., Sullivan, A., Melkus, G. D., & Grey, M. (2004). A nurse-coaching intervention for women with Type 2 diabetes. *The Diabetes Educator, 30*, 795–804.

CHAPTER EIGHT

Development of a Middle Range Theory of Quality of Life of Stroke Survivors Derived From King's Conceptual System

Jenecia Fairfax

In addition to mortality, morbidity, and patient satisfaction, health-related quality of life (HRQOL) is an outcome of health care as well as a consequence of illness or injury. Health care professionals, including nurses, recognize that illness and injury can have profound effects on a person's quality of life. Quality of life (QOL) is therefore viewed as an important health care outcome (Frey, 2001; Fuhrer, 1994). A stroke, which hits the individual suddenly and, in its wake, leaves traumatic and disabling sequelae is frequently viewed as a personal disaster, by both the individual and the family. The HRQOL of stroke survivors is an important area of study using a nursing framework that needs to be done.

When nurse researchers use nursing conceptual frameworks and theories to do nursing research, they contribute to the science of nursing by adding to the knowledge base. The development and testing of theories derived from conceptual frameworks and grand theories builds the knowledge base for nursing, provides evidence of credibility for one of nursing's grand-level theories, gives direction for future research, and can be used to develop nursing interventions. Nursing interventions based on research provide evidence for the validity and efficacy of the intervention.

This would lead to the development of practice theories that are conceptually based and empirically tested. The purpose of this chapter is to describe the development of a middle range theory of QOL of stroke survivors derived from King's conceptual system (1981).

THEORY DEVELOPMENT APPROACH

Middle range theories can be constructed by means of several theory development strategies (Meleis, 1997; Walker & Avant, 1995). Theoretical substruction as explicated by Dulock and Holzemer (1991) was used to move from the highest level of abstraction (the theoretical constructs) to the lowest level of abstraction (the scores of the empirical indicators). At the highest level of abstraction are the three theoretical constructs of King's (1981) conceptual system: the social system, the interpersonal system, and the personal system. The next level of abstraction is the theoretical concepts, which are relevant for understanding the constructs. The subconcepts, derived from the concepts, are less abstract but still not measurable. The empirical indicators are operationalization of the subconcepts and are more concrete and measurable. Finally, the measure scores indicate the level of measurement.

DESCRIPTION OF THE MIDDLE RANGE THEORY

The middle range theory of QOL of stroke survivors was derived from King's conceptual system using the concepts of interaction, perception, self, and health. These concepts were defined according to King (1981). The concepts of social support, perceptual integrity, perception of level of disability, and HRQOL were substructed from the foregoing concepts. Definitions of these concepts and the relationship among them constitute the conceptualization of the middle range theory of the quality of life of stroke survivors. The vertical arrows in Figure 8.1 indicate the level of abstraction, and horizontal arrows indicate the relationship among the constructs, concepts, and subconcepts.

THEORY LINKAGE WITH SELECTIVE
LITERATURE REVIEW

Interaction

Interaction in King's (1981) conceptual system includes both process and content. The process of human interaction as defined by King derives from

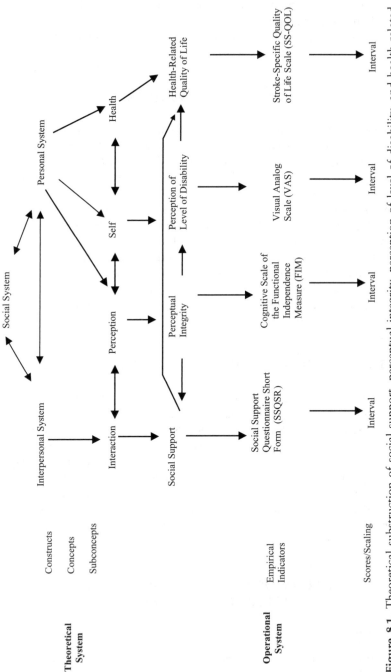

Figure 8.1. Theoretical substruction of social support, perceptual integrity, perception of level of disability, and health-related quality of life as derived from King's (1981) conceptual system.

social psychology. The process model includes perception, judgment, and actions of individuals, as well as reaction, interaction, and transaction among individuals. Interactions occur between or among two or more persons. Each interaction involves both verbal and nonverbal communication that is characterized by values and is goal-directed. Individuals bring personal knowledge, needs, goals, expectations, perceptions, and experiences that influence the interaction. King (1981) identified interaction as being universal and reciprocal. She stated, "a concept of perception is fundamental in all human interaction" (p. 61). Two other concepts that were also identified as being fundamental to interaction are communication (the informational component) and transaction (the valuational component). Communication is defined as information exchange. Interaction also involves the exchange of material goods, services, or both.

Interaction is essential to the development of relationships. The result of interaction in relationships is growth, change, and personal development. Interactions may have either a positive or a negative influence on health (King, 1981 p. 88).

Social support is conceptualized as human interaction based on King's (1981) view of interaction. It is a multidimensional construct derived from stress and coping theory. There is no single definition of social support to date. In one of the earliest definitions of social support, Weiss (1974) proposed that social support included the provision of attachment, social integration, and nurturance, as well as obtaining guidance through social relationships. Later definitions of social support included affirmation, affection, and aid (Cobb, 1976; House, 1981; Kahn, 1979). Cohen and Syme (1985) attempted to integrate multiple perspectives, definitions, and outcomes and broadly defined social support as the resources provided by other persons. This definition allows for the possibility that support may have negative as well as positive effects on health and well-being. Diamond and Jones (1983), in an attempt to integrate the multiple definitions into a broad theoretical definition of social support, identified four points on which various definitions converge: (a) communication of positive affect, (b) a sense of social integration, (c) reciprocity of directedness as a factor in the continuance of support and satisfaction in interaction, and (d) the provision of tangible aid.

Although there is some diversity in the definitions of social support, it is conceptualized as a component of social interaction with family, friends, neighbors, and others with whom one has personal contact. Consistent with King's (1981) view of the content and character of interaction are the elements of (a) reciprocity, (b) exchange of aid and communication, and (c) mutuality (p. 84). The quality of interactions influences health; therefore, the quality of social support as a component of interaction can also be expected to influence health. Social support as a human environment interaction based on King's concept of interaction has been used by other researchers (Frey, 1989) as well. For this study, social support is operationally defined as individuals' assessment of their perceived social support and satisfaction with it. The empirical indicators will be the scores on the Social Support Questionnaire Short Form (SSQSR; Sarason, Sarason, Shearin, & Pierce 1987). The SSQSR has known test–retest reliability and construct validity. The level of measurement is interval.

Perception

King (1981) defined perception as

> a process of organizing, interpreting, and transforming information from sense data and memory. It is a process of human transactions with environment. It gives meaning to one's experience, represents one's image of reality, and influence behavior. (p. 24)

Perception is universal, subjective, personal, and selective for each person. The individual's view of the world is derived from experiences provided by the perception of others and objects in the environment. Perception is selective in that each individual determines what stimuli are permitted to enter from the environment. The experiences of each person vary depending on spatial–temporal relationships, the integrity of the nervous system, level of development, and the context in which perceptions are experienced. Awareness of past events, values, and needs are factors that serve to organize one's perception. Role—status in the family, in the world of work, and in recreation—influences the individual's perceptions. Because perceptions are based on the individual's background of experiences, they are uniquely personal.

An internally altered nervous system (i.e., sensory stimulation, overload, or deprivation) and some personality factors may alter perceptions. The concept of perception is essential to understanding persons as systems and the influence perception has on human interaction. Because of the influence perception has on human interactions, it is a process of human transactions with the environment.

Perception is defined as the act of perceiving or of receiving impressions by the senses, that act or process of the mind, that makes known an external object. *Perceptual* is defined as involving perception (*American Heritage College Dictionary,* 2000, p. 1014). *Integrity* is the state of being unimpaired (*American Heritage College Dictionary,* 2000, p. 706). Perceptual integrity is therefore the state of unimpaired functioning of bodily systems or organs that are involved in sensing or perceiving the world.

Stroke sequelae may result in impairments of a number of body systems that could impair perception; such impairments may include neglect of involved extremities, homonymous hemianopia, loss of depth perception, double vision, nystagmus, dysphasia, dysgraphia, aphasia, perseveration, confusion, shortened attention span, loss of mental acuity, short-term memory loss, impulsivity, and problems conceptualizing and generalizing (Schnell, 1997). These impairments can cause major changes in the individual. Stroke survivors also suffer from depression with reported rates varying from 22% to 53% (Aström, Adolfsson, & Asplund, 1993; Herrmann, Black, Lawrence, Szekely, & Szalai, 1998; Kauhanen et al., 1999; Pohjasvaara et al., 1998; Swartzman, Gibson, & Armstrong, 1998). Depression poststroke was also associated with generalized anxiety disorder, abnormal illness behavior, and cognitive impairment with the domains of memory, nonverbal problem solving, attention, and psychomotor speed being the most likely to be affected (Clark & Smith, 1998).

In a review of the literature, Swartzman and colleagues (1998) identified depression, anxiety, emotional lability and disinhibition, catastrophic reaction and aggression, and indifference reactions as behavioral changes that occur poststroke. Pound, Gompertz, and Ebrahim (1998) found that stroke survivors reported feelings of unhappiness, difficulty talking (especially with strangers), poor memory, and confusion.

King (1981) concurred that an internally altered nervous system and illness may alter perceptions (p. 25). Research has shown that impairments experienced by the stroke survivor can change the integrity of the nervous system and may cause personality changes. These changes alter the stroke survivor's perceptions. Perceptual integrity involves unimpaired functioning of bodily systems or organs that are involved in sensing or perceiving the world. The subconcept of perceptual integrity may therefore be derived from perception. Perceptual integrity is operationally defined as individuals' assessment of their cognitive functioning as measured by the Functional Independence Measure (FIM; Uniform Data System for Medical Rehabilitation, 1993). The FIM has undergone extensive testing and revision. Psychometric properties reported for the FIM include face and construct validity, discriminant validity, interrater reliability, and precision (Hall, Hamilton, Gordon, & Zasler, 1993). Items on the cognitive subscales include comprehension, expression, social interaction, problem solving, and memory—the empirical indicators of perceptual integrity. Scores are at the level of interval measurement.

Self

Self is dynamic with values and beliefs that help one to maintain balance in life. Self is perceived in relation to others and objects in the environment. Interactions with others give one a sense of self. Positive interactions enhance self, whereas negative interactions diminish self. Each person is unique in genetic inheritance, experiences, and perceptions of the external world. Individuals acquire values, needs, and goals through growth and development that give them an awareness of personal separateness while recognizing the influence of others and their reactions to the self. Self is goal-oriented with activities directed toward personal fulfillment. King (1981) defined self as a composite of thoughts and feelings that constitute a person's awareness of individual existence and a conception of who and what he or she is. Persons' self is the sum total of all they can call their own. It includes among other things, a system of ideas, attitudes, values and commitments, and one's total subjective environment. The self constitutes a person's inner world as distinguished from the outer world consisting of all other people and things. The self is the individual as known to the individual. It is that to which we refer when we say "I" (pp. 27–28).

Self is defined as "the total, essential, or particular being of a person; the individual. The essential qualities distinguishing one individual from another. One's consciousness of one's own being or identity" (*American Heritage College Dictionary*, 2000, p. 1236).

In five qualitative studies, stroke survivors reported a loss of sense of self (Doolittle, 1991; Folden, 1994; Mumma, 1986; Secrest & Thomas, 1999). Stroke survivors were reported to focus not on what functions they had left but rather on what losses they had experienced and what the loss of functions meant to them (Doolittle, 1991; Folden, 1994; Haggstrom, Axelsson, & Norberg, 1994; Mumma, 1986; Secrest, & Thomas, 1999). In the preliminary development of an instrument to measure disability perception, Laman and Lankhorst (1994) found a difference between objective disability and perception of disability (subjective). These researchers also indicated that coping mechanisms might influence the impact of a disability. Health care providers' perceptions of the patient's functional level were reported to be higher than the patients', which was significant (Mattie, Campbell, Crisler, & Woodruff, 1992; Mattie, Crisler, Campbell, & Woodruff, 1991). These studies note that survivors' perceptions of their disabilities are different from those of health care providers.

According to King (1981), self is a composite of thoughts and feelings that constitute people's awareness of their individual existence and a conception of who and what they are. The stroke survivor's perception of level of disability is their assessment of their functionality, their awareness of their individual existence, and may therefore be derived from self. The Visual Analog Scale (VAS), developed by Price, McGrath, Raffi, and Buckingham (1983), is a subjective measurement of functioning and is therefore a reliable measure of the stroke survivor's perception of level of disability. The VAS is at the interval level of measurement.

Health

King (1981) defined health as "dynamic life experiences of a human being, which implies continuous adjustment to stressors in the internal and external environment through optimal use of one's resources to achieve maximum potential for daily living" (p. 5). Health is a process of growth and development that is not always smooth and without conflict. Health relates to the way in which individuals deal with the stresses of growth and development while functioning within their sociocultural groups.

King (1990) noted that the characteristics of health are genetic, subjective, relative, dynamic, environmental, functional, cultural, and perceptual. The ability to maintain a level of health that enables one to perform the activities of daily living (ADLs) that lead to a relatively useful, satisfying, productive, and happy life is one of life's challenges (King, 1981, 1990). Health is a function of persons interacting with their environment. Environment is a function of balance between internal and external interactions.

Health is also a functional state in the life cycle, and illness indicates some interference in this cycle. Functioning, like health, involves performance of ADLs in a manner that allows the individual to lead a relatively useful, satisfying, productive, and happy life. Functioning or performance according to King (1981) depends on harmony and balance in the individual's environment. Health and illness are both dimensions in the life span of human beings whose meanings are influenced by culture, definitions of health, and environment.

King (1981) indicated that measurement of health is a worldwide issue. The traditional indicators of health, such as mortality and morbidity, are not adequate because they do not recognize the social, emotional, or economic consequences of illness. King suggested that measurement of health should include attributes that are essential for human beings to function in their roles, environmental factors, and the developmental process.

Health has a multiplicity of definitions. *Health* is defined as the overall condition of an organism at a given time with soundness, especially of body and mind. A condition of optimal well-being has been suggested (*American Heritage College Dictionary*, 2000, p. 1236). The World Health Organization (1980) defined health as "a state of complete physical, mental and social well-being and not merely the absence of disease." In addition, health was defined as:

A state of dynamic balance in which an individual's or a group's capacity to cope with all the circumstance of living is at an optimum level. A state characterized by anatomical, physiological, and psychological integrity, ability to perform personally valued family, work, and community roles; ability to deal with physical, biological, psychological and social stress; a feeling of well-being; and freedom from the risk of disease and untimely death. (*Stedman's Medical Dictionary*, 1997, p. 382)

There are multiple definitions of health, many related to the discipline defining it. For nursing, health is viewed as a multidimensional phenomenon that is more than the absence of disease or illness (Smith, 1981). Smith (1983) proposed four models of health: the clinical model, the role performance model, the adaptive model, and the eudemonistic model. The clinical model has the narrowest view. Health is viewed as the absence of signs and symptoms of illness (Smith, 1983). The other models can be viewed as an expansion of the clinical model with the eudemonistic model embracing the concerns of the other three models and therefore is the most comprehensive. The adaptive model is most closely related to King's (1981) conceptualization of health. Health is viewed in relation to a person's interaction with the environment. King viewed health from a social role and general systems perspective. Health includes adaptive and functional potential and performance. Health is implied as a factor in life that allows one to function in one's usual role (King, 1994).

King did not define QOL; however, she stated that "the conceptual system is timeless and is not culture bound. It can be used at anytime in any culture because it provides structure to observe interacting elements in the environment that enhance or impinge on quality of life" (King, 1994, p. 30).

There is great diversity in the definitions of HRQOL. A conceptual formulation that has emerged in clinical settings defines HRQOL "functionally by patients' perceptions of performance in four areas: physical and occupational, psychological, social interaction, and somatic sensation" (Schipper, Clinch, & Olweny, 1996, p. 11). This conceptualization includes the essence of most definitions. Underlying this conceptualization is the subjective nature of HRQOL, interpersonal relationships within and outside the family, and transactions between the person and the environment, all of which are influenced by sociocultural factors. HRQOL is a narrower subset of the overall concept of QOL. It looks at QOL only in the health context. HRQOL includes the domains of physical, psychological, social, spiritual, and role functioning, as well as general well-being of QOL. Most definitions of QOL include the individual's degree of satisfaction or perception of satisfaction with life (Andrews, 1974; Hornquist, 1982; Oleson, 1990; Zahn, 1992).

Health according to King (1981) includes people's ability to function in their usual roles and performance of ADLs in a manner that allows individuals to lead a relatively useful, satisfying, productive, and happy life, which are both congruent with the conceptualization of HRQOL. Therefore, HRQOL is substructed from health.

HRQOL is operationally defined as people's assessment of their energy, language, mood, personality, thinking, vision, mobility, upper extremity function, performance of self-care, family and social roles, and work and productivity as measured by the Stroke-Specific Quality of Life scale (SS-QOL; Williams, Weinberger, Harris, Clark, & Biller, 1999). This instrument was developed specifically to measure HRQOL in stroke patients. There are only preliminary results regarding reliability and validity of the SS-QOL at this time. The total and subscales scores are the empirical indicators. The level of measurement is interval.

ASSUMPTIONS AND PROPOSITIONS

King's (1981) conceptualizations and characterizations of relationships among the personal and interpersonal systems make it possible to make inferences about interaction, perception, self, and health. The following assumptions, derived from King's conceptual system for nursing, serve as the basis for the proposed model of the theory of quality of life of stroke survivors (TQOLSS):

1. Perceptions of individuals determine their reality.
2. Perception influences the interactions of individuals.
3. Human interaction influences individual health.
4. Perception influences, through interaction, individuals' health.
5. Social support is a human interaction and therefore influences individual health.
6. Health of individuals as a personal system is a multidimensional phenomenon.
7. Health has biological, psychological, social, and functional dimensions.
8. Health of individuals has structural and functional elements.

Propositions for this model are as follows:

1. Perception affects all interactions, gives an individual a sense of self and others, and affects assessment of one's HRQOL.
2. Social support (a type of interaction) affects the stroke survivor's HRQOL.

HYPOTHESES

The proposed model to be tested hypothesizes that perceptual integrity (cognition) has both a direct and indirect effect on HRQOL, that perception of level of disability has a direct effect on HRQOL, and that social support has both a direct and indirect effect on HRQOL. The hypotheses were based on the foregoing assumptions. The model will be tested in a

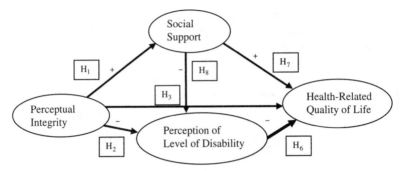

Figure 8.2. Middle range theory of health-related quality of life of stroke survivors. H1–H8 = Hypotheses 1, 2, 3, 6, 7, and 8 from text.

population of stroke survivors in a Midwestern inner city. The hypotheses to be tested are as follows:

1. Perceptual integrity has a direct and positive effect on social support.*
2. Perceptual integrity has a direct and negative effect on perception of level of disability.*
3. Perceptual integrity has a direct and positive effect on the stroke survivor's HRQOL.*
4. Perceptual integrity has an indirect effect on the stroke survivor's HRQOL through perception of level of disability.
5. Perceptual integrity has an indirect effect on the stroke survivor's HRQOL through social support.
6. Perception of level of disability has a direct and negative effect on the stroke survivor's HRQOL.*
7. Social support has a direct and positive effect on the stroke survivor's HRQOL.*
8. Social support has a direct and negative effect on perception of level of disability.*

(* These hypotheses are mapped in Figure 8.2.)

SUMMARY

Previous research on stroke survivors' QOL was not based on a nursing framework. The development and testing of theories derived from conceptual frameworks and grand theories builds the knowledge base for nursing and provides evidence of credibility for one of nursing's grand-level theories. Nursing interventions based on research provide evidence for the validity and efficacy of the intervention. This would lead to the development of practice theories that are conceptually based and empirically tested. A theory of stroke survivors' QOL derived from King's (1981) conceptual system was developed using substruction. Empirical testing of this theory will contribute to the science of nursing by providing evidence of credibility for King's conceptual system and providing the basis for nursing interventions in the care of stroke survivors.

REFERENCES

American Heritage College Dictionary. (2000). Boston: Houghton Mifflin.

Andrews, F. M. (1974). Social indicator of perceived life quality. *Social Indicators Research, 1,* 279–284.

Aström, M., Adolfsson, R., & Asplund, K. (1993). Major depression in stroke patients: A 3-year longitudinal study. *Stroke, 24,* 976–982.

Clark, M. S., & Smith, D. S. (1998). The effects of depression and abnormal illness behavior on outcome following rehabilitation from stroke. *Clinical Rehabilitation, 12,* 73–80.

Cobb, S. (1976). Social support as a moderator of life stress. *Psychosocial Medicine, 38,* 300–313.

Cohen, S., & Syme, S. L. (1985). Issues in the study and application of social support. In S. Cohen & S. L. Syme (Eds.), *Social support and health* (pp. 3–22). Orlando, FL: Academic Press.

Diamond, M., & Jones, S. L. (1983). Social support: A review and theoretical integration In P. L. Chinn (Ed.), *Advances in nursing theory development* (pp. 235–249). Rockville, MD: Aspen.

Doolittle, N. D. (1991). Clinical ethnography of lacunar stroke: Implications for acute care. *Journal of Neuroscience Nursing, 23,* 235–240.

Dulock, H. L., & Holzemer, W. L. (1991). Substruction: Improving the linkage from theory to method. *Nursing Science Quarterly, 4,* 83–87.

Folden, S. L. (1994, Fall). Managing the effects of a stroke: The first months. *Rehabilitation Nursing,* 79–85.

Frey, M. A. (1989). Social support and health: A theoretical formulation derived from King's conceptual framework. *Nursing Science Quarterly, 2,* 138–148.

Frey, M. A. (2001). Health-related quality of life: Promises and pitfalls. *Journal of Child and Family Nursing, 4,* 63–67.

Fuhrer, M. (1994). Subjective well-being: Implications for medical rehabilitation outcomes and models of disablement. *American Journal of Physical Medicine and Rehabilitation, 73,* 358–364.

Haggstrom, T., Axelsson, K., & Norberg, A. (1994). The experience of living with stroke sequelae illuminated by means of stories and metaphors. *Qualitative Health Research, 4,* 321–337.

Hall, K. M., Hamilton, B. B., Gordon, W. A., & Zalser, N. D. (1983). Characteristics and comparisons of functional assessment indices: Disability Rating

Scale, Functional Independence Measure, and Functional Assessment Measure. *Journal of Head Trauma Rehabilitation, 8*, 60–74.

Herrmann, N., Black, S. E., Lawrence, J., Szekely, C., & Szalai, J. P. (1998). The Sunnybrook Stroke study: A prospective study of depressive symptoms and functional outcomes. *Stroke, 29*, 618–624.

Hornquist, J. O. (1982). The concept of quality of life. *Scandinavian Journal of Social Medicine, 10*, 57–61.

House, J. S. (1981). *Work stress and social support.* Reading, MA: Addison-Wesley.

Kahn, R. (1979). Aging and social support. In M. Riley (Ed.), *Aging from birth to death: Interdisciplinary perspectives* (pp.189–199). Boulder, CO: Westview Press for American Association for the Advancement of Science.

Kauhanen, M. L., Korpelainen, J. T., Hiltunen, P., Brusin, E., Mononen, H., Maatta, R., et al. (1999). Poststroke depression correlates with cognitive impairment and neurological deficits. *Stroke, 30*, 1875–1880.

King, I. M. (1981). *A theory for nursing: Systems, concepts, process.* Albany, NY: Delmar.

King, I. M. (1990). Health as the goal of nursing. *Nursing Science Quarterly, 3*, 123–128.

King, I. M. (1994). Quality of life and goal attainment. *Nursing Science Quarterly, 7*, 29–32.

Laman, H., & Lankhorst, G. J. (1994). Subjective weighting of disability: An approach to quality of life assessment in rehabilitation. *Disability and Rehabilitation: An International Multidisciplinary Journal, 16*, 198–204.

Mattie, K. B., Campbell, L., Crisler, J. R., & Woodruff, C. (1992). The impact of selected demographic variables and disability types on perceptions of clients functioning level. *Journal of Applied Rehabilitation Counseling, 23*, 29–34.

Mattie, K. B., Crisler, J. R., Campbell, L., & Woodruff, C. (1991). Clients' functioning level as perceived by clients and rehabilitation professionals. *Journal of Applied Rehabilitation Counseling, 22*(2), 3–6.

Meleis, A. I. (1997). *Theoretical nursing: Development & progress* (3rd ed.). Philadelphia: Lippincott.

Mumma, C. M. (1986). Perceived losses following stroke. *Rehabilitation Nursing, 11*, 3

Oleson, M. (1990). Subjectively perceived quality of life. *Image: Journal of Nursing Scholarship, 22*, 187–190.

Pohjasvaara, T., Leppävuori, A., Siira, I., Vataja, R., Kaste, M., & Erkinjuntti, T. (1998). Frequency and clinical determinants of poststroke depression. *Stroke, 29*, 2311–2317.

Pound, P., Gompertz, P., & Ebrahim, S. (1998). A patient-centered study of the consequences of stroke. *Clinical Rehabilitation, 12*, 338–347.

Price, D. D., McGrath, P. A., Raffi, A., & Buckingham, B. (1983). The validation of visual analogue scales as ratio scale measures for chronic and experimental pain. *Pain, 17*, 45–56.

Sarason, I. G., Sarason, B. R., Shearin, E. N., & Pierce, G. R. (1987). A brief measure of social support: Practical and theoretical implications. *Journal of Social and Personal Relationships, 4*, 497–510.

Schipper, H., Clinch, J. J., & Olweny, C. L. M. (1996). Quality of life studies: Definitions and conceptual issues. In B. Spilker (Ed.), *Quality of Life and Pharmoeconomics in Clinical Trials* (2nd ed., pp. 11–23). Philadelphia: Lippincott.

Schnell, S. S. (1997). Nursing care of clients with cerebrovascular disorders. In J. M. Black & E. Matasarrin-Jacobs (Eds.), *Medical-surgical nursing: Clinical management for continuity of care* (5th ed., pp. 771–833). Philadelphia: Saunders.

Secrest, J. A., & Thomas, S. P. (1999). Continuity and discontinuity: The quality of life following stroke. *Rehabilitation Nursing, 24,* 240–246.

Stedman's medical dictionary. (1997). Baltimore: Williams & Wilkins.

Smith, J. (1981). The idea of health: A philosophical inquiry. *Advances in Nursing Science, 3*(4), 43–50.

Smith, J. (1983). *The idea of health: Implications for the nursing profession.* New York: Teachers College Press.

Swartzman, L. C., Gibson, M. C., & Armstrong, T. L. (1998). Psychological considerations in adjustment to stroke. *Physical Medicine and Rehabilitation: State of the Art Review, 12,* 19–41.

Uniform Data System for Medical Rehabilitation. (1993). *Guide for the Uniform Data Set for Medical Rehabilitation.* UB Foundation Activities. Amherst, NY.

Walker, L. O., & Avant, K. C. (1995). *Strategies for theory construction in nursing* (3rd Ed.). Norwalk, CT: Appleton & Lange.

Weiss, R. (1974). The provision of social relationships. In Z. Rubin (Ed.), *Doing unto others* (pp. 17–26). Englewood Cliffs, NJ: Prentice Hall.

Williams, L. S., Weinberger, M., Harris, L. E., Clark, D. O., & Biller, J. (1999). Development of a Stroke-Specific Quality of Life Scale. *Stroke, 30,* 1362–1369.

World Health Organization. (1980). *International classification of impairments, disabilities, and handicaps.* Geneva, Switzerland: World Health Organization.

Zahn, L. (1992). Quality of life: Conceptual and measurement issues. *Journal of Advanced Nursing, 17,* 795–800.

CHAPTER NINE

Development and Initial Testing of a Theory of Patient Satisfaction With Nursing Care

Mary B. Killeen

Patient satisfaction information becomes increasingly more important to today's outcomes-oriented health care environment. The patient satisfaction survey is one mechanism for translating diverse consumer preferences into improved provider performance in an intensely competitive health care environment. Valid measurement of patient satisfaction has become a serious financial issue in hospitals for two reasons. First, unfavorable patient satisfaction ratings may prompt high-cost decisions. Changes in physical plants including new construction are often prompted by competition with other providers. Second, satisfaction surveys may affect a hospital's standing as a provider of managed care within various health plans. Patient satisfaction data are important to employer purchasers of health care plans who must decide which health plans to keep and drop (Weisman & Kock, 1989). Ultimately, hospitals could lose dollars and contracts with health plans based on patient satisfaction data that may not be valid. The focus of hospital surveys on hotel-like amenities may be short-sighted. Rather, the best overall predictor of consumer satisfaction with the hospitalization service encounter has been found to be satisfaction with nursing care (Abramowitz, Cote, & Betty, 1987; McDaniel & Nash, 1990; Press & Ganey, 1990). Hospital surveys could be better predictors of patient loyalty if more attention was paid to patient satisfaction with nursing care.

There is a critical need for valid and reliable instruments to measure satisfaction with professional nursing in hospitals separate from the usual hospital satisfaction surveys. However, knowledge of patient satisfaction in the discipline of nursing has suffered from a lack of conceptual clarity (Eriksen, 1995) and paucity of reliable and valid measures in the hospital setting (McDaniel & Nash, 1990). Furthermore, methodological problems have contributed to the difficulty of reliably and validly measuring patient satisfaction in health care and in nursing. The mounting importance of standardized measurement of nursing-sensitive outcomes, including the theory of patient satisfaction with nursing care (PSNC), in computerized information systems for managerial decision making is highlighted by the national goal to measure quality care (American Nurses Association, 1995; Agency for Healthcare Research and Quality, 2002; National Quality Forum, 2004). At a time when demand for patient satisfaction data is high among nurse administrators, it is surprising that a comprehensive instrument for measurement of consumer attitudes toward professional nursing care in the hospital setting does not currently exist in the literature.

A theory was developed by the author to address the need for a valid and reliable patient satisfaction instrument guided by a nursing theoretical framework based on Imogene King's conceptual system (1981). The purpose of this chapter is to explicate the middle range theory of the PSNC. The specific aim is to examine the concept and theory of PSNC for consistency with King's conceptual system.

THEORY DEVELOPMENT APPROACH

The conceptual model concepts and propositions used to guide the concepts of the theory and subsequent research were derived from King's (1981) conceptual system and Eagly and Chaiken's (1993) attitude model. The theoretical approach was theory derivation (Walker & Avant, 1983). Because patient satisfaction is accepted as an attitude (Ware, Snyder, Wright, & Davis, 1983), the concepts of the Eagly and Chaiken's (1993) attitude model were transposed from the field of social psychology to patient satisfaction in the field of nursing and reformulated within King's (1981) conceptual system as cognitive, affective, and behavioral patient-consumer perceptions and response concepts. Additional concepts were developed from the patient satisfaction literature and reformulated using King (1981) to represent the influencers of patient satisfaction with nursing care, that is, the individual patient-consumer and the nursing situation.

Philosophic Orientation and Boundaries of the PSNC Theory

King's conceptual system (1981) provides the broad philosophic orientation for the middle range theory of patient satisfaction with nursing care. Composed of three open systems in a dynamic interacting conceptual system—personal systems, interpersonal systems, and social systems—King's work has contributed to a theoretical base for the discipline of nursing. King's conceptual system includes a focus on the development of a relationship between patient and nurse. Patient satisfaction with nursing care is an outcome of the interpersonal interaction process between the patient and nurse. Patient satisfaction has been accepted by the nursing profession as a nursing-sensitive outcome of care (American Nurses Association, 1995; Lang & Clinton, 1984; Lang & Marek, 1992, Megivern, Halm, & Jones, 1992). The philosophic orientation of King's conceptual system is a fitting choice for the theory of PSNC.

The focus of the theory of PSNC is the patient-consumer view of the nursing profession. Traditionally, health care professionals have not viewed a patient as a consumer. However, an individual may be a consumer of nursing services as with other services. In the marketing perspective of this theory, it is reasonable to view a patient as a consumer and to label him or her as a particular consumer type using the term *patient-consumer* (Soffer, 1978). The nurse's perception of the patient or of nursing, although important, does not enter into the theory of PSNC. Furthermore, patient evaluation of hospital amenities commonly found in patient satisfaction hospital surveys is not intended to be part of the nursing-focused PSNC theory.

DESCRIPTION OF THE MIDDLE RANGE THEORY OF PSNC

Concept of Patient Satisfaction

Patient satisfaction has been described as a concept that is difficult to conceptualize and measure (Eagly & Chaiken, 1993; Ware et al., 1983). Therefore, it was necessary to first seek a robust conceptualization for the concept of patient satisfaction of nursing care (see Figure 9.1).

The construct, Attitude of Satisfaction, includes the constructs of Perception, Satisfaction, and Attitude. At the construct level, Satisfaction is an Attitude influenced by Perception. Antecedents–processes and consequences–responses are correlates rather than components of attitudes (Eagly & Chaiken, 1993). Rather than defining the Attitude of Satisfaction directly, it was considered an unmeasurable, intervening construct. Patient-consumer perceptions are derived from the antecedents–processes of an attitude. Patient-consumer responses are derived from

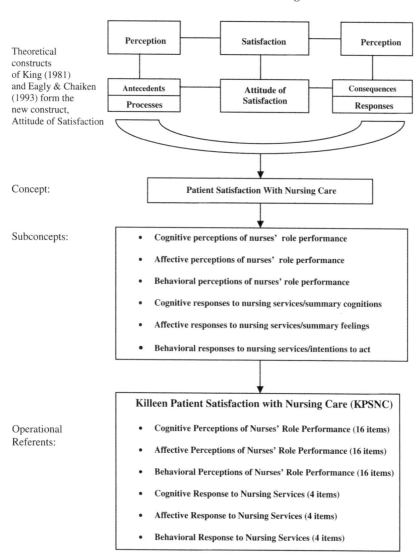

Figure 9.1. Conceptualization of the concept of patient satisfaction with nursing care.

responses–consequences of attitude. For the concept of patient satisfaction with nursing care, subconcepts are three patient perceptions of nurse role performance (cognitive, affective, and behavioral) and three patient responses to nursing services (cognitive, affective, and behavioral). These six subconcepts are proxy concepts for the unobservable construct of Attitude of Satisfaction and together represent the concept of patient satisfaction with nursing care. The concept of patient satisfaction with nursing care is described further in the section on theory linkage with King's work. The theoretical definition of the concept of PSNC is as follows: the patient-consumer's perceptions of nurses' role performance and responses to the experience of receiving nursing services. The Killeen Patient Satisfaction With Nursing Care (KPSNC) instrument measures the six subconcepts that form the concept of patient satisfaction with nursing care.

The patient-consumer perceptions and responses subconcepts, definitions, and examples are as follows:

1. Theoretical (Th): *Cognitive perceptions of nurses' role performance:* patient-consumer evaluations of nurses' role performance based on knowledge-type information from direct personal experience during a specific hospitalization (i.e., a patient's factual report of his or her experience with professional nursing care).
   Operational (Op): The patient-consumer's total score on the Cognitive Perceptions of Nurses' Role Performance instrument items.

2. (Th): *Affective perceptions of nurses' role performance:* patient-consumer evaluations of nurses' role performance based on feelings and emotions–type information and fulfilled and unfulfilled need experiences from direct personal experience during a specific hospitalization (i.e., a patient's feelings about his or her experience with professional nursing care).
   (Op): The patient-consumer's total score on the Affective Perceptions of Nurses' Role Performance instrument items.

3. (Th): *Behavioral perceptions of nurses' role performance:* patient-consumer evaluations of nurses' role performance based on own behavior (self-perception) in terms of interactions with nurses during a specific hospitalization (i.e., a patient's perception of his or her behavior in relation to his or her experience with professional nursing care).
   (Op): The patient-consumer's total score on the Behavioral Perceptions of Nurses' Role Performance instrument items.

4. (Th): *Cognitive response to nursing services:* patient-consumer summary impressions evaluation based on his or her judgment about the totality of experiences with the services provided by nurses during a specific hospitalization.
   (Op): The patient-consumer's total score on the Cognitive Response to Nursing Services (CRNS) instrument items.

5. (Th): *Affective response to nursing services:* patient-consumer summary feelings evaluation based on liking or disliking the services provided by nurses during a specific hospitalization.

(Op): The patient-consumer's total score on the Affective Response to Nursing Services (ARNS) instrument items.

6. (Th): *Behavioral response to nursing services:* patient-consumer summary intentions to act evaluation based on intentions to live a healthy lifestyle or to reuse or recommend a hospital because of the services provided by nurses during a specific hospitalization. (Op): The patient-consumer's total score on the Behavioral Response to Nursing Services (BRNS) instrument items.

Theory of PSNC

Theoretical system of the theory of PSNC

The theoretical system of the theory of PSNC is displayed in Figure 9.2. Besides patient satisfaction with nursing care, the two other main concepts of the theory of PSNC are individual patient-consumers and nursing

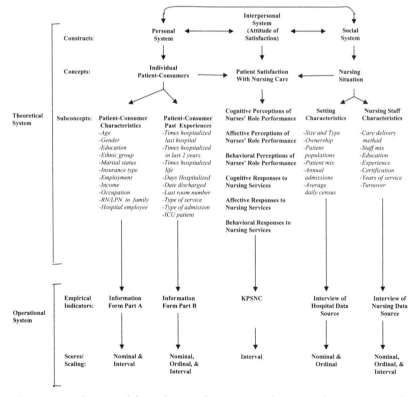

Figure 9.2. Theoretical formulation of patient satisfaction with nursing care derived from King's interacting systems framework.

situation. The three concepts are derived from King's (1981) conceptual system constructs of personal, interpersonal, and social systems that are interacting. King's interpersonal system in this theory conceptualization borrows from Eagly and Chaiken's (1993) attitude theory, which is described under the section on theory linkage to King's work. The two concepts of individual patient-consumers and nursing situation influence the concept of patient satisfaction with nursing care.

The concept of individual patient-consumer is defined as the recipient of care who interacts in the role of patient-consumer with caregivers within the health care system including the nursing situation environment. Subconcepts of individual patient-consumers are patient past experiences and patient characteristics. Essential variables of each are listed in Figure 9.2. Past experiences and sociodemographic characteristics of the individual influence perceptions and responses to nursing care. Individuals' perceptions are aggregated in the evaluation of patient satisfaction in organizations, but it is important to remember that the individual is the focus in the theory.

Nursing situations are primarily located within health care systems, such as the hospital. The concept of nursing situation is defined as the environment in which nursing care occurs, which includes the specific health care or other setting characteristics and nursing staff characteristics. Subconcepts of nursing situations are setting characteristics and nursing staff characteristics. Essential variables of each are shown in Figure 9.2.

Operational system of the theory of PSNC

Operational concepts of the theory of PSNC and their measurement are shown in Figure 9.2. Empirical indicators include an information form, the KPSNC tool, and interviews. The purpose of the information form is the collection of data for the variables that might suggest characteristics associated with patient satisfaction with nursing care. The information form collects data on the most recent hospitalization experience and is organized into two sections: Part A and Part B. The 10 items for patient characteristics (nominal and interval levels of measurement) and the 12 items for patient past experiences (nominal, ordinal, and interval) are listed in Figure 9.2. The KPSNC instrument is a 60-item, interval-level instrument that is described in the methodology section.

Data on the setting and nursing staff characteristics as listed in Figure 9.2 were obtained through various interviews with hospital and nursing sources. Data are at the nominal, ordinal, and interval levels of measurement.

THEORY LINKAGE TO KING'S WORK

King's Conceptual System

King's conceptual system for nursing provided the overall conceptual framework for the development of a middle range theory of patient satisfaction (see Figure 9.2). King defined perception as "a process of organizing, interpreting, and transforming information from sense data and memory" (1981, p. 24). King confirmed the existence of a relevant relationship, stating that she viewed "*satisfaction* may be the result of one's *perception.*" Moreover, King stated that "*perception* is a comprehensive concept and encompasses cognitive, affective, and behavioral aspects." King believes that "perceptions and attitudes are different" and that "an attitude is a result of experiences" (I. M. King, personal communication, January 4, 1994). Following King's clarification of satisfaction influenced by perceptions, a need for a clearer understanding of the nature of patient satisfaction was sought in the social psychology literature. Is patient satisfaction an opinion, a sentiment, a global impression, or an attitude? After an extensive review, the evidence for patient satisfaction formation as an attitude was based on Eagly and Chaiken's (1993) attitude model.

Eagly and Chaiken's Attitude Model

Eagly and Chaiken (1993) presented the idea that an attitude, as an inferred state, is formed as "a product of cognitive, affective, and behavioral processes" (p. 15). Therefore, stimuli that denote the attitude object are observable antecedents of an unobservable attitude. Antecedents include cognitive, affective, and behavioral informational processes. Responses that express evaluation and therefore reveal people's attitudes are observable consequences of an attitude. Evaluative responses can be divided into three classes: cognitive, affective, and behavioral (Figure 9.3).

Theoretical perspectives and empirical findings in the attitude research area support the model of correlates of attitude approach in this PSNC theory. The assumption that attitudes derive from a process of cognitive learning is implicit in much of attitude research (Eagly & Chaiken, 1993). For example, as people gain direct or indirect information about the attitude object, they form beliefs according to expectancy–value theory (Fishbein & Ajzen, 1975).

Affective perceptions as one basis of attitude formation appeared in the classical conditioning model of attitude change (Eagly & Chaiken, 1993). From this perspective, the latent attitude of patient satisfaction is

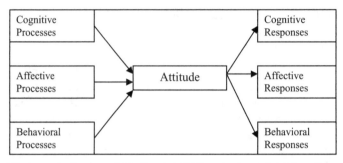

Figure 9.3. Eagly and Chaiken's (1993) attitude model. *Note*. From *The Psychology of Attitudes* (pp. 10, 15), by A. H. Eagly and S. Chaiken, 1993, New York: Harcourt Brace Jovanovich, Inc. Copyright 1993 by Harcourt Brace Jovanovich, Inc. Adapted with permission.

a product of the pairing of an attitude object (i.e., a registered nurse—a conditioned stimulus) with a stimulus (e.g., caring act) that elicits an affective response (unconditioned stimulus). Need fulfillment can also be a stimulus of affective perceptions (Eagly & Chaiken, 1993).

Behavioral perceptions derive from research by Bem (1967a, 1967b, 1972), who determined that attitudes are determined primarily by previous behaviors. He proposed a theory of self-perception explaining that people tend to infer attitudes that are consistent with their prior behavior. For example, if a patient recalls smiling at a nurse, that person believes he or she was favorably disposed toward some aspects of that nurse's care.

"Evaluative responses of the cognitive type are thoughts or ideas about the attitude object" (Eagly & Chaiken, 1993, p. 11). They may be overt (verbal statements of beliefs) or covert (inferred or perceived). The attributes associated with the attitude object (e.g., a registered nurse) "express positive or negative evaluation and therefore can be located by psychologists on an evaluative continuum" (p. 11).

"Evaluative responses of the affective type consist of feelings, needs, emotions, and sympathetic nervous system activity that people experience in relation to attitude objects" (Eagly & Chaiken, 1993, p. 11). Like cognitive responses, they may range from extremely positive to extremely negative. Eagly and Chaiken took the position, with others, that evaluation and affect are distinct. Evaluation is treated as an intervening state between stimuli and responses elicited by stimuli. Affect is "one type of responding by which people express their evaluations" (p. 12).

"Evaluative responses of the behavioral (or conative) type consist of the overt actions that people exhibit in relation to the attitude object" (p. 12). Also, behavioral responses can be regarded as including *intentions* to act.

On the basis of Eagly and Chaiken's (1993) synergistic viewpoint of attitude, "the different classes of evaluative responses impinge on one another and exist in an interactive, cooperative relation" (p. 666). They stated, "experience in any one of these domains—cognitive, affective, or behavioral—tends to elicit responses in the other domains" (p. 667). Eagly and Chaiken's extensive review showed that discriminate validity of the three classes has been demonstrated "only sometimes." Therefore, the total set of perceptions and responses instruments may determine the more abstract evaluation of professional nursing that is formed by patient-consumers rather than each component being consistently separable on an empirical basis.

Linkage of Eagly and Chaiken's (1993) Attitude Model to King's Conceptual System

Eagly and Chaiken (1993) defined an attitude as "a psychological tendency that is expressed by evaluating a particular entity with some degree of favor or disfavor" (p. 1). The nature of satisfaction is concluded to be that of an attitude based on King (I. M. King, personal communication, January 4, 1994) and a thorough review of the literature. The antecedents to attitude are processes based on information, experience, or stimuli that denote an attitude object (Eagly & Chaiken, 1993). The consequences of attitudes are evaluative responses according to Eagly and Chaiken. King's concept of perception is consistent with Eagly and Chaiken's processes and responses concepts. The part of King's definition of perception that is consistent with antecedents or processes is "a process of organizing, . . . and transforming information" (1981, p. 24). The part of King's definition of perception that is consistent with the consequences or evaluative responses is "interpreting . . . information from sense data and memory" (p. 24).

Eagly and Chaiken (1993) further divided processes and responses into cognitive, affective, and behavioral classes. This is consistent with King's view of individuals as thinking, feeling, reacting human beings. Eagly and Chaiken's attitude model directly links with King's conceptual system concept of perception. The new, middle range concepts of cognitive, affective, and behavioral perceptions and responses are derived from King's conceptual system concept of perception. The Eagly and Chaiken model provides additional support for the six concepts that form the middle range theoretical structure used to guide the content for instrument development. With the use of the tripartite view of attitudinal responding and attitude formation (Eagly & Chaiken, 1993), perceptions and responses are defined and measured independently and yet together comprise, at a higher level of abstraction, the single construct of attitude. It is possible that adding emotional and behavioral perceptions and responses of patient-consumers may provide more insight than cognitive perceptions and responses alone in deciding attitudes toward nurses and nursing services. Furthermore, the use of diverse human perceptions and responses—that is, cognitive, affective, and behavioral—is more holistic and fitting with the nursing profession's social contract with the public (American Nurses Association, 2001) than cognitive consumer perceptions and responses alone. The theory of Eagly and Chaiken and the relationship between perception and satisfaction are further explicated by the linkages of King's concepts with the concepts in the Killeen theory of PSNC.

King's Concepts and the Theory of PSNC

The concept of patient satisfaction with nursing care in the theory of PSNC incorporates King's concepts of perceptions, communications, expectations, mutual goals of nurse and patient, decision making, and the nurse and patient as a system of interdependent roles. The specific linkages between King's concepts from her conceptual system and the concepts and subconcepts of the theory of PSNC are shown in Table 9.1.

Individuals

Individuals are personal systems in King's conceptual system (King, 1981). "Persons exhibit some common characteristics, such as the ability to

Table 9.1. Linkages Between King's (1981) Concepts and Theory of PSNC Concepts

King's concepts	Components of the study concepts (bold face)
Individuals	Thinking, feeling, acting **individual patient-consumers**
Perception	**Cognitive, affective, and behavioral perceptions**
Role	**Nurses' role performance** as perceived by patient-consumers
Decision making	**Cognitive, affective, and behavioral patient-consumer responses of intentions** to act as a consequence of experiencing nursing care
Nursing situation	The environment of professional nursing and all its **hospital and staff characteristics**
Past experiences	**Past experiences with nurses and other characteristics of the patient-consumer**
Goal attainment	PSNC representing an outcome of effective nursing care (i.e., goal attainment)

Note. PSNC = Patient Satisfaction with Nursing Care.

perceive, to think, to feel, to choose between alternative courses of action, to set goals, to select the means to achieve goals, and to make decisions" (p. 19). King identified individuals as thinking, feeling, reacting human beings able to participate in transactions and decision making related to health care services.

Perception

Perception, a basic concept in King's conceptual system, is the "process of organizing, interpreting, and transforming information from sense data and memory" (King, 1981, p. 24). King believes cognition, feelings, and intentions are encompassed within the concept of perception (I. M. King, personal communication, January, 4, 1994). Perception therefore is intentionally subjective and consistent with the cognitive, affective, and behavioral dimensions in the PSNC theory.

Role

Roles are characterized by King (1981) as dynamic, as involving interpersonal relationships, and as a way to give and receive information. King differentiated role expectations and role performance as two components in the broad concept of role that influence transactions. Role behaviors expected of nurses by patients are explicated as "those of care giver, teacher, friend, and advocate" (p. 94). King's patient-oriented role names are used to guide dimensions of the instrument to mean the nurse professional role performance of skilled caregiver; patient educator; therapeutic, caring relationship provider; and patient advocate.

Decision making

Decision making is a personal process that involves subjective behaviors according to King (1981). Because King (1981) believed decision making is individual, situational, and goal-directed, it can be said to be based on one's summary of impressions, feelings, and intentions to act.

Behavior usually is considered something quite different from intentions. However, decision making in King's conceptual system is analogous to behavioral intentions in the theory of PSNC. The concept of behavioral intentions is considered behavior because (a) it is behavior that is verbalized and (b) it is used in the sense of conation, "indicating how a person does, would or plans to act with respect to the object" (Ajzen, 1989, p. 244). The three subconcepts of behavioral responses to nursing care represent one's intention to reuse or recommend nursing services. This implies the individual's willingness to carry out positive health-related behaviors in the future. Evidence of intentions to use services associated with satisfaction is found in Pascoe's (1983) review of the literature on patient satisfaction in primary health care. "Findings consistently indicate that dissatisfaction is associated with intention to switch services and self-report of having terminated services" (p. 198). Miller, Johnson, Garrett, Wikoff, and McMahon (1982) use behavioral intentions as client outcomes at the time of discharge to predict future behavior in maintaining health goals. In this theory, the definition of behavioral intentions also includes intentions to achieve health-related goals consistent with King's (1981) emphasis on client goals.

Nursing situation

King (1981) described characteristics, functions, and behaviors of nurses in all types of nursing situations. She defined a nursing situation as "the immediate environment, spatial and temporal reality, in which nurse and client establish a relationship to cope with health states and adjust to changes in activities of daily living if the situation demands it" (p. 2). She usually included client goals and goal setting when discussing a nursing situation. Essential variables in nursing situations include geographic place, perceptions, communications, expectations, and mutual goals of nurse and patient, as well as the nurse and patient as a system of interdependent roles. Nursing situations are primarily located within health care systems, such as the hospital.

Past experiences

Past experiences in the theory of PSNC refer to past experiences with nurses and the health care system. "Each (person) brings past experiences, present needs, expectations, and goals that influence perceptions in the interactions" (King, 1981, p. 84). Past experiences and health system environmental factors, including temporal–spatial relationships, influence perceptions of both the caregiver and recipient of care (1981).

Goal attainment

Goal attainment is central to many of King's concepts. Because goal attainment is a product of the nurse–patient interaction process and is equated with effective nursing care (King, 1981), the nursing-sensitive outcome of patient satisfaction with nursing care may be considered central to goal attainment between nurses and patient-consumers.

Summary of Theory Linkage to King's Work

King's concepts and terms are important to the systemization of patient-consumer perceptions and responses to professional nursing. The concept of *role* as *role performance* within King's systemization of *perception* formed the basis for the perceptions subconcepts. The subconcepts of behavioral responses, based on *decision making,* was expanded to add cognitive and affective concepts consistent with King's (1971, 1981) view of individuals as thinking, feeling, and acting human beings. King confirmed the identification of these selected concepts that are linked to the theory's conceptual definitions (I. M. King, personal communication, April 16, 1994).

SELECTED LITERATURE REVIEW

Although hospitals emphasize the importance of patient satisfaction surveys, the significance, validity, and usefulness of the patient satisfaction concept has been seriously questioned in the literature (Hunt, 1977; Pascoe & Attkisson, 1983; Ware, Davies-Avery, & Stewart, 1978; Willson & McNamara, 1982). Researchers of satisfaction with medical care have identified the need to address both systems and methodological issues underlying the measurement of patient satisfaction. The need for improved methods and increased reliability and validity of patient satisfaction measures is particularly acute (Lebow, 1974; Locker & Dunt, 1978; Ware et al., 1978; Willson & McNamara, 1982). Nurse researchers have called for further research to develop patient satisfaction measures related to professional nursing (Hinshaw & Atwood, 1981; Mahon, 1997; Ventura, Fox, Corley, & Mercurio, 1982). Merkouris, Ifantopoulos, Lanara, and Lemonidou (1999), in an extensive literature review on patient satisfaction with nursing, additionally identified a lack of valid and reliable instruments.

Descriptive studies in the nursing literature on patient-oriented dimensions of nurses' role performance exist in the form of two instruments that operationally use nurse provider dimensions of professional nursing for patients to evaluate. Risser (1975) developed an instrument, the Risser Patient Satisfaction Scale, for use in the ambulatory setting that used three content dimensions of patient attitude toward nurses and professional nursing: (a) technical–professional area; (b) educational relationship area; and (c) trusting relationship area. One item was modified in the adaptation of the tool for use in the acute care setting. Construct validity was not estimated.

LaMonica, Oberst, Madea, and Wolf (1986) used Risser's (1975) definition of satisfaction with care and her conceptualization of three aspects of performance in developing their satisfaction instrument. Results from repeated investigations of the Risser instrument (Hinshaw & Atwood, 1982; Risser, 1975; Ventura et al., 1982) and the LaMonica Oberst Patient Satisfaction Scale (LOPSS) (LaMonica et al., 1986; Munro,

Jacobsen, & Brooten, 1994) show no reliable differences among the subscales except for the responses of two of Hinshaw and Atwood's heterogeneous subsamples. Therefore, the likelihood of separate dimensions being measured by these two well-known nursing patient satisfaction instruments, the Risser Patient Satisfaction Scale and the LOPSS, is questionable. No other satisfaction instruments were found that indicate separate dimensions of nurses' role performance.

A search of the patient satisfaction with professional nursing literature revealed no published, tested instruments that used a nursing conceptual system to organize their construction. Risser's (1975) operational definition of patient satisfaction, which is still used, was based mainly on experiential data and not on a conceptual system or theoretical definition. It is important for operational adequacy that research instruments accurately reflect the theory in a given study (Fawcett & Downs, 1986). According to Lynn (1986), using conceptual domains is the first step in instrument development. The theory proposed here uses King's conceptual system to guide instrument development. This conceptualization may address the demand for greater understanding of patients' assessments of nursing behaviors and, eventually, improved patient satisfaction methodology.

In conclusion, it is evident from the literature that the existing measures of patient satisfaction with professional nursing do not provide an adequate basis for today's health care decisions related to the nursing-sensitive outcome of patient satisfaction.

METHODOLOGY

Theory Development Process

The development of the PSNC theory included several steps. The development of the concept of patient satisfaction with nursing care (Figure 9.1) and the theory of patient satisfaction with nursing care (Figure 9.2) were described in the previous sections.

In the next step, the patient-consumer perceptions of role performance of nurses subconcepts had to be explicated in relation to King. Roles based on King (1981) were compared with roles in Risser and LaMonica instrument dimensions and found to be congruent except for the role of "advocate," which is missing in their instruments (see Table 9.2).

Consequently, the three perceptions instruments were designed to measure patient-consumer perceptions of nurses' role performance in four subscales, thereby identifying role dimensions responsible for favorable or unfavorable patient-consumer perceptions.

Table 9.2. King's Roles and Nursing Literature Instrument Dimensions

King's roles	Nursing literature instrument dimensions
Caregiver	Technical–professional
Teacher	Educational relationship
Friend	Trusting relationship; Intrapersonal
Advocate	—

Formalization of the theory of PSNC

Relevant concepts from the middle range theory of PSNC are presented with explicit propositions about their dimensions and connections. Five of King's concepts or terms, *individuals* (characteristics), *past experiences, role performance, decision making* (responses), and *nursing situation* are influencers of the concept of patient satisfaction with nursing care in the theory of PSNC.

1. Characteristics of patient-consumers (individuals) influence patient satisfaction with nursing care.
2. Past experiences of patient-consumers influence patient satisfaction with nursing care.
3. Nurses' role performance as perceived by patient-consumers influences patient satisfaction with nursing care.
4. Decision making by patient-consumers influence their responses to nursing services and patient satisfaction with nursing care.
5. Nursing situations influence patient satisfaction with nursing care.

Assumptions

Several assumptions are made explicit for the middle range theory of PSNC.

1. Patient-consumers evaluate nurses and nursing services based not only on their rational beliefs but also on affective and behavioral perceptions and responses.
2. Role performance of nurses is the actual object of patient-consumer perceptions and responses.
3. Patient-consumers respond to professional role behaviors of professional nurses.
4. Patient-consumers can separate nurses' role performance and environmental influences of the setting.
5. Performance of roles by registered nurses is "professional nursing care" as defined by state nurse practice acts.

Summary of theory development process

Problems in the attitude literature suggest that there is no overwhelming empirical evidence for one view of the theoretical nature of patient satisfaction and a new direction in defining its meaning may be justified. Six subconcepts, rather than one hypothetical patient satisfaction construct, may more clearly specify the nature and meaning of patient satisfaction for the discipline of nursing. King's conceptual system was identified as one having utility and robustness for a conceptualization to guide patient satisfaction research. The PSNC theory generation process involved constructing the theory using ideas and concepts in reconfigurations to support explication of patient satisfaction, specifically with nursing care. Evaluation of the PSNC theory followed generation of the theory. Testing began with a content validity process to validate precise operational definitions of the subconcepts of patient satisfaction with nursing care.

Theory Testing: Content Validity Process

Item generation and refinement

Some suitable items that performed well in a psychometric sense were chosen from existing hospital and nursing satisfaction with care instruments. Using the structure of the theory of PSNC, an initial pool of 364 items was initially developed, resulting in a blueprint of the concept of PSNC. Item development packets consisting of 229 items, and directions for the pretest were sent to 13 individuals who reviewed the items and completed item development packets. The reviewers were encouraged to edit existing items and add new items and place an asterisk in front of those items they preferred. An additional 135 items were generated by the 13 participants.

The composition of reviewers included two patients based on the belief that their ideas would keep the language patient-oriented. The process of reduction of items was aided by the elimination of items marked redundant or weak by the reviewers. As a result, 221 items were prepared for review by the content validity judges. Finally, an expert in education theory in nursing was asked to verify the cognitive, affective, and behavioral classification of the items.

Judgment of content validity

The content validity of the perceptions and response instruments was evaluated using the Waltz and Bausell (1981) quantifiable technique as delineated by Lynn (1986). Three panels of experts (expert nurses, King experts, and patients) were selected as judges of the subject matter of the instruments. The content domain, patients' perceptions of nurses' roles and responses to nursing services, was separated into six definitions and four roles, each of which appeared at the top of the appropriate page in the content validity tool.

The quantification of content validity used was the Content Validity Index (CVI), which is derived from rating each item using a modification of Lynn's (1986) four-option rating scale (1 = *inconsistent*; 2 = *neutral*; 3 = *consistent*; 4 = *very consistent*). The actual CVI is the proportion of items that receive a rating of 3 or 4 by the experts (Waltz & Blausell, 1981). The proportion needed to establish content validity beyond the .05 level of significance is 1.00 for three or fewer judges (Lynn, 1986), which is the criterion for the rating of individual items in this study. For each instrument as a whole to be considered content valid, an acceptable level of interrater agreement among judges of .80 or greater is needed (Waltz, Strickland, & Lentz, 1984). To ensure that potential items had not been overlooked related to the content domain, each judge was asked to identify any area(s) that may have been omitted from the instruments. Suggestions for item improvement and for improvement of the instruments and materials were also requested from the experts.

Content validity judges

The major criterion for selection of the content domain panel of judges was expert-level involvement in delineation of professional nurses' roles in hospital settings. The profession's view of roles of registered nurses in hospitals is the content area assumed to be known by nurse administrators, leaders in the nursing profession, and researchers of nurses' roles. Two to three of each of the following were sought to ensure broad knowledge of the content domain: (a) nurse administrator, (b) leader in professional organization, and (c) nurse researcher. Based on these assumptions, a purposive panel of eight experts with diverse characteristics was selected to be content domain judges of the perceptions and response items. However, only three of the nurse experts returned fully completed materials. Likewise, five judges were selected based on their expertise in King's (1981) systems conceptual system. Three returned usable materials.

For the third panel, two "expert patients" were asked to participate, and both returned the materials. Because the instruments are based on professional roles as viewed by the profession but are intended for patients to answer, it is important to uncover if the explicated roles are relevant to patients' perceptions. The directions to the patient experts were the same as those sent to the professional role judges, that is, based on relevance to the definitions provided.

Content validity testing

Judges were furnished with a specific set of instructions for evaluation of the items based on the content validity criteria. The target population (hospital inpatient) point of view was considered by instruction to the judges that the nurses' role behaviors must be observable by patients. Directions were clear on the judges' role: delineation of the full content domain. The theoretical definitions were provided to the content domain panel, who were told to match items to concepts by judging their relevance; the King panel was asked to evaluate the theoretical relevance of the items to King's (1981) conceptual system and to answer the question, "Are the items consistent with King's conceptual system?" and the patient panel was asked to rate how much they liked or disliked each item being included in a patient satisfaction survey.

Content validity results. Ninety-three (93) of the 221 items were rated 100% content valid by the two- to three-member panels (a rating of 3 or 4). Taking the eight experts as a whole, the Lynn (1986) criteria of 88% was used to fill in items needed for a broad representation of nurses' activities within the role subscales of the perceptions instruments. Once the CVI was derived for the individual 132 pilot items (72%–100%) and no area(s) were identified that had been omitted from the instruments, the content validity process was completed for the pilot instruments. The CVI for the pilot instrument was 82% for the King expert panel and 72% for the nurse experts and patient experts panels. For the final 60-item instrument, the overall CVI was 83%. Because the derived CVI of 83% surpassed the required 80% content validity (Waltz et al., 1984), the content validity of the KPSNC was found acceptable for use with acute-care patients.

STRENGTHS AND LIMITATIONS OF THE MIDDLE RANGE THEORY OF PSNC

Evaluative Criteria for Theory Generation

Logical adequacy involves looking for contradictions or discontinuities represented among the proposed relationships. The theoretical perspective contains five levels of abstraction referring to three constructs: satisfaction, perception, and attitude. King's conceptual system does not propose positive or negative relationships among the constructs of interacting systems, so the "rule of signs" does not apply between the construct and concept levels. The propositions do not specify positive or negative relationships. There was no lack of connections between concepts and empirical indicators. The propositions connecting concepts and referents are represented at each level of abstraction. Overall, the theoretical perspective is clearly represented, highly specific and logically adequate to support a comparative descriptive, quasi-experimental, or experimental study once the measures are validated.

Empirical adequacy and empirical correspondence are demonstrated in the theory of PSNC. Viewing the substruction confirms that an operational indicator exists for every relevant concept resulting in empirical adequacy. An operational definition and indicator is present for each relevant concept in the theoretical structure. The unit of analysis in the theoretical analysis and the empirical indicators are focused on the individual except for the nursing situation concept and indicators. Despite the units of analysis being mixed, the nursing situation concept is consistent with the social system construct of King that represents the environment. At the analysis level, the patient data will be aggregated to identify if differences exist for groups of patients with various aspects of the nursing situation (environment).

The clarity of presentation, precision, parsimony, and substantive adequacy of the theory are considered in an overall assessment. Figures 9.1 and 9.2 together present the theory in a clear manner. The theoretical precision is noteworthy, giving the state of conceptualization and measurement of patient satisfaction. The precision with which the operational indicators are identified strengthens the content validity and potential construct validity of the KPSNC instrument. The theory development description presented by the author is lengthy and could be compressed in future written descriptions. The immediate clinical relevance of the theory is not fully known.

APPLICATION TO THE CLINICAL PROBLEM

The assessment of patient-consumer perceptions and responses to professional nursing using the KPSNC is proposed as an improved method of measuring the patient perspective of nursing beyond the current use of patient satisfaction surveys in hospital settings.

The author has found this theory to be robust through the use of theory-derived instruments in three studies. The dissertation work (Killeen, 1996) involved two pilot studies to refine and shorten the KPSNC instrument. These two pilots and the main instrumentation testing involved 2,800 subjects in five diverse hospital settings in the state of Michigan. In a study on comfort management of chronically and terminally ill clients, the conceptual blueprint was used to develop an adapted instrument titled Patient Satisfaction With Comfort Management (Killeen, 2002). In response to the need for a nursing focus in patient satisfaction in the ambulatory setting, an instrument modification of the KPSNC was done (Patient Satisfaction With Ambulatory Professional Nursing) in a large ambulatory setting (Killeen, Quigley, & Ashby, 2004).

Use of the KPSNC for nurse development and quality assessment tools by nursing managers is important to the nation's health care. Additional revisions and testing of the instruments may result in evaluation of professional nursing in organizations by assessing levels and types of nurses' roles using the role titles in the theory. Managers' use of the theory for continuous quality improvement, based on the degree to which each nurse role is associated with overall satisfaction, could lead to better decisions to improve the level and effectiveness of professional nursing care.

Consumer influence is visible in hospital settings in the form of "patient satisfaction surveys" found in quality assessment monitoring and internal marketing studies. Use of the KPSNC as a measure of satisfaction with nursing as either a proxy or a complement for a measure of satisfaction with hospital care appears to be indicated.

Consumer perceptions of and demands for quality in health services play a major role in organizational survival of hospitals. Beginning in 1994, the Joint Commission on Accreditation of Healthcare Organizations required all institutions to have a mechanism in place to measure patient satisfaction. Thus, the ability to define, measure, and influence patient-consumer perceptions and responses to professional nursing as an observable facet of the quality of care is critical for hospitals.

Research on the image of nursing (Kalish & Kalish, 1987) suggests that the public's expectations of nurses often fail to reflect the goal of nursing as a profession described by King (1981): "to help individuals maintain their health so they can function in their roles" (pp. 3–4). Patient satisfaction information, as provided by data from use of the KPSNC, is needed by the nursing profession to decide where to target efforts in educating the public about nurses and professional nursing practice.

FUTURE RECOMMENDATIONS

The discipline of nursing needs knowledge of measurement of patient-consumer perceptions and responses to identify the relationships of these perceptions and responses to professional nurses' behaviors. With a theoretical foundation for patient satisfaction, work on measurement can proceed. The next step is secondary analysis of data in instrumentation studies using the KPSNC and its revisions for testing of the relationships among the concepts of the theory of PSNC. If the relationships are found to be consistent, hypotheses testing in quasi- and true experimental research should follow. Some research questions might include the following:

1. Do patients who have been assigned nurses with high levels of competency (education, experience, certification, years of service) have higher levels of satisfaction than those with nurses of mid- to low levels of competency?
2. Which care delivery methods and staff mix levels are associated with high satisfaction levels with nursing care?
3. If patients have high satisfaction levels with nursing care, are they more likely to attain health goals than patients with mid- to low satisfaction levels?

Additional testing and refinement of the KPSNC has been done, and more will be done. Items identified as statistically problematic must be examined in light of their theoretical contribution to the overall instrument and relevant subscales. Cognitive testing with former patients in focus groups should be done to build on psychometric evaluation. The subscales should be revised with each testing to comprise a minimum number of items. The revised instrument should be reviewed by nursing theory experts to reexamine its content validity. Finally, further psychometric testing using a multistate sample of recently discharged hospital patients should be conducted.

The importance of the concept of patient satisfaction with professional nursing within a conceptual system should be examined along with other nursing concepts by nurse scientists and graduate-level nursing students. Introduction to the literature on patient and consumer satisfaction should be required to provide future nurse leaders with a foundation in this area of evidence-based practice.

SUMMARY

In summary, the theory of patient satisfaction with nursing care provides a conceptual foundation for development and testing of the KPSNC instrument in hospitals and other settings. The details of this theory should inspire nurse leaders to test all or parts of the theoretical relationships in their settings. All nurses need to understand the importance of nursing theory to our profession. Creative efforts to demonstrate how theory guides research studies and how the findings from the theory driven research provide answers to clinical problems need to be supported and rewarded in health care systems. In addition to adding to knowledge in the discipline of nursing about patient satisfaction with nursing care, the theory may be used to feedback knowledge dynamically to King's conceptual system and to refine the global perspective of her work on an ongoing basis as our profession moves forward in construction of its theory base.

REFERENCES

Abramowitz, S., Cote, A. A., & Berry, E. (1987). Analyzing patient satisfaction: A multianalytic approach. *Quality Review Bulletin, 13*, 122–130.

Agency for Healthcare Research and Quality. (2002, February). What is AHRQ? Retrieved December 7, 2006, from http://www.ahrq.gov/about/whatis.htm.

Agency for Health Care Policy and Research. (1990, February). *Program note: Medical treatment effectiveness research* (pp 1–10). Washington, DC: U.S. Department of Health and Human Services.

Ajzen, I. (1989). Attitude structure and behavior. In A. R. Pratkanis, S. J. Breckler, & A. G. Greenwald (Eds.), *Attitude structure and function* (pp. 241–274). Hillsdale, NJ: Erlbaum.

Alexander, M. A. (1989). Evaluation of a training program in breast cancer nursing. *The Journal of Continuing Education in Nursing, 21*, 260–266.

Allanach, E. J., & Golden, B. M. (1988). Patients' expectations and values clarification: A service audit. *Nursing Administration Quarterly, 12*, 17–22.

American Nurses Association. (1976). *Code for nurses' with interpretative statements*. Washington, DC: Author.

American Nurses Association. (1980). *Nursing: A social policy statement*. (ANA publication code: NP-63 35M). Washington, DC: Author.

American Nurses Association. (1995). *Nursing care report card for acute care*. Washington, DC: American Nurses Publishing.

American Nurses Association. (2001). *Nursing's social policy statement* (2nd ed.). Washington DC: American Nurses Publishing.

Bem, D. J. (1967a). Self-perception: An alternative interpretation of cognitive dissonance phenomena. *Psychological Review, 74*, 183–200.

Bem, D. J. (1967b). Self-perception: The dependent variable of human performance. *Organizational Behavior and Human Performance, 2*, 105–121.

Bem, D. J. (1972). Self-perception theory. In O. Berkowitz (Ed.), *Advances in experimental social psychology* (Vol. 6, pp. 2–62). New York: Academic Press.

Eagly, A. H., & Chaiken, S. (1993). *The psychology of attitudes*. Orlando, FL: Harcourt Brace Jovanovich.

Eriksen, L. R. (1995). Patient satisfaction with nursing care: Concept clarification. *Journal of Nursing Measurement, 3*, 59–76.

Fawcett, J., & Downs, F. S. (1986). *The relationship of theory and research*. Norwalk, CT: Appleton-Century-Crofts.

Fishbein, M., & Ajzen, I. (1975). *Belief, attitude, intention and behavior: An introduction to theory and research*. Reading, MA: Addison-Wesley.

Hinshaw, A. S., & Atwood, J. R. (1982). A patient satisfaction instrument: Precision by replication. *Nursing Research, 31,* 170–175, 191.

Hunt, H. K. (1977). CS/D—Overview and future research directions. In H. K. Hunt (Ed.), *Conceptualization and measurement of consumer satisfaction and dissatisfaction* (pp. 455–488). Cambridge, MA: Marketing Science.

Kalish, P. A., & Kalisch, B. J. (1987). *The changing image of the nurse.* Menlo Park, CA: Addison-Wesley.

Killeen, M. B. (1996). Patient-consumer perceptions and responses to professional nursing care: Instrument development. *Dissertation Abstracts International* (University Microfilms No. DAO 72699).

Killeen, M. B. (2002, April). *Development of comfort management as a proposed NIC and validation of three NOCs as useful clinical tools in a pilot study on comfort management of end-of-life and chronically ill patients.* Paper presented at the 2002 NNN Conference, Chicago, IL.

Killeen, M. B. (2003). Comfort management as a proposed NIC and validation of three NOCs for end-of-life and chronically ill patients [abstract]. *International Journal of Nursing Terminologies and Classifications, 14* (Suppl. 4), 19.

Killeen, M. B., Quigley, P., & Ashby, R. (2004, February). *Satisfaction with professional nursing care in the ambulatory setting.* Poster presented at the First Regional Magnet Nursing Conference, Tampa, FL.

King, I. M. (1971). *Toward a theory for nursing: General concepts of human behavior.* New York: Wiley.

King, I. M. (1981). *Toward a theory for nursing: Systems, concepts, process.* New York: Wiley.

LaMonica, E. L., Oberst, M. T., Madea, A. R., & Wolf, R. M. (1986). Development of a patient satisfaction scale. *Research in Nursing and Health, 9,* 43–50.

Lang, N. M., & Clinton, J. F. (1984). Assessment of quality of nursing care. In H. Werley & J. Fitzpatrick (Eds.), *Annual Review of Nursing Research* (Vol. 2, pp. 135–164). New York: Springer Publishing Company.

Lang, N. M., & Marek, K. D. (1992, October). Outcomes that reflect clinical practice. *Proceedings of the State of the Science conference* (NIH Publication No. 93-411). National Center for Nursing Research, September 11–13, 1991.

Lebow, J. (1974). Consumer assessments of the quality of medical care. *Medical Care, 12,* 328–327.

Locker, D., & Dunt, D. (1978). Theoretical and methodological issues in sociological studies of consumer satisfaction with medical care. *Social Science & Medicine, 12,* 283–292.

Lynn, M. R. (1986). Determination and quantification of content validity. *Nursing Research, 35,* 382–385.

McDaniel, C., & Nash, J. G. (1990). Compendium of instruments measuring patient satisfaction with nursing care. *Quality Research Bulletin, 16,* 182–188.

Mahon, P. Y. (1997). Review of measures of patient satisfaction with nursing care. *Image: Journal of Nursing Scholarship, 29,* 196.

Megivern, K., Halm, M. A., & Jones, G. (1992). Measuring patient satisfaction as an outcome of nursing care. *Journal of Nursing Care Quality, 6,* 9–24.

Merkouris, A., Ifantopoulos, J., Lanara, V., & Lemonidou, C. (1999). Patient satisfaction: A key concept for evaluating and improving nursing services. *Journal of Nursing Management,* 719–728.

Michigan Board of Nursing and Michigan Nurses Association. (1992). *Legal & professional regulation of nursing practice in Michigan.* Okemos: Michigan Nurses Association.

Miller, P., Johnson, N., Garrett, M. J., Wikoff, R., & McMahon, M. (1982). Health beliefs and adherence to the medical regimen of ischemic heart disease patients. *Heart and Lung, 11,* 332–339.

Munro, B. H., Jacobsen, B. S., & Brooten, D. A. (1994). Re-examination of the psychometric characteristics of the LaMonica–Oberst Patient Satisfaction Scale. *Research in Nursing & Health, 17,* 119–125.

National Quality Forum. (2004). *National priorities of healthcare quality measurement and reporting.* Retrieved February 15, 2005, from http://www. qualityforum.org/webprioritiespublic.pdf

Pascoe, G. C. (1983). Patient satisfaction in primary health care: A literature review and analysis. *Evaluation and Program Planning, 6,* 185–210.

Pascoe, G. C., & Attkisson, C. C. (1983). The Evaluation Ranking Scale: A new methodology for assessing satisfaction. *Evaluation and Program Planning, 6,* 335–347.

Press, I., & Ganey, R. F. (1990). What experiences contribute to satisfaction with the hospital? *Michigan Hospitals, 26,* 17–21.

Risser, N. L. (1975). Development of an instrument to measure patient satisfaction with nurses and nursing care in primary care settings. *Nursing Research, 24,* 45–52.

Soffer, A. (1978). Consumer rights in medicine. *Archives of Internal Medicine, 138,* 95.

Ventura, M. R., Fox, R. N., Corley, M. C., & Mercurio, S. M. (1982). A patient satisfaction measure as a criterion to evaluate primary nursing. *Nursing Research, 31,* 226–230.

Walker, L. O., & Avant, K. C. (1983). *Strategies for theory construction in nursing.* Norwalk, CT: Appleton-Century-Crofts.

Waltz, C. F., & Bausell, R. B. (1981). *Nursing research: Design, statistics, and computer analysis.* Philadelphia: Davis.

Waltz, C. F., Strickland, O. L., & Lenz, E.R. (1984). *Measurement in nursing research.* Philadelphia: Davis.

Ware, J. E., & Davies, A. R. (1983). Behavioral consequences of consumer dissatisfaction with medical care. *Evaluation and Program Planning, 6,* 291–297.

Ware, J. E., Davies-Avery, A., & Stewart, A. L. (1978). The meaning and measurement of patient satisfaction. *Health & Medical Care Services Review, 1,* 2–15.

Ware, J. E., & Snyder, M. K. (1975). Dimensions of patient attitudes regarding doctors and medical care services. *Medical Care, 13,* 669–682.

Ware, J. E., Snyder, M. K., Wright, R., & Davies, A. R. (1983). Defining and measuring patient satisfaction with medical care. *Evaluation and Program Planning, 6,* 247–263.

Weisman, E., & Koch, N. (1989). Special patient satisfaction issue [editorial]. *Quality Review Bulletin, 15*(6), 166–167.

Willson, P., & McNamara, J. R. (1982). How perceptions of a simulated physician–patient interaction influence intended satisfaction and compliance. *Social Science Medicine, 16,* 1699–1704.

CHAPTER TEN

Relationships Among Basic Empathy, Self-Awareness, and Learning Styles of Baccalaureate Prenursing Students Within King's Personal System

Barbara A. May

Empathy is an important concept in nursing because it is related positively to client and nurse outcomes (Holt-Ashley, 1987; Olson, 1995; Reid-Ponte, 1992). Most nursing studies of empathy have concentrated on the interaction process or the interpersonal relationship between the nurse and client. However, because perceptions of the nurse can influence the interaction process (King, 1981), it is important to study the characteristics of nurses that may influence their perceptions. A middle range nursing theory of empathy, derived from the personal system of King's conceptual system, was formulated (Alligood & May, 2000). This chapter presents a study that examined and tested that middle range theory of relationships among empathy, self-awareness, and learning styles.

STATEMENT OF THE PROBLEM

Although the importance of empathy in nurse–client interactions has been discussed extensively in the literature (Forsyth, 1979; Gould, 1990), problems in conceptualizing empathy and methodological problems have resulted in conflicting findings (Gagan, 1983; Olsen, 1991). Some researchers have even questioned the conceptual fit of empathy for nursing (Gordon, 1983; Morse et al., 1992). Additionally, in a nurse–client interaction, empathy is more than saying the appropriate words; it is also a feeling within a person that provides understanding of others. However, over the past 50 years, most nursing studies have focused only on the training and learning of empathic behaviors and skills (Clay, 1984; Cox, 1989; Henderson, 1989; Hodges, 1991; Kalisch, 1973; LaMonica, 1983; Layton, 1979; Norris, 1986; Reynolds & Presly, 1988; Young-Mason, 1991).

To address these issues, Alligood (1992) discussed the importance of recognizing two types of empathy: basic and trained. Whereas basic empathy was defined as a universal human trait, trained empathy was defined as a clinical skill state. She suggested further studies be conducted for theoretical clarification of both types. A recent study supported two types of empathy, and the researchers recommended that measurement of empathy be based on this differentiation (Evans, Wilt, Alligood, & O'Neil, 1998). Findings from a phenomenological study by Baillie (1996) also supported two types of empathy. Nurse participants in this study reported that nurses' empathy built on their natural ability to empathize. The significance of Alligood's (1992) differentiation of two types of empathy is that nursing has focused on the wrong type and must shift its emphasis from trained empathy to basic empathy. This change shifts the focus from interpersonal skill acquisition to intrapersonal development. Thus, this study was proposed to develop an understanding of the nature of the intrapersonal trait of basic empathy.

Empathy and self-awareness are viewed as integral to therapeutic relationships. However, although the concept of empathy has been discussed for many years, the concept of self-awareness is relatively new in nursing literature (Rawlinson, 1990). Nurse educators have recognized the importance of self-awareness and incorporated the concept into the curriculum, but methods of teaching self-awareness have been called into question (Burnard, 1984; Cook, 1999). Although self-awareness has been suggested as an important antecedent to understanding other people (Jay, 1995; Jerome & Ferraro-McDuffie, 1992; Smith, 1995), little is known about the concept or its relationship to other variables because few empirical studies have been conducted.

Learning styles have been studied extensively in nursing (Brazen & Roth, 1995; Cavanagh, Hogan, & Ramgopal, 1995; Daly, 1996; Duncan, 1996; L. C. Hodges, 1988; Jambunathan, 1995; Keane, 1993; Merritt, 1983; Rakoczy & Money, 1995). Most of these studies have been descriptive in nature, identifying preferences on the basis of demographics, educational level, or specialty areas, or they have focused on the relationship between a given learning style and various characteristics of the student or nurse. Cross (1976) noted that learning styles have a broad influence on many aspects of personality and behavior, such as perception, memory, problem solving, interests, and social behavior. Although theoretical linkage between empathy and learning styles has been suggested in the literature (Lange, 1979), few, if any, studies have been conducted to provide empirical support for this relationship. Some authors (McCarthy & Schmeck, 1988) have proposed that increasing self-acceptance will permit greater self-awareness and lead ultimately to a cognitive style characterized by greater versatility, flexibility, and adaptation in overall functioning, but no studies were found to support this relationship empirically.

THEORETICAL FRAMEWORK

King's conceptual system is the conceptual model from which a middle range theory of basic empathy, self-awareness, and learning styles was derived. Personal systems concepts from King's conceptual system that are meaningful to this middle range theory are perception, self, body image, and learning. Using interpretive hermeneutics, a nursing theory of empathy within King's personal system was formalized (Alligood & May, 2000). That theory proposed that empathy organizes perception, facilitates awareness of self and others, and affects learning.

Perception is a major concept in the personal system because "it is through perception that an individual comes to know self, to know other persons, and to know objects in the environment" (King, 1981, p. 19). Based on King's ideas, perception was proposed as a dimension of sensory perception and a way of knowing that organizes, interprets, and transforms information into meaningful understanding (Alligood, Evans, & Wilt, 1995; Alligood et al., 1998). Because perception is an awareness of persons and is related to the concept of self, perception includes an awareness of one's self (Alligood & May, 2000). Therefore, basic empathy and self-awareness are both related to perception.

King (1981) stated that "Knowledge of self is a key to understanding human behavior, because self is the way I define me to myself and to others" (p. 26). Furthermore, "awareness of self helps one to become a sensitive human being who is comfortable with self and with relationships with others" (p. 28). Therefore, empathy has been proposed as an affective dimension of human sensitivity as discussed by King (Alligood & May, 2000) and is related to self-awareness.

Body image was defined by King (1981) as "a person's perceptions of his own body, others' reactions to his appearance, and is a result of others' reactions to self" (p. 33). Perceptions about the self as a social entity that have an effect on others is a form of self-awareness that is called social awareness. Body image relies heavily on empathy because the reaction of others, which may be positive or negative, occurs as people see others reacting to them (Alligood et al., 1995). Therefore, empathy promotes social awareness (Alligood & May, 2000).

The concept of learning as formulated by King (1986, 1992) described learning as a self-activity requiring active participation on the part of the learner. Additionally, learning is individual and learners bring to learning situations their personal interests, needs, and past experience, and each individual has a different learning style. Perception is essential for learning and is influenced by feelings and emotions. The relationship of perception and empathy has been proposed to be fundamental concerning how nurses learn nursing (Alligood et al., 1995, 1998, 1999). Empathy is a feeling attribute that influences learning as well as affecting the organization of perceptions, which in turn affects learning (Alligood & May, 2000). If self-awareness is learning about the self by bringing thoughts, feelings, strengths, and weaknesses to a conscious level, and if self-awareness is learned rather than taught (Burnard, 1984), then self-awareness is also related to learning.

PURPOSE

This study was designed as descriptive correlational research at the factor-relating level of theory development. The specific concepts of perception, body image, self, and learning from King's conceptual system were examined. The purpose of this study was to explore the relationships among basic empathy, self-awareness, and learning styles of prenursing baccalaureate student nurses and to test the middle range theory derived from the nursing theory of empathy within King's conceptual system.

RESEARCH QUESTIONS AND HYPOTHESIS

On the basis of the middle range theory of personal system empathy (Alligood & May, 2000), the following research question was asked: What is the nature of the relationships among basic empathy, self-awareness, and learning styles of baccalaureate prenursing students? In addition, a secondary research question was asked: What is the nature of the relationships among basic empathy, self-awareness, learning styles, and psychosocial personal characteristics related to the concept of growth and development, which includes (a) age; (b) birth order; (c) highest educational level achieved; (d) previous training in communication skills, human relationships skills, or counseling skills; (e) previous education in communication skills, human relationships skills, or counseling skills; and (f) both previous training and education in communication skills, human relationships skills, or counseling skills of baccalaureate prenursing students? The study hypothesis was that there are relationships among basic empathy, self-awareness, and learning styles of baccalaureate prenursing students.

METHOD

The study was conducted with freshman, sophomore, and junior undergraduate students with a declared nursing major enrolled at public institutions in southeastern states. To be eligible for the study, students had to meet the following criteria: (1) be enrolled as an undergraduate prenursing student, (2) have just begun their didactic or clinical courses in nursing, (3) not be a registered nurse, and (4) be 18 years of age or older and willing to complete the research instruments. The sample was a nonprobability convenience sample of full-time or part-time baccalaureate prenursing students. There were two dependent variables and 12 independent variables. A sample size of 20 subjects per variable was determined necessary for the analysis (Stevens, 1996). Thus, a minimum sample size of 280 was required.

A total number of 424 students from eight sites chose to participate. One-way analysis of variance was used to ensure that there were no significant differences for participants on the basis of site.

The sample size was adjusted to a total of 380 after data from participants who were associate or diploma nurses were removed. Data were also removed from participants if more than 15% of the data were missing for one variable or for scores that were determined to be outliers. With a sample size of 380, a small effect size can be detected in the population with a power of .95 at the .05 level of significance (Kraemer & Theimann, 1987).

Measurement Instruments

The Hogan Empathy Scale (HES; Hogan, 1969) and the Emotional Empathic Tendency Scale (EETS; Mehrabian & Epstein, 1972) were used to measure basic empathy in this study. The HES was selected because it was designed to assess trait empathy by the degree to which individuals perceived the inner experience of others. Because the HES is a dichotomous instrument, the index of reliability was determined to be .69, which is satisfactory and similar to what other researchers have found (Bussa, 1993; Forsyth, 1979; Koch, 1991). The EETS was selected because it was developed specifically to measure the emotional response to the perceived emotional experiences of others. A Cronbach's alpha of .79 was computed for the EETS in this study. This reliability coefficient was similar to that found by Koch (1991), which indicated that the EETS had good reliability for this sample.

The revised Private and Public Self-Consciousness subscales (Scheier & Carver, 1985) were used to assess self-awareness in this study. They were designed to measure an individual's beliefs, aspirations, values and feelings, and qualities of the self from which impressions are formed in other people's eyes. In this study, Cronbach's alphas of .67 and .81 were computed for the Private and Public Self-Consciousness subscales.

Learning styles were measured by the Learning Styles Questionnaire (LSQ; Honey & Mumford, 1992). The LSQ was selected for this study because it focused on observable behavior rather than the psychological basis for that behavior and was developed from an experiential learning theory. This is in agreement with King (1986), who, in her definition of learning, stated that learning can be evaluated in observable behaviors and inferred from behavioral manifestations. Additionally, the experiential learning theory and King's conceptual system emphasize the holistic view of man and the importance of the individual (Joyce-Nagata, 1996). Furthermore, both experiential learning and a systems approach view learning as a dynamic and lifelong process with active involvement (Honey & Mumford, 1992; King, 1986).

Based on the experiential learning cycle, learners are classified into four learning styles: activists, reflectors, theorists, and pragmatists. Activists are characterized as being open-minded to new ideas and ventures. On the other hand, reflectors are seen as careful and cautious in their approach to new ideas; whereas theorists adopt a rational and logical approach to problems or new situations, pragmatists tend to be practical and realistic in their thinking and are less interested in theory or basic principles. Therefore, activists tend to have lots of experience, reflectors do lots of reviewing, theorists reach conclusions, and pragmatists make plans. For some individuals, no strongly preferred style emerges, and these individuals are called *all rounders* because they adopt a variety of styles (Honey & Mumford, 1992). Again, because this is a dichotomous scale, an index of reliability was computed for the four subscale learning styles: activist, .85; reflector, .84; theorists, .78; and pragmatist, .75.

Procedure

Before implementation of the study, permission was obtained from the institutional review board of the researcher's affiliating university. The deans or associate deans of the selected schools of nursing were contacted to obtain permission to use their school as a site for the study. A date and time was arranged with faculty members at each site to meet with the nursing students to explain the study and administer the research instruments. The instruments were administered during a class or orientation session. To ensure confidentiality, no names were attached to any data. Each participant received a packet in a manila envelope containing four numerically coded instruments, a numerically coded personal information questionnaire, two pencils, and a written general explanation of the study. It took approximately 15 to 30 minutes for participants to complete the instruments. To maintain confidentiality, students were asked to return the completed instruments in the manila envelope.

Data Analysis

Descriptive statistics, frequencies, and measures of central tendency were computed on the study variables. Canonical correlation was used to address the research questions and to test the research hypothesis. Canonical correlation is used when there is more than one independent variable and more than one dependent variable because it gives a better understanding of all the relationships (Munro, 1997). Reliability of the study instruments was determined with Cronbach's alpha coefficients and the index of reliability.

Study Results

Descriptive statistics were computed to describe the sample characteristics and demographic variables. Although students from eight sites from two southeastern states participated, more than half of the sample (57%) was from three sites. Ages of participants ranged from 18 to 50 with more than half of the sample (63.1%) between the ages 18 and 22 years ($M = 23.6$ years). As expected, the sample was predominantly female, Caucasian, single, childless, and had an annual family income of less than $60,000. Although 282 participants in the study had only a high school education, 97 participants had a college degree. The majority of the sample was firstborn or lastborn children. Furthermore, the majority of the sample reported previous education or previous training in communication skills, human relationships skills, or counseling skills. Only 72 participants had no education or training in these skills.

Table 10.1. Canonical Correlational Analysis Among Basic
Empathy Variables (Set 1) and Self-Awareness, Learning
Styles, and Psychosocial Factors (Set 2)

	Canonical Variate	
Variable Sets	1	2
Set 1		
Basic Empathy		
HES	.477*	.879*
EETS	.928*	−.371*
Set 2		
Private self-awareness	.517*	.127
Public self-awareness	.413*	−.387*
Learning styles		
Activist	.092	.671*
Reflector	−.128	−.724*
Theorist	−.474*	−.345*
Pragmatist	−.719*	.038
All rounder[a]	−.013	.121
Psychosocial factors		
Age	−.168	.100
Birth order[b]	.075	.075
Educational level[c]	−.101	.179
Previous education[d]	.089	.117
Previous training[d]	−.078	.170
Canonical correlation	.444	.368
Variance explained	19.7%	13.6%

Note. *structure coefficients > .30.
[a] 1 = yes, 0 = no.
[b] 1 = first born and only child; 0 = middle child and last born.
[c] 1 = high school or GED; 0 = college degree.
[d] 1 = yes; 0 = no.

A canonical correlation was computed to analyze the relationships
between a set of scores of basic empathy and a set of scores of self-
awareness, learning styles, and psychosocial factors. The overall relationships among basic empathy, self-awareness, and learning styles was significant beyond the .001 alpha level using Bartlett's test of Wilk's lambda.
The canonical correlation analysis is reported on Table 10.1.

Because there cannot be more canonical correlation coefficients than
there are variables in the smaller set (the two dependent measures of
basic empathy), two canonical correlation coefficients were produced.
Correlation coefficients greater than .30 are meaningful (Munro, 1997).
Therefore, the first canonical variate indicated that students who reported
higher levels of self-awareness (both private and public) and who were
less theoretical and pragmatic in their learning styles had higher levels

of basic empathy. The second canonical variate indicated that students, who reported lower levels of public self-awareness were more activist and less theoretical and reflective in their learning styles, and had higher levels of basic empathy as measured by the HES. The selected psychosocial personal characteristics were not significantly related to basic empathy, self-awareness, and learning styles. The hypothesis was supported: There were significant relationships among basic empathy, self-awareness, and learning styles of baccalaureate prenursing students.

DISCUSSION

The advancement of nursing science is dependent on the extension and testing of nursing theories. In this regard, a middle range theory of basic empathy, self-awareness, and learning styles, derived from a nursing theory of personal system empathy conceptualized within King's conceptual system, was proposed and was tested. According to King (1981), concepts in the personal system are related because individuals react holistically to their experiences. This study provides additional support for the relationships among personal system concepts of perception, self, body image, and learning. Also, King observed that knowledge about the concepts of the personal system helps one to understand individuals. The findings of this study add to the knowledge about personal systems and thus, greater knowledge about student nurses. Furthermore, King stated that individuals' perceptions of self and body image are reflected in their personal behavior. Thus, student nurses will be better able to facilitate empathic therapeutic relationships with their clients when they are aware of and use their own intrapersonal empathy and self-awareness. Knowledge gained from the findings about relationships among basic empathy, self-awareness, and learning styles can assist nurse educators to recognize and value basic empathic responses of student nurses.

Whereas most previous studies have focused on the interpersonal system to explore the concept of empathy, little research has been devoted to the personal system. Thus, this study represented a beginning exploration of the concept of basic empathy within the intrapersonal system. Findings from the study provide initial support for the nursing theory of personal system empathy, which was derived from King's (1981) conceptual system. Results of the present study suggest that basic empathy is related to self-awareness and learning as proposed by the nursing theory of personal system empathy. Basic empathy was related to self-awareness (private or self, and public, or body image) and related to all four learning styles (activist, reflector, theorist, and pragmatist).

The findings of this study revealed that diversity exists in basic empathy levels of baccalaureate prenursing students. As a group, basic empathy levels were in the moderate range. Similar findings have been reported by other researchers (Anderson, 1990; Brunt, 1985; Forsyth, 1979; Gold & Rogers, 1995; Mehrabian & Epstein, 1972). Although both private and public self-awareness levels were higher than levels reported by other researchers (Carmon, 1992; Scheier & Carver, 1985), the levels in this sample reflected diversity as well. Therefore, nursing students do come into the education setting with different levels of basic empathy and self-awareness that nurse educators must take into consideration.

Nurse educators must also take learning styles into consideration. As a group, the highest mean score for the four learning styles was the reflector learning style and the lowest mean score was the activist learning style. This is similar to findings of other researchers (Cavanagh et al., 1995; Dux, 1989; Honey & Mumford, 1992).

Conclusions

The implications of this study for nursing education need to be considered. The findings provide initial support for significant relationships among basic empathy, self-awareness, and learning styles of baccalaureate prenursing students. Consequently, there is a need for more emphasis in the curriculum on students' personal development of basic empathy through facilitation of self-awareness. Developing a greater sense of awareness of who one is as a person and as a health professional, which includes feelings, thoughts, needs, and behavior, is important in gaining a clear understanding of how individual behaviors affect nurse–client relationships.

The proposal that there is a need to shift the focus of educational efforts to facilitation of intrapersonal empathy is further supported by this study. New methods must be considered to enhance and facilitate the use of students' natural empathic responses. Often psychomotor skills are emphasized more than affective skills in nursing education. Facilitating basic empathy leads to a greater commitment by nursing programs to strengthen the affective aspects in students' learning. To be an empathic health provider, development of affective skills that foster the therapeutic use of *self* is imperative. King (1981) observed that individuals are open systems interacting with the environment whose perceptions influence their interactions and their health. The significant relationships among basic empathy, self-awareness, and learning styles within a nursing framework have implications for the development of nurses, nursing research, and nursing education.

REFERENCES

Alligood, M. R. (1992). Empathy: The importance of recognizing two types. *Journal of Psychosocial Nursing, 30*(3), 14–17.

Alligood, M. R., Evans, G. W., & Wilt, D. L. (1995). King's interacting systems and empathy. In M. A. Frey & C. L. Sieloff (Eds.), *Advancing King's systems framework and theory of nursing* (pp. 66–78). Thousand Oaks, CA: Sage.

Alligood, M. R., Evans, G. W., Wilt, D. L., Seavor, C., May, B., & Witucki, J. (1998, February). *Conceptualization of nursing empathy using hermeneutics.* Paper presented at the Southern Nursing Research Society, Fort Worth, TX.

Alligood, M. R., Evans, G. W., Wilt, D. L., Seavor, C., May, B., & Witucki, J. (1999). Conceptualization of nursing empathy using hermeneutics. *King International Nursing Group: King's Systems Update, 2*(1), 1.

Alligood, M. R., & May, B. A. (2000). A nursing theory of personal system empathy: Interpreting a conceptualization of empathy in King's interacting systems. *Nursing Science Quarterly, 13*, 243–247.

Anderson, M. L. (1990). *The influence of psychiatric nursing professionals on empathy of psychiatric nursing students.* Unpublished doctoral dissertation, Texas A&M University, College Station.

Baillie, L. (1996). A phenomenological study of the nature of empathy. *Journal of Advanced Nursing, 24*, 1300–1308.

Brazen, L., & Roth, R. A. (1995). Using learning style preferences for perioperative clinical education. *AORN Journal, 61*, 189–195.

Brunt, J. H. (1985). An exploration of the relationship between empathy and technology. *Nursing Administration Quarterly, 9*(4), 69–78.

Burnard, P. (1984). Developing self-awareness. *Nursing Mirror, 158*(21), 30–31.

Bussa, G. (1993). Influence of development and demographics on empathy in traditional and non-traditional nursing students. (Doctoral dissertation, University of Southern Mississippi, 1993). *Dissertation Abstracts International 54-05A*, 1634.

Carmon, B. W. (1992). Relationship between self-awareness, social anxiety, and perceptual empathy in undergraduate nursing students. (Master's thesis, University of Alaska, Anchorage, 1992). *Masters Abstracts International, 32-03*, 936.

Cavanagh, S. J., Hogan, K., & Ramgopal, T. (1995). The assessment of student nurse learning styles using the Kolb Learning Styles Inventory. *Nurse Education Today, 15*, 177–183.

Clay, M. (1984). Development of an empathic interaction skills schedule in a nursing context. *Journal of Advanced Nursing, 9*, 343–350.

Cook, S. H. (1999). The self in self-awareness. *Journal of Advanced Nursing, 29*, 1292–1299.

Cox, H. (1989). Drama in the arts lab: Building empathy skills. *Australian Nurses Journal, 19*, 14–15.

Cross, K. P. (1976). *Accent on learning.* San Francisco: Jossey-Bass.

Daly, R. C. (1996). Nurse manager learning styles in a learning environment. *Seminars for Nurse Managers, 4*, 107–121.

Duncan, G. (1996). An investigation of learning styles of practical and baccalaureate nursing students. *Journal of Nursing Education, 35*, 40–42.

Dux, C. (1989). An investigation into whether nurse teachers take into account the individual learning styles of their students when formulating teaching strategies. *Nurse Education Today, 9*, 186–191.

Evans, G. W., Wilt, D. L., Alligood, M. R., & O'Neil, M. (1998). Empathy: A study of two types. *Issues in Mental Health Nursing, 19*, 1–9.

Forsyth, G. L. (1979). Exploration of empathy in nurse–client interaction. *Advances in Nursing Science, 2*, 33–42.

Gagan, J. M. (1983). Methodological notes on empathy. *Advances in Nursing Science, 5*, 65–72.

Gold, J. M., & Rogers, J. D. (1995). Intimacy and isolation: A validation study of Erikson's theory. *Journal of Humanistic Psychology, 35*, 78–86.

Gordon, M. (1983). A philosophical analysis of caring in nursing. *Journal of Advanced Nursing, 8*, 289–295.

Gould, D. (1990). Empathy: A review of the literature with suggestions for an alternative research strategy. *Journal of Advanced Nursing, 15*, 1167–1174.

Henderson, M. C. (1989). A comparison of two approaches to empathy training. *Nurse Educator, 14*, 23–36.

Hodges, L. C. (1988). Students entering professional nursing: Learning styles, personality type and sex-role identification. *Nurse Education Today, 8*, 68–76.

Hodges, S. A. (1991). An experiment in the development of empathy in student nurses. *Journal of Advanced Nursing, 16*, 1296–1300.

Hogan, R. (1969). Development of an empathy scale. *Journal of Counseling and Clinical Psychology, 33*, 307–316.

Holt-Ashley, M. (1987). Relationships of empathy training to empathic level of nurses and patient satisfaction with nursing care. (Doctoral dissertation, Texas Women's University, 1987). *Dissertation Abstracts International, 47–02B*, 569.

Honey, P., & Mumford, A. (1992). *The manual of learning styles* (3rd ed.). Maidenhead, England: Honey.

Jambunathan, J. (1995). Using Kolb's LSI to study learning styles of junior baccalaureate nursing students. *Nurse Educator, 20*, 7.

Jay, T. (1995). The use of reflection to enhance practice. *Professional Nurse, 10*, 593–595.

Jerome, A. M., & Ferraro-McDuffie, A. R. (1992). Nurse self-awareness in therapeutic relationships. *Pediatric Nursing, 18*, 153–156.

Joyce-Nagata, B. (1996). Students' academic performance in nursing as a function of student and faculty learning style congruency. *Journal of Nursing Education, 35*, 69–73.

Kalisch, B. J. (1973). What is empathy? *American Journal of Nursing, 73*, 1548–1552.

Keane, M. (1993). Preferred learning styles and study strategies in a linguistically diverse baccalaureate nursing student population. *Journal of Nursing Education, 32*, 214–221.

King, I. M. (1981). *A theory for nursing: Systems, concepts, process.* Albany, NY: Delmar.

King, I. M. (1986). *Curriculum and instruction in nursing.* Norwalk, CT: Appleton-Century-Crofts.

King, I. M. (1992). King's theory of goal attainment. *Nursing Science Quarterly, 5*, 19–26.

Koch, M. M. (1991). Assessment of medical student empathy and their correlates. (Doctoral dissertation, University of Southern California, 1991). *Dissertation Abstracts International, 52–1119,* 3827.

Kraemer, H. C., & Theimann, S. (1987). *How many subjects: Statistical power analysis in research.* Newbury Park, CA: Sage.

LaMonica, E. L. (1983). Empathy can be learned. *Nurse Educator, 8,* 19–23.

Lange, C. M. (1979). *Identification of learning styles.* New York: National League for Nursing.

Layton, J. M. (1979). The use of modeling to teach empathy to nursing students. *Research in Nursing and Health, 2,* 163–176.

McCarthy, P., & Schmeck, R. R. (1988). Students' self-concepts and the quality of learning in public schools and universities. In R. R. Schmeck (Ed.), *Learning strategies and learning styles* (pp. 131–156). New York: Plenum Press.

Mehrabian, A., & Epstein, N. (1972). A measure of emotional empathy. *Journal of Personality, 40,* 525–543.

Merritt, S. L. (1983). Learning style preferences of baccalaureate nursing students. *Nursing Research, 32,* 367–372.

Morse, J. M., Anderson, G., Bottorff, J. L., Yonge, O., O'Brien, B., Solberg, S. M., et al. (1992). Exploring empathy: A conceptual fit for nursing practice? *Image: Journal of Nursing Scholarship, 24,* 273–280.

Munro, B. H. (1997). *Statistical methods for heath care research* (3rd ed.). Philadelphia: Lippincott.

Norris, J. (1986). Teaching communication skills: Effects of two methods of instruction and selected learner characteristics. *Journal of Nursing Education, 25,* 102–106.

Olsen, D. P. (1991). Empathy as an ethical and philosophical basis for nursing. *Advances in Nursing Science, 14,* 62–75.

Olson, J. K. (1995). Relationships between nurse-expressed empathy, patient-perceived empathy and patient distress. *Image: Journal of Nursing Scholarship, 27,* 317–322.

Rakoczy, M., & Money, S. (1995). Learning styles of nursing students: A 3-year cohort longitudinal study. *Journal of Professional Nursing, 11,* 170–174.

Rawlinson, J. W. (1990). Self-awareness: Conceptual influences, contributions to nursing, and approaches to attainment. *Nurse Education Today, 10,* 111–117.

Reid-Ponte, P. (1992). Distress in cancer patients and primary nurses' empathy skills. *Cancer Nursing, 15,* 283–292.

Reynolds, W. J., & Presly, A. S. (1988). A study of empathy in student nurses. *Nurse Education Today, 8,* 123–130.

Scheier, M. F., & Carver, C. S. (1985). The Self-Consciousness Scale: A revised version for use with general populations. *Journal of Applied Social Psychology, 15,* 687–699.

Smith, C. (1995). Learning about yourself helps patient care: Using self-awareness to improve practice. *Professional Nurse, 10,* 390–392.

Stevens, J. (1996). *Applied multivariate statistics for the social sciences.* (3rd ed.). Mahwah, NJ: Erlbaum.

Young-Mason, J. (1991). The secret sharer as a guide to compassion. *Nursing Outlook, 39,* 62–63.

CHAPTER ELEVEN

A Theory of Health Perception

Understanding the Menopause Transition

Nancy C. Sharts-Hopko

Women's experience of menopause is increasingly a compelling concern as the baby boom generation transits this life stage. It has been most interesting and enlightening to revisit the issues around menopause a quarter of a century after this author's original research was conducted, to reflect on what factors have changed and what have remained the same. From the 1960s to the early 2000s, debate raged between the obstetrical and gynecological community and social scientists about whether the menopause transition should be construed as a deficiency disease in need of pharmaceutical intervention or as a social construct learned by women that influences their self-perceptions as they age.

Much of the menopause literature from that time until recently, including studies of American women as well as those of other nationalities (Bravata, Rastegar, & Horwitz, 2002; Brody, Farmer, & White, 1984; Ekstrom, Esseveld, & Hovelius, 2003; Lam, Leung, Haines, & Chung, 2003; Salkovskis, Wroe, & Rees, 2004; Wilson, 1968), has focused on efforts to convince midlife women to adhere to hormone replacement therapy (HRT) regimens, which purportedly offered a wide array of benefits. A major shift occurred since mid-2002 with growing evidence that hormone replacement therapies are, themselves, associated with life-threatening adverse effects and that their capacity to protect women from various illnesses associated with aging such as cardiovascular disease, stroke, osteoporosis, and Alzheimer's disease is limited to nonexistent (Diamanti-Kandarakis, 2004; McGinley, 2004). In its wake, more holistic approaches to menopause are emerging from within the biomedical community.

At the time this study was conceived, King's conceptual system (1981) provided a way of understanding women's health as a subjective experience of inner and interpersonal processes within a social context having to do with one's ability to fulfill one's roles. Health, for King (1981, 1990), is the way individuals deal with the stresses of growth and development while functioning within their cultural context; it represents a cultural value.

The last 4 decades have brought U.S. women a dramatic rescripting of gender roles, thus altering the social context in which women experience menopause at the same time as medical perspectives on appropriate management of menopause have shifted. This chapter explores whether the theory, first developed and tested in the early 1980s for the purpose of understanding women's experience of the menopause transition, has been consistent with more recent empirical evidence.

THEORY DEVELOPMENT APPROACH

Walker and Avant (1995) described a process for theory synthesis that entails these general steps: (a) identification of one focal concept or variable, or a framework of several focal concepts; (b) a careful and thorough review of literature examining relationships of variables related to the focal concept or among the focal concepts; and (c) organization of relational statements about the one or more focal concepts and examination of the relational statements for patterns.

In the case of this investigation, an exhaustive review of literature focused on women's experience of menopause. In the late 1970s and early 1980s, it was still possible to obtain and review nearly everything that had been published in English related to women's menopause experience. The main bodies of literature about the menopause experience were found in (a) medicine, (b) anthropology, (c) the social sciences, (d) the psychoanalytic literature, and (e) women's studies. Up to that point, the discipline of nursing had generally ignored menstruation and menopause research, and it was this curious gap that aroused the investigator's interest in this phenomenon.

Factors that were repeatedly found to bear on women's experience of menopause in the review of literature are depicted in Figure 11.1. Based on consideration of the direction of a factor's relationship with menopause

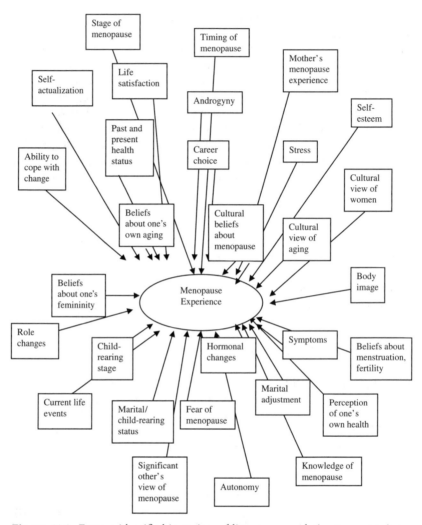

Figure 11.1. Factors identified in review of literature as relating to women's experience of menopause.

experience as well as similarities of types of factor, these factors appeared to cluster into five categories, depicted in Figure 11.2: (a) the occurrence and stage of menopause; (b) life stress; (c) sex-role typing; (d) perception of one's own health, and (e) menopause experience, including symptoms as well as attitudes toward menopause. Content validation for this clustering of factors was provided by fellow doctoral students and faculty members during the development of the research proposal.

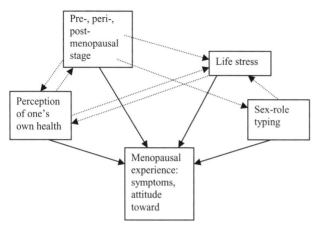

Figure 11.2. Theoretical framework for a study of women's perceived health status during the menopause transition.

DESCRIPTION OF THE MIDDLE RANGE THEORY

The original literature review led to the formulation of proposed relationships among menopausal stage, current life change, attitude toward women's roles and perceived health status among women aged 40 to 55 with age statistically controlled. King's conceptual system provided the investigator direction in identifying essential concepts from the review of literature that would be useful in understanding women's experience of menopause, and it provided a clear articulation of the assumptions held by the investigator about the nature of these variables and their interrelationships.

It was hypothesized that (a) the later the menopausal stage, the more positive the perceived health status of women aged 40 to 55, as what was an unknown, anticipated experience becomes known; (b) current life change, which represents an energetic challenge, and stress, is negatively correlated with perceived health status in women aged 40 to 55; and (c) nontraditional attitude toward women's roles is positively correlated with perceived health status in women aged 40 to 55, because less traditional women are less completely invested in their childbearing and childrearing capacity.

Relationships to perceived health status of additional factors suggested by the literature, including childbearing history, menopausal symptoms, use of hormone replacement therapy, perception of mother's menopause experience, perception of partner's attitude toward menopause, economic level, educational level, perceived timing of menopause as "on-time" or "off-time" were examined (Neugarten, 1979). Together, these variables account for physical processes as well as the social and cultural context in which women experience the menopause transition, consistent with King's conceptual system (2001).

Assumptions included that women do not become ill as they approach age 49, the average age of menopause; that the transitional experience called menopause, experienced by all women in middle age, like pregnancy, is not a condition of ill health or disease; and that middle age is not "old age" or the beginning of decline.

THEORY LINKAGE TO KING'S WORK

In King's (1981, 2001) conceptual system, individuals are viewed as open systems existing within a cultural context. Although the study was not intended to provide support for King's conceptual system, concepts within the conceptual system that were of particular relevance to this research include perception, self, growth and development, time, health, role, and stress. King's understanding (1981, 1990, 2001) of the relevance of the concepts of perception and role, the nature of self, people's growth and development as they move through time, and stress to health provided the theoretical basis, corroborated by the review of literature, for the specific relationships posited among the study variables.

Individuals, or personal systems, are ever diversifying, unified, and in continual interaction with their internal and external environments, including specifically their culture. Individuals have perspectival perception of their own unique realities. Self is a dynamic internal construct reflecting one's experience with others and the environment. Personal systems experience growth and development, a unidirectional flow of events through the life process subject to influences by genetics, experience, and the environment. Time is the way individuals experience and perceive the succession of events in their lives. Menopause is a developmental transition that occurs over time in stages. Health, for King, is the way individuals respond to the stresses of growth and development within their cultural context; it represents a cultural value. Personal systems play out sets of learned behaviors, or roles, in interaction with others; these roles are dynamic and reciprocal. Individuals are characterized by varying degrees of stress, or energy exchange between the personal system and internal and external environments, which is experienced as a dynamic, personal, and subjective state.

Menopause is one developmental event, occurring over time in middle adulthood among women. The experience of menopause may demand that the woman reformulate her view of herself. Self-evaluation occurs against a backdrop of learned or perceived social standards. Role is a situational set of behaviors that are learned. Perception of self throughout a health transition such as menopause is viewed by King (1981) as being influenced by role and role expectations of others. Women experience menopause within a cultural and interpersonal context. It is likely that concurrent upheaval in women's lives will be negatively related to how they experience menopause. Within the King model, stress is viewed as an energy response of an individual to elements in the environment that has the capacity to alert perception of reality. Additionally, as the anthropological and social science literature has suggested, women's experience of menopause may be heavily influenced by the extent to which they are invested in the childbearing and childrearing role (Flint, 1975; Wright, 1981).

Tallying of menopausal symptoms has consistently been an unsatisfactory measure of women's experience of menopause (Banger, 2002; Bloch, 2002; Hardy & Kuh, 2002; Reynolds, 2002). What is more important to how women perceive themselves and their menopause experience is women's perception of their health during the menopause transition. Symptoms will be perceived and experienced as ill health to the extent that they disrupt one's fulfillment of one's role, self-perception, and experience of the perceptions of others. The meaning women attribute to such experiences influences their view of their own health, their help-seeking behavior, and probably other aspects of their evaluation of self and of feminine identity. Meaning may be learned from the culture in general, and significant interpersonal relationships such as those with their mothers or spouses.

SELECTIVE LITERATURE REVIEW

A comprehensive review of the medical, psychoanalytic, anthropological, social science, and women's studies literature provided the basis for this research. At the time this study was undertaken in the late 1970s, the medical and also the psychoanalytic literature, in professional as well as popular publications, reflected an overriding assumption that menopause is a deficiency disease or a series of losses requiring intervention and the compelling issue was how to foster women's compliance with hormone replacement therapy (Campbell & Whitehead, 1977; Leppert, 1981). Generally speaking, the medical literature did not directly bear on the research at hand but did reflect an important contextual factor for midlife women—one clear voice in society about the meaning and nature of menopause.

It was also apparent that anthropological and cross-cultural studies within the social sciences tended to describe positive or neutral experiences of menopause (Flint, 1975; Kaufert, 1980; Skultans, 1970; Wright, 1981), whereas studies of U.S. women, particularly White women, were more likely to document negative expectations about aging in general, aging in women, and menopause in particular—an observation that carries through to the present time (Avis et al., 2001; Bart, 1972; Chim et al., 2002; Meyer, 2001; Sampselle, Harris, Harlow, & Sowers, 2002; Wilbush, 1981). The women's studies literature was beginning to articulate the relationship between societal expectations of women and their own experiences (Bart, 1972; Dreyer, Woods, & James, 1981).

METHODOLOGY

Participants

It was determined that for the design proposed, 248 subjects were required (Cohen, 1977, pp. 413–444). After institutional review board approval of the study, 249 women aged 40 to 55 were recruited from community groups using nonprobabilistic strategies. Exclusion factors included history of mastectomy, hysterectomy, oophorectomy or medical menopause, prior mental illness, current chronic illness or disability, failure to complete eighth grade, and being foreign-born. The sample was intended to include well American women experiencing a natural menopause transition.

Instruments

Eighty-three women represented each menopausal stage, by self-report of menstrual characteristics. In addition, they were asked to rate where they were in terms of premenopause, perimenopause or postmenopause. Premenopause was defined as the time before midlife change in the quality or frequency of menstruation. Perimenopause was the time from onset of menstrual change until 12 months after the last menstrual period. Postmenopause was operationally defined as the time after menses has ceased for 12 months (Brown, Mishra, & Dobson, 2002). Menopausal stage is related to King's concepts of growth and development and of time. Growth and development is explained holistically as a physical and social phenomenon (King, 1981, p. 30). The unidimensional nature of time is evidenced by processes of growth and development (p. 43). Participants completed four instruments and a personal data form that included items related to their health history and menopause experience as well as items designed to provide gross validation of the instruments.

Perceived Health Status (PHS) was an investigator-created instrument that combined three existing tools targeting physical, emotional, and social dimensions of well-being: the Health Perceptions Questionnaire (HPQ; Ware, 1976); the Affect Balance Scale (ABS; Bradburn, 1969); and the Life Satisfaction Index (LSI; Campbell, Converse, & Rodgers, 1976). The PHS reflects King's concepts of health and perception. King viewed health as dynamic, requiring continuous adjustment to internal and external stressors (King, 1981, p. 5). Perception is a process of human transaction with the environment that gives meaning to one's experiences and influences one's behavior (p. 24). Because of the importance of interpersonal interactions in the experience of health in King's conceptual system and because of her understanding of health as one's perception of one's ability to fulfill social roles, a multidimensional instrument was used to assess perceived health status.

The HPQ (Ware, 1976), which focuses on physical health, includes 32 items each scored from 1 (*poor health*) to 5 (*good health*) for a total range of 32 to 160. An example of an item is, "Most people get sick a little easier than I do." One-year test–retest reliability has been reported to be .88 ($N = 1200$). The HPQ correlates significantly with subsequent use of outpatient services as well as other indicators of health.

The ABS (Bradburn, 1969) assesses psychological well-being using two dimensions, positive affect and negative affect, each with five items scored *yes* or *no*. One of the positive items is, "During the past few weeks did you ever feel particularly excited or interested in something?" One of the negative items is, "During the past few weeks did you ever feel so restless that you couldn't sit for long in a chair?" Each positive item is rated $+1$ if the response is "yes," and each negative item is rated -1 if the response is "yes." The total score ranges from -5 to $+5$. Three-month test–retest reliability was found to be .76 ($N = 200$) by the developer of the instrument, and correlations from .61 to .90 have been demonstrated with other morale measures.

The LSI, a measure of satisfaction with social linkages, included seven items each rated from 1 (*least satisfying*) to 5 (*most satisfying*) for a total range of 7 to 35. Campbell and associates (1976) reported a test–retest reliability greater than .70, item-total correlations of at least .70, and a correlation of the global satisfaction item with the total LSI score of .57. One example of an item on this instrument is, "On the whole, how satisfied are you with the work you do?"

The Menopause Symptom Checklist (MSC; Neugarten & Kraines, 1965) was used precisely because of its questionable validity. That is, it had been widely used in studies of women's menopause experience, yet its originators had never reported demonstrations of validity. Although the tool included symptoms popularly attributed to menopause, Neugarten and Kraines demonstrated that the only symptom significantly more common among menopausal women than women of other age groups was hot flashes. The aim in including this measure was to determine the extent to which menopause symptoms were important to women's health perceptions as they progressed through the menopause transition, thus challenging the prevalent assumptions found in the medical and psychoanalytic literature at the time.

The MSC (Neugarten & Kraines, 1965) includes 28 items popularly attributed to menopause, each rated *not in the last 12 months, a few times in the last 12 months*, or *frequently in the last 12 months*. In addition, the respondent is asked to go back and check those symptoms that have caused worry. Symptoms are scored 1 point if they have not occurred, 2 points if they have occurred a few times, and 3 points if they have occurred frequently, and an additional point is added if they have caused worry. Scores range from 28 to 112. Sample symptoms include "pounding of the heart," "can't concentrate," and "hot flashes." The authors of the instrument have never published reliability data, although in this study an alpha coefficient of .83 was demonstrated. This variable relates to King's concepts of health and perception, in that the experience of symptoms contributes to the meaning that women ascribe to menopause and thus their self-evaluation of their health during that transition, as well as their appraisal of their status as normal or not (King, 1981, pp. 5, 24).

The Life Experiences Survey (LES; Sarason, Johnson, & Siegel, 1978) was a modification of the Schedule of Recent Events (SRE; Holmes & Rahe, 1967). Rather than preassigning a stress impact score for each current life event, as on the SRE, the LES allowed participants to add novel stressors and also to score each stressor's impact for themselves. This instrument reflects King's conceptualizations about perception and stress. Stress, viewed by King as individual, personal, and subjective, is a dynamic state of human interaction with the environment in which energy is exchanged (King, 1981, p. 98). Forty-seven standard events plus up to three novel stressors were scored from 0 to +/−3. Sample items include the following: "New job," "female: pregnancy," and "trouble with employer." The total LES score was the sum of absolute values of the total positive and negative scores, and ranged from 0 (*no stress*) to 150 (*high stress*). Sarason and associates reported a test–retest reliability of .82 and favorable correlations with the SRE.

The Index of Sex Role Orientation (ISRO; Dreyer et al., 1981) was designed to differentiate women who hold their family roles as most important from women who value themselves most as individuals. For King, role is a set of expected behaviors related to one's position in a social system, associated with specific rights and obligations (1981, p. 93) and self-appraisal of health is related to the ability to fulfill one's role. Sixteen items were scored from 1 (*most traditional*) to 5 (*most modern*) for a range of 16 to 80. Sample items include the following: "Most women who want a career should not have children," and "A woman should have exactly the same job opportunities as a man." The originators of the instrument achieved a split-half reliability coefficient of .92 and test–retest reliability of .62. They were able to sort members of feminist versus church groups with better than 95% accuracy on the basis of score.

RESULTS

Results of various analyses have been reported previously (Sharts Engel, 1984, 1987; Sharts-Hopko, 1995). Significant relationships were observed among menopausal stage, current life change, attitude toward women's role, and perceived health status though the relationship between menopausal stage and PHS was negative rather than positive, as predicted, and that between ISRO and PHS was geometric rather than linear.

Age, which was entered into a hierarchical regression first as a control variable, was not significantly related to PHS. The global LES (Sarason et al., 1978) score as well as both the negative and positive LES scores were significantly related to PHS. In addition, an interaction between LES and ISRO (Dreyer et al., 1981) boosted variance accounted for in PHS. When all of the independent variables that were significantly related to the dependent variable PHS, including menopausal stage; positive LES; negative LES; ISRO; $ISRO^2$; LES × ISRO; perception of mother's menopause; perception of life partner's attitude toward menopause; MSC (Neugarten & Kraines, 1965); perceived timing of menopause as early, on-time, or late; and years of education were hierarchically regressed in the order listed after age, R^2 equaled .51 (df 13, 81) when cases with missing data were deleted ($n = 95$). The independent variables that demonstrated a significant relationship to the dependent variable, perceived health status, the measures that were used, and the direction of the relationships are depicted in Table 11.1.

The missing data resulted from the wording of one stem item: "If you are in menopause or the change of life now, or if you have finished with it. . . ." Many of the participants in this study incorrectly estimated their progression through the menopause transition, an observation that has also been reported more recently by several investigators (Jones, 1997; Taffe, Garamszegi, Dudley, & Dennerstein, 1997). Despite that problem, and particularly because relationships are more difficult to observe in smaller samples, accounting for more than half of variance in the dependent variable is notable in a descriptive correlational study.

One important observation about this research is that the inclusion of well, native-born American women who were undergoing a natural menopause transition limited the variance in PHS as well as the independent variables. Moreover, although recruitment of the sample

Table 11.1. Independent variables, instruments, and direction of relationship to the dependent variable, Perceived Health Status

Independent variable	Measure	Direction of relationship
Menopausal stage	Self-rating	−
Current life stress, total	Life Events Survey (LES)	−
Positive current life change	LES—Positive	+
Negative current life change	LES—Negative	−
Attitude toward women's roles	Index of Sex Role Orientation (ISRO)	+
	ISRO^2	+
	LES × ISRO	+
Perception of mother's menopause	Likert scale of same	+
Perception of significant other's attitude toward menopause	Likert scale of same	+
Menopausal symptoms	Menopause Symptom Checklist (MSC)	−
Perceived timing of menopause	On-time (+)/Off-time (−)	+
Educational level	Self report: years of schooling	+

occurred in diverse community settings, the sample overwhelmingly comprised well-educated Caucasian women who scored in the less traditional range on ISRO (Dreyer et al., 1981). In turn, these limitations restricted the opportunity for demonstrating relationships among the variables that have real-world utility. The experience of socially privileged, more liberal women who are likely to identify and mobilize an array of resources as they experience menopause may not illuminate how the full spectrum of American women, particularly those who are poorer, less well educated, more marginalized, and more respectful of authority structures perceive this health transition and make decisions related to it. The way women perceive a health transition is integrally related to their actions (King, 2001).

APPLICATION TO THE CLINICAL PROBLEM

The research reported here, completed more than 20 years ago, provided empirical evidence to support a theory positing that perceived health status of midlife women transitioning through menopause is, to a significant extent, a function of menopausal stage, current life stress, attitude toward women's roles, menopausal symptoms, perception of their mother's menopause, perception of their life partner's perception of menopause, educational level, and perceived timing of menopause as on-time or off-time. Age, which was controlled statistically, was not a factor. Menopausal stage was related to perceived health status negatively rather than positively, and it would be useful to explore the nature of this relationship in greater depth. Nevertheless, the broader understanding that growth and development bears on perceived health status was supported. It must be acknowledged that nearly half of the variance in PHS was not accounted for by the middle range theory. Still, consistent with King's conceptual system, it is useful to regard menopause as a physical transition experienced within a social context and to regard women's health perceptions as being influenced by the meaning they ascribe to the event. How women perceive their health during the menopause transition is relevant because health perceptions factor into how women make decisions about self-care and treatment options (Bravata et al., 2002; Ekstrom et al., 2003; Loppie & Keddy, 2002).

Recent scholarship has much to say in support of this theory. Although this study did not support a positive relationship between menopausal stage and perceived health status, recent research suggests that women do tend to experience reduced anxiety and a more positive attitude about menopause as they actually progress through the transition (Bertero, 2003; George, 2002; Papini, Intrieri, & Goodwin, 2003; Sampselle et al., 2003). Even so, the debate as to whether menopause is associated with an increased occurrence of depression continues (Banger, 2002; Bosworth et al., 2001).

Recent research provides confirmation that current life stress, conceptualized either as significant life events or as hassles versus uplifts, bears on women's experience of menopause (George, 2002). Although women may conceive of menopause as a medical event, the way they experience it is influenced by other concurrent issues such as caring for elderly relatives, change in employment or financial status, changing relationships with children, illness in the family, death of family or friends, and changes in relationships including divorce (Ballard, Kuh, & Wadsworth, 2001).

It is a reflection on how the women's movement has progressed that whether midlife women are more oriented toward home and family versus external commitments is no longer a major theme in the women's health literature. One indirect clue as to how this issue affects midlife women is found in a study entailing in-depth interviews with a diverse sample of 16 Texas women. For these women, menopause was fairly inconsequential because other things going on in their lives were of much greater importance or were more stressful (Winterich & Umberson, 1999). This is in sharp contrast to the 1960s portrayal of menopausal women as devoid of any role (Wilson, 1968).

Not surprisingly, recent literature indicates that symptoms that women experience bear on their health perceptions and well-being. Bosworth and associates (2001) reported an association between climacteric symptoms, such as sleep disruption, mood swings and memory problems, and depressive symptoms. An instrument that was developed to assess the health perceptions of midlife women correlates significantly with the General Health Questionnaire (Hunter, 1992). This line of research has taken an interesting turn because it appears that women's body-image and self-esteem contribute to perceived severity of and ability to cope with menopausal symptoms (Bloch, 2002; Reynolds, 2002).

Bernice Neugarten (1979) theorized that people live their lives with a preconceived "schedule" for when significant life events will occur; and these events are more or less stressful depending on whether, for a given individual, they occurred "on-time," when anticipated, or "off-time," either earlier or later than expected. Premature menopause, or premature ovarian failure, is that which occurs before the age of 40. Recent studies of early menopause confirm that it may be associated with anger, depression, disruption, sadness, resignation, perception of self as old, envy of still-fertile women, and depersonalization (Boughton, 2002; Orshan, Furniss, Forst, & Santoro, 2001; Pasquali, 1999). No studies of women's experience of later-than-expected menopause have been located, although Hvas (2001), having studied 393 Danish women, found that the majority described positive aspects of menopause including cessation of menses, premenstrual syndrome or pregnancy fears, and freedom from various family obligations. It is conceivable that the last woman in a social group to experience menopause might envy her peers or feel out of step.

That significant others in one's life, which in this study included one's life partner and one's mother, influence attitudes toward menopause, and women's symptoms are, in turn, influenced by these attitudes, were findings of a recent study of 169 married couples (Papini et al., 2003). Certainly women are influenced by their perceptions of society's attitude toward aging (Ballard et al., 2001; Banister, 2000; Ransdell, Wells, Manore, Swan, & Corbin, 1998). White American women in particular see menopause as an indicator that they are moving far from society's youthful ideal (Sampselle et al., 2002), and women who have greater body dissatisfaction are more likely to use HRT (McLaren, Hardy, & Kuh, 2003). Women may see menopause as a time-limited physiological event that might require medical attention, but what it represents is life-stage progression and the need to reexamine meaning in one's life (Jones, 1997).

One major theme in a qualitative study of 70 Australian women aged 45 to 70 was the sociocultural context in which women experience menopause (Berger & Forster, 2001). As the authors noted, culture provides for the transmission of values, attitudes, and meanings about middle age and where women derive the meaning of their experiences. It is consistent with this observation that a woman is likely to absorb attitudes about menopause from her mother. In the early 1980s, it was, and still is, the author's assumption that all of the factors that the original and recent reviews of literature identified as relevant to the experience of menopause have emerged as an interplay between women and influential others in their social and cultural world.

FUTURE RECOMMENDATIONS

One issue that warrants acknowledgment is that worldwide, menopause research has increasingly tended to embrace the dominant U.S. medical perspective that menopause is a health alteration requiring management, particularly in Western cultures (Cousins & Edwards, 2002; Salkovskis et al., 2004). Still, alternative perspectives continue to be reported in the United States and elsewhere.

The issue of the direction of the relationship between menopausal stage and perceived health status needs to be explored; the original study uncovered an inverse relationship, and more recent research suggests that the original hypothesis may have support. It may be that the explosion in information about menopause that is available to the public, as evidenced by a visit to a large bookstore or an Internet search, has altered the way that this developmental transition impacts perceived well-being. Still, it does have an impact.

Although research conducted since this study was first reported has provided support for the theory of health perceptions as a means for understanding the menopause transition, its utility requires further testing, particularly among women representing diverse socioeconomic and cultural groups within and outside of the United States. The dynamic found in this study among the concepts of perception, self, growth and development, time, health, role, and stress that provided a means of understanding how women experience menopause suggests that these concepts should be explored in relation to other developmental transitions in both men and women throughout the life span.

SUMMARY

As detailed in this chapter, the theory of health perception appears, so far, to have been substantiated as a means for understanding the menopause transition by subsequent research. That is, more recent research has provided support that perceived health status of midlife women transitioning through menopause is related to menopausal stage, current life stress, attitude toward women's roles, menopausal symptoms, perception of their mother's menopause, perception of their life partner's perception of menopause and perceived timing of menopause as on-time or off-time. Consistent with King's conceptual system (1981, 1990, 2001), menopause is a physical transition experienced within a social context and women's health perceptions are influenced by the meaning they ascribe to the event. This is true despite a major shift in thinking about recommended medical management of menopause with HRT (Diamanti-Kandarakis, 2004; McGinley, 2004). Over time it will be important to see whether a natural, holistic perspective on menopause as a physical event ascribed meaning by women within a social and cultural context gains momentum or whether medical science perseveres in developing a product that will be as enthusiastically promoted as HRT has been since the 1960s.

REFERENCES

Avis, N. E., Stellato, R., Crawford, S., Bromberger, J., Ganz, P., Cain, V., et al. (2001). Is there a menopausal syndrome? Menopausal status and symptoms across racial/ethnic groups. *Social Sciences and Medicine, 52,* 345–356.

Ballard, K. D., Kuh, D. J., & Wadsworth, M. E. J. (2001). The role of the menopause in women's experiences of the "change of life." *Sociology of Health & Illness, 23,* 397–424.

Banger, M. (2002). Affective syndrome during perimenopause. *Maturitas, 41*(Suppl. 1), S13–S18.

Banister, E. M. (2000). Women's midlife confusion: "Why am I feeling this way?" *Issues in Mental Health Nursing, 21,* 745–764.

Bart, P. (1972). Depression in middle-aged women. In J. M. Bardwisk (Ed.), *Readings on the psychology of women* (pp. 134–142). New York: Harper & Row.

Berger, G., & Forster, E. (2001). An Australian study on the sociocultural context of menopause: Directions for contemporary nursing practice. *Contemporary Nurse, 11,* 271–282.

Bertero, C. (2003). What do women think about menopause? A qualitative study of women's expectations, apprehensions and knowledge about the climacteric period. *International Nursing Review, 50,* 1090–118.

Bloch, A. (2002). Self-awareness during the menopause. *Maturitas, 41,* 61–68.

Bosworth, H. B., Bastian, L. A., Kuchibhatla, M. N., Steffens, D. C., McBride, C. M., Skinner, C. S., et al. (2001). Depressive symptoms, menopausal status, and climacteric symptoms in women at midlife. *Psychosomatic Medicine, 63,* 603–608.

Boughton, M. A. (2002). Premature menopause: Multiple disruptions between the woman's biological body experience and her lived body. *Journal of Advanced Nursing, 37*, 423–430.

Bravata, D. M., Rastegar, A., & Horwitz, R. I. (2002). How do women make decisions about hormone replacement therapy? *American Journal of Medicine, 113*, 22–29.

Bradburn, N. M. (1969). *The structure of psychological well-being.* Chicago: Aldine.

Brody, J. A., Farmer, M. E., & White, L. R. (1984). Absence of menopausal effect on hip fracture occurrence in white females. *American Journal of Public Health, 74*, 1397–1398.

Brown, W. J., Mishra, G. D., & Dobson, A. (2002). Changes in physical symptoms during the menopause transition. *International Journal of Behavioral Medicine, 9*, 53–67.

Campbell, A., Converse, P. E., & Rodgers, W. L. (1976). *The quality of American life: Perceptions, evaluations, satisfactions.* New York: Russell Sage Foundation.

Campbell, S., & Whitehead, M. (1977). Oestrogen therapy and the menopausal syndrome. *Clinics in Obstetrics and Gynaecology, 4*, 31–47.

Chim, H., Tan, B. H. I., Ang, C. C., Chew, E. M. D., Chong, Y. S., & Saw, S. M. (2002). The prevalence of menopausal symptoms in a community in Singapore. *Maturitas, 41*, 275–282.

Cohen, J. (1977). *Statistical power analysis for the behavior sciences* (Rev. ed.). New York: Academic Press.

Cousins, S. O., & Edwards, K. (2002). Alice in menopauseland: The jabberwocky of a medicalized middle age. *Health Care for Women International, 23*, 325–343.

Diamanti-Kandarakis, E. (2004). Hormone replacement therapy and risk of malignancy. *Current Opinions in Obstetrics and Gynecology, 16*, 73–78.

Dreyer, N. A., Woods, N. F., & James, S. A. (1981). ISRO: A scale to measure sex-role orientation. *Sex Roles, 7*, 173–182.

Ekstrom, H., Esseveld J., & Hovelius B. (2003). Associations between attitudes toward hormone therapy and current use of it in middle-aged women. *Maturitas, 46*, 45–57.

Flint, M. (1975). The menopause: Reward or punishment? *Psychosomatics, 16*, 161–163.

George, S. A. (2002). The menopause experience: A woman's perspective. *Journal of Obstetrical, Gynecological and Neonatal Nursing, 31*, 77–85.

Hardy, R., & Kuh, D. (2002). Change in psychological and vasomotor symptom reporting during the menopause. *Social Science & Medicine, 55*, 1975–1988.

Holmes, T. H., & Rahe, R. H. (1967). The social readjustment rating scale. *Journal of Psychosomatic Research, 11*, 213–218.

Hunter, M. (1992). The women's health questionnaire: A measure of mid-aged women's perceptions of their emotional and physical health. *Psychiatry and Health, 7*, 45–54.

Hvas, L. (2001). Positive aspects of menopause: A qualitative study. *Maturitas, 39*, 11–17.

Jones, J. B. (1997). Representations of menopause and their health care impli-cations: A qualitative study. *American Journal of Preventive Medicine, 13*, 58–65.

Kaufert, P. A. (1980). The perimenopausal woman and her use of health services. *Maturitas, 2*, 191–205.

King, I. (1981). *A theory for nursing: Systems, concepts, process.* New York: Wiley.

King, I. (1990). Health as the goal for nursing. *Nursing Science Quarterly, 3*, 123–128.

King, I. (2001). Imogene King's theory of goal attainment. In M. Parker (Ed.), *Nursing theories and nursing practice* (pp. 275–286). Philadelphia: Davis.

Lam, P. M., Leung, T. N., Haines, C., & Chung, T. K. H. (2003). Climacteric symptoms and knowledge about hormone replacement therapy among Hong Kong Chinese women aged 40–60 years. *Maturitas, 45*, 99–107.

Leppert, P. (1981). Doctor, will menopause really change my life? *Ladies' Home Journal, 98*, 40–42.

Loppie, C., & Keddy, B. (2002). A feminist analysis of the menopause discourse. *Contemporary Nurse, 12*, 92–99.

McGinley, A. M. (2004). Health beliefs and women's use of hormone replacement therapy. *Holistic Nursing Practice, 18*, 18–25.

McLaren, L., Hardy, R., & Kuh, D. (2003). Women's body satisfaction at midlife and lifetime body size: A prospective study. *Health Psychology, 22*, 370–377.

Meyer, V. F. (2001). The medicalization of menopause: Critique and consequences. *International Journal of Health Services, 31*, 769–792.

Neugarten, B. (1979). Time, age and the life cycle. *American Journal of Psychiatry, 136*, 887–894.

Neugarten, B. L., & Kraines, R. J. (1965). Menopausal symptoms in women of various ages. *Psychosomatic Medicine, 27*, 266–273.

Orshan, S. A., Furniss, K. K., Forst, C., & Santoro, N. (2001). The lived expe-rience of premature ovarian failure. *Journal of Obstetric, Gynecologic and Neonatal Nursing, 30*, 202–208.

Papini, D. R., Intrieri, R. C., & Goodwin, P. E. (2003). Attitude toward menopause among married middle-aged adults. *Women and Health, 36*, 55–68.

Pasquali, E. A. (1999). The impact of premature menopause on women's experi-ence of self. *Journal of Holistic Nursing, 17*, 346–364.

Ransdell, L. B., Wells, C. L., Manore, M. M., Swan, P. D., & Corbin, C. B. (1998). Social physique anxiety in postmenopausal women. *Journal of Women and Aging, 10*, 19–39.

Reynolds, F. (2002). Exploring self-image during hot flushes using a semantic differential scale: Associations between poor self-image, depression, flush frequency and flush distress. *Maturitas, 42*, 201–207.

Salkovskis, P. M., Wroe, A. L., & Rees, M. C. (2004). Shared decision making, health choices and the menopause. *Journal of the British Menopause Society, 10* (Suppl. 1), 13–17.

Sampselle, C. M., Harris, V., Harlow, S. D., & Sowers, M. (2002). Midlife devel-opment and menopause in African American and Caucasian women. *Health Care for Women International, 23*, 351–363.

Sarason, I. G., Johnson, J. H., & Siegel, J. M. (1978). Assessing the impact of life changes: Development of the life experiences survey. *Journal of Consulting and Clinical Psychology, 46,* 932–946.

Sharts Engel, N. C. (1984). On the vicissitudes of health appraisal. *Advances in Nursing Science, 7,* 12–23.

Sharts Engel, N. C. (1987). Menopausal stage, current life change, attitude toward women's roles and perceived health status among 40–55-year-old women. *Nursing Research, 36,* 353–357.

Sharts-Hopko, N. C. (1995). Using health, personal, and interpersonal system concepts within King's systems framework to explore perceived health status during the menopause transition. In M. A. Frey & C. L. Sieloff (Eds.), *Advancing King's systems framework and theory of nursing* (pp. 147–160). Thousand Oaks, CA: Sage.

Skultans, V. (1970). The symbolic significance of menstruation and the menopause. *Man, 5,* 639–651.

Taffe, J., Garamszegi, C., Dudley, E., & Dennerstein, L. (1997). Determinants of self rated menopause status. *Maturitas, 27,* 223–229.

Walker, L. O., & Avant, K. C. (1995). *Strategies for theory construction in nursing* (3rd ed.). Norwalk, CT: Appleton & Lange.

Ware, J. E. (1976). Scales for measuring general health perceptions. *Health Services Research, 11,* 396–415.

Wilbush, J. (1981). What's in a name? Some linguistic aspects of the climacteric. *Maturitas, 3,* 1–9.

Wilson, R. A. (1968). *Feminine forever.* New York: Evans.

Winterich, J. A., & Umberson, D. (1999). How women experience menopause: The importance of social context. *Journal of Women and Aging, 11,* 57–73.

Wright, A. L. (1981). On the calculation of menopause symptoms. *Maturitas, 3,* 55–63.

CHAPTER TWELVE

The Theory of Group Power Within Organizations—Evolving Conceptualization Within King's Conceptual System

Christina Leibold Sieloff

Historically, the literature (Ashley, 1973, 1975; Reverby, 1987; Roberts, 1996, 2000) provides evidence that members of the nursing profession have been oppressed. As a result, nurses have tended to demonstrate oppressed group behaviors (Farrell, 2001; Roberts, 1996, 2000) such as (a) horizontal violence and (b) devaluing of the profession. In addition, nursing groups, within organizations, have tended to act as if they have little power.

In contrast, King, as early as 1981, identified that power was a positive resource that could be used by all nurses to assist them in achieving goals. These goals could include both nurse–patient goals that have been mutually identified or nursing group goals that have been established by the nurses within a group.

It is important for nursing groups, within organizations, to achieve goals set with patients and with other nurses. If these goals or outcomes cannot be achieved, nurses and nursing as a profession could be portrayed as ineffectual and a potential financial drain on a health care organization. Therefore, it is important that nursing groups not only recognize their power but also act to use that power in the achievement of goals or outcomes.

The theory of group power within organizations (TGPO), initially developed as the theory of nursing departmental power, was designed to assist nursing groups to improve their power levels. By using the theory, and the associated instrument (Sieloff–King Assessment of Group Power Within Organizations [SKAGPO]), a nursing group could assess its initial level of power, its power capacity, and its actualized power or ability to use power. Variables within the TGPO can also provide guidance to nursing groups as they develop plans to increase both their power capacity and their actualization of power.

The purpose of this chapter is to describe the evolution of a middle range theory of group power, developed from within Imogene King's conceptual system (1981). The initial development of the theory of nursing departmental power (TNDP) is briefly described. The initial development of the related instrument, the Sieloff–King Assessment of Departmental Power (SKADP) is explored. Psychometric testing of the SKADP, and its subsequent revisions, is discussed. Revisions in the middle range theory, resulting from the psychometric testing of the related instrument, are also reviewed.

THEORY DEVELOPMENT APPROACH

The power of a nursing department, within a health care organization, became a focus of interest when nursing departments, although often the largest department within a health care organization, frequently did not have the necessary power to achieve the department's goals. To understand why this lack of nursing power occurred within organizations, the business and health care literature, related to power and nursing, were reviewed.

Within the business literature, the strategic contingencies theory of power (SCTP; Hickson, Hinings, Lee, Schneck & Pennings, 1971a) was identified as a theory that could provide conceptual assistance to understand a nursing department's apparent lack of power within organizations. The SCTP states that three concepts (centrality, coping with uncertainty, and substitutability) contributed to a department's power within an organization.

Within the nursing and health care literature, King's (1981) conceptual system was identified as a nursing framework that identified power as a major concept, discussed within the context of a social system. In addition, King defined power positively, as the ability to achieve goals, identifying power as a potential resource for nurses within organizations.

Reformulation and synthesis were then used by this researcher as strategies to combine concepts and their relationships from the SCTP (Hickson et al., 1971a) within King's (1981) conceptual system. Key concepts within the SCTP (centrality, coping with uncertainty, and substitutability) were reformulated with King's conceptual system as position, controlling the effects of environment forces, and role (Sieloff, 1995). These concepts, along with the concept of resources, were proposed to contribute to a nursing department's power capacity.

However, before a nursing department's power capacity could be actualized, additional variables were proposed to intervene. These variables were identified to assist in explaining why nursing departments, with large power capacities, seemed to actualize very little power. These intervening variables were identified as (a) chief nurse executive's (CNE's) power ability, composed of the CNE's knowledge, skill, and importance placed on power by the CNE; and (b) departmental goals (Sieloff, 1995).

SELECTIVE LITERATURE REVIEW RELATED TO THE LACK OF POWER WITHIN NURSING AND KING'S CONCEPTUAL SYSTEM

The following selective literature review briefly examines (a) oppressed groups, (b) the lack of empirical evidence related to nursing group power, and (c) variables that constitute the theory of group power within organizations. These variables include (a) controlling the effects of environmental forces, (b) position, (c) resources, (d) role, (e) power perspective, (f) chief nurse executive's power competency, (g) communication competency, and (h) goals and outcomes competency.

Oppressed Groups

There has been extensive literature published on the oppressed nature of the profession of nursing. As a result of this ongoing, historical oppression, nurses, individually and in groups, tend to exhibit more oppressed group behaviors and demonstrate an associated powerlessness.

As power is defined as the "capacity to achieve goals" (King, 1981, p. 127), one may then conclude that nurses, demonstrating a lack of power, or powerlessness, would tend to have difficulty achieving their goals. This premise has been supported by numerous observations made by this researcher in a variety of clinical settings.

Lack of Empirical Evidence Related to Nursing Group Power

Reviews of the literature, from 1986 until recently, have continued to demonstrate a lack of specific strategies to improve nursing's power outside the legislative arena. The majority of literature has been found to focus on oppressed group behaviors of nurses and nonempirically based discussions of power and how nurses might act to improve their personal power.

Controlling the Effects of Environmental Forces

The health care environment has constantly changed, and continues to do so today. Forces within the environment and organizations affect how health care is planned and provided. The status quo no longer exists, and change has become the norm.

Changes in health policy at both the state and federal levels result in changes not only at the local level but also within each health care organization. Similarly, within each health care organization, such changes affect all levels of the organization and staff.

As a result, all health care organizations, and groups with those organizations, are continuously coping with uncertainty. The SCTP (Hickson, et al., 1971a) proposed that the ability to cope with uncertainty was a source of power for all departments within an organization. Although the SCTP did not focus specifically on health care organizations, the researcher's communications with Dr. Hickson (personal communication, October 30, 1992) supported the application of the concepts of the SCTP to health care organizations. Reformulation of the key concepts from the SCTP, and their relationships, within King's (1981) conceptual system, resulted in the concept of *coping with uncertainty* being reconceptualized as *controlling the effects of environmental forces*. This concept was defined as "effectively managing the potential negative consequences that result from the effect of changing health care trends on the ability of an [organization] to achieve its goals" (Sieloff, 1996, p. 31).

If a nursing group is able to anticipate, prepare for, and adjust to the effects of environmental forces, the TGPO proposes that the nursing group's power will be enhanced. In addition, if a nursing group is also able to assist the overall organization to anticipate, prepare, and adjust for the effects of environmental forces, the nursing group's power will be further enhanced.

Position

Within the SCTP (Hickson, et al., 1971a), the centrality of an organizational department, within an organization, was proposed to be a key variable in determining the power of a department. This concept, *centrality*, was reconceptualized within King's (1981) conceptual system, as *position*, and defined as "the centrality of a nursing [group] within the communication network of a health care suprasystem" (Sieloff, 1995, p. 57).

Within health care organizations today, communications have become increasingly complex. Patients use cell phones to contact the staff working with them. Computerized charting is replacing paper medical records. Futuristic views of health care propose that all of an individuals' health records could be recorded on a single card that individuals would carry with them in case of emergency. Because communication is a key concept within King's (1981) conceptual system, the centrality of a nursing group, within an organization's communication system, was proposed to be a key variable in determining a nursing group's level of power.

To have a high degree of centrality within an organization, a nursing group must have access to sufficient information to function efficiently. In addition, to ensure that a nursing group receives sufficient information, the organization must also recognize the centrality of a nursing group's functioning within an organization. As a result, a powerful nursing group would be perceived by the organization as (a) having expertise that is valued within the organization, (b) providing care that is viewed as central to the delivery of quality services by other organizational groups, and (c) being contacted by other groups within the organization for input on patient care.

Resources

Resources continue to be a critical component of an organization's success. Within any organization, resources are also critical if an organizational group is to meet its goals successfully.

Role

The SCTP (Hickson, et al., 1971a) proposed that a department's degree of substitutability was another key element determining whether a department was powerful. If an organization could easily obtain substitute workers for a department without disrupting the organization's work, that department had minimal power. If, however, an organization could not easily obtain substitute workers for a department and, without the presence of those workers, the organization's work was significantly disrupted, that department had power.

This concept of *substitutability* was reconceptualized within King's (1981) conceptual system as role, and defined as "the degree to which the work of a health care suprasystem is accomplished through the work of a nursing [group]" (Sieloff, 1995, p. 58). All nursing groups would seem to have a high level of this variable because without registered nurses, most health care organizations would fail to function.

Power Perspective

Many nursing management texts continue to focus on French and Raven's (1959) definition, and sources, of power, a focus that tends to present power as a negative concept. This focus contributes to a lack of interest, on the part of nurses, in the concept of power. Two major nursing authors who conceptualized power as a positive concept, and a resource for nurses, are King, with publications beginning in 1981, and Chinn, with publications beginning in 1995. However, when reviewing the general nursing literature, the view of power has remained less than positive. If a nurse leader perceives power as negative, that leader will not seek to use power on behalf of a nursing group. In contrast, if a nurse leader perceives power as positive, that leader is more likely to aid the group in using its power.

Chief Nurse Executive's Power Competency

The literature on systems identifies that the leader of a system, in this case, a nursing group or nursing department, serves as a boundary spanner for that group or department, interacting with other systems on the group's or department's behalf. As a result, a CNE's, or nursing group leader's, competency in relation to power is a key variable, contributing to the ability of a group to use its power. This concept, the CNE power competency, was defined as ability of a nursing group leader to communicate effectively with other organizational groups and, by doing so, enhance the power of a nursing group.

To demonstrate a high level of CNE power competency, a nurse leader must begin by fostering and maintaining the support of key individuals within the nursing group. Beyond the nursing group, the nurse leader must also demonstrate an understanding of how others within the organization use power and use collaboration with other groups within the organization to achieve goals. Finally, a nurse leader must be actively involved in administrative decision making for the overall organization.

Communication Competency

As mentioned earlier in relation to the concept of position, communication is a key concept within King's (1981) conceptual system. Hence, it is important that a nursing group be competent in relation to communication processes. This concept, *communication competency*, was defined as the knowledge and skills related to the giving of information from one group to another group. Basic to the development of this relevant knowledge and skills is the recognition that the power of a nursing group is enhanced through communication with other organizational groups. Thus, if a nursing group does not value or facilitate communication, its power will be limited.

In addition, communication competency also refers to a nursing group's representation on decision-making groups within the health care organization. Such groups would include both multidisciplinary committees and key organizational decision-making groups (e.g., executive councils). Such representation must, if the highest level of power is to be obtained, include voting privileges on all groups.

Goals and Outcomes Competency

The existence of goals was identified within King's (1981) conceptual system as a key antecedent of power. Without goals, there would be no power. Hence, for a nursing group to have power, it is critical that the group be competent in relation to goals and outcomes. This concept, *goals and outcomes competency,* was defined as the knowledge and skill of a group in relation to the process of achieving "events that are valued, wanted or desired" (King, 1981, p. 145) by a group.

To have the highest level of power, in relation to the goals and outcomes competency, a nursing group would need to have clearly defined goals. These goals would have been developed with all registered nurses having the opportunity for input. In addition, because cost containment continues to be a key focus within all health care organizations, a nursing group's goals should address the effective use of resources. Furthermore, because registered nurses should be considered a resource for a health care organization, a nursing group's goals should provide for the development of the registered nurses' clinical competence.

METHODOLOGY

Evolving Instrumentation

Initial psychometric testing of the Sieloff–King assessment of departmental power

The focus of the initial research was the development and initial psychometric testing of an instrument designed to test the TNDP, the SKADP. Initially, 442 items were developed as a result of a review of the literature. The number of items was reduced to 125, and these items were then reviewed by 10 content validity judges, five experts in power, including Dr. J. Pfeffer, and five experts in King's conceptual system, including Dr. King. The content validity index (CVI) for the SKADP was 87.36% (pilot study instrument) and 80.6% (final instrument; 78% being the minimum acceptable for 10 judges; Lynn, 1986). As a result of a pilot testing of 88 items, 40 items were selected for inclusion in the final instrument.

The finalized SKADP instrument (Sieloff, 1996) was then psychometrically tested. The instrument's Cronbach's alpha was .91, and the split half was .76 ($n = 206$).

To estimate the criterion-related concurrent validity of the SKADP, Hickson et al.'s (1971b) instrument "About Your Own and Other Departments" (AYOOD) was used as the criterion instrument. In all psychometric tests of the SKADP and SKAGPO, departments used in the AYOOD instrument were changed, with permission of the original primary author, to reflect the major departments within a health care organization setting (D. J. Hickson, personal communication, October 30, 1992).

Criterion-related validity was examined using the correlation of the SKADP with (a) the overall revised AYOOD (Hickson et al., 1971b), (b) 26 questions of the revised AYOOD that specifically addressed nursing, and (c) one question of the AYOOD that specifically inquired about the power level for nursing. The SKADP correlated with the (a) overall AYOOD (.33, $p = .01$), (b) 26 questions of the AYOOD (.49, $p = .01$), and (c) the nursing-specific question of the AYOOD (.47, $p = .01$).

Finally, a principle components factor analysis, with a varimax rotation, of the SKADP suggested the need for further instrument revision, identifying six factors with loadings of more than three items, and one item with an eigen value over 1. Four variables remained stable (controlling the effects of environmental forces, position, resources, and role). One item (labeled group goals), with an eigen value over one, was retained because of its theoretical contribution to the instrument. The variable, CNE's power ability, consisted of two, rather than three, variables. "Review of the related items, their factor loadings, and their contributions to the instrument and subscale alphas, resulted in the regrouping of the items into two revised factors: power competence and power perspective" (Sieloff, 2003, p. 185).

Revision of the instrument

In the initial research, several subjects declined to participate due to organizational changes that had resulted in the elimination of nursing departments within their organizations. In addition, at that time, organizations were also involved in restructuring and reengineering (Kerfoot, 1990), resulting in different organizational structures than had previously existed, for example, matrices and project teams.

These changes prompted the researcher to review the initial instrument. To ensure that all selected subjects would be able to participate and to reflect the previously recognized changes in organizations, the wording used in the SKADP was revised to change the word *department* to *group*, change the word *hospital* to *organization*, and rename the instrument the Sieloff–King Assessment of Group Power Within Organizations (SKAGPO).

The SKAGPO (Sieloff, 1999) was the resulting revision of the SKADP (Sieloff, 1996). Research, involving the psychometric testing of the SKAGPO, replicated the initial research with a stratified random sampling of 600 CNEs from hospitals across the United States.

In this research, the instrument's Cronbach's alpha was .92 ($n = 334$). The split-half analysis, with the equal length Spearman–Brown Correction formula, was .92 ($n = 334$). In relation to the instrument's criterion-related validity, the correlation between the chief nurse executives' scores on the SKAGPO and the executives' scores on a criterion (AYOOD—abbreviated form; Hickson et al., 1971b) was calculated. The resulting correlation was .625 ($p = .1, n = 321$), providing support for the criterion-related validity of the SKAGPO.

After reviewing the results of the principle components factor analysis with a varimax rotation, the researcher identified that five of the proposed variables remained stable (controlling the effects of environmental forces, position, power perspective, resources, and role).

> The items constituting the proposed subscale, power competence, [however] loaded on three separate factors, with the exception of one item loading on the factor, role. Following a review of the three factors items' loading, and the theoretical focus of each item, the three factors were retained and labeled: a) CNE's power competency, b) communication competency, and c) goals and outcomes competency. (Sieloff, 2003, p. 186)

Confirmatory factor analysis of the SKAGPO

The final research related to the further refinement of the SKAGPO involved structural equation modeling (SEM) to analyze the relationships between the proposed variables of the middle range theory (confirmatory factor analysis). The goal was to determine statistically whether the relationships in the proposed model were compatible with the data variance and covariance matrix. Various goodness of fit tests, or fit indices, were used to determine whether the proposed model covariance structure was different from the observed relationships.

Factor loadings for the SKAGPO's subscales (e.g., standardized regression weights) ranged from .43 to .89. Data regarding the overall fit of the final proposed model were: $\chi^2 = 504.7$, $df = 291$, $p \leq .00$, Goodness of Fit Index = .9, Normed Fit Index = .86, Incremental Fit Index (IFI) = .94, Comparative Fit Index (CFI) = .94, and Root Mean Square Error of Approximation (RMSEA) = .05. In summary, fit indices of the final

Table 12.1. Theoretical Definitions of the Concepts Comprising the Theory of Nursing Departmental Power: Initial Conceptualization

Concept	Definition
CNE's knowledge of power	The level of information held by a CNE regarding power (Evans [Sieloff], 1989)
CNE's power ability	CNE's knowledge of power, skill in utilizing power, and the importance placed on power by a chief nurse executive (Sieloff, 1995)
CNE's skill in utilizing power	The level of expertise held by a chief nurse executive in implementing power strategies (Evans [Sieloff], 1989)
Control of effects of environmental forces	Effectively managing the potential negative consequences that result from the effect of changing health care trends on the ability of a hospital to achieve its goals (Evans [Sieloff], 1989)
Departmental goals	"Events that [a nursing department has determined are to be] valued, wanted or desired" (King, 1981, p. 145)
Importance placed on power by the CNE	A CNE's perception of the positive or negative aspects of power (Evans [Sieloff], 1989)
Position	"The centrality of [the] nursing department within the communication network of a [hospital]" (Sieloff, 1995, p. 57)
Power (actualized)	Theoretical—implementation of the capacity of a group to achieve its goals (Sieloff, 1996)
Power (capacity)	Capacity of a group to achieve its goals (Sieloff, 1996)
Resources	Any commodity that the nursing department can use for goal achievement (Maas, 1988)
Role	"Degree to which the work of a [hospital] is accomplished through the efforts of [the] nursing department" (Sieloff, 1995, p. 58)

Note. CNE = chief nurse executive.

proposed model suggested "an adequate fit" to the data. The $\chi^2:df$ ratio was less than three, IFI and CFI indices were relatively close to .95, and the RMSEA was indicative of a slightly better than average fit (Byrne, 2001; Hair, Anderson, Tathan, & Black, 1998).

As the result of this research, support was demonstrated for the relationships proposed between the variables of the SKAGPO. Because the SKAGPO variables and relationships mirror the concepts and relationships of the TGPO, beginning statistical support has been provided for the theories' concepts and relationships.

Evolving Theoretical Concepts

The theoretical concepts, originally proposed in the TNDP, have also evolved over time. This evolution is evident in Tables 12.1 to 12.4. Table 12.1 details the original concepts and their theoretical definitions, and

Table 12.2. Theoretical Definitions of the Concepts Comprising the Theory of Nursing Departmental Power: Following Initial Psychometric Testing of the SKADP

Concept	Definition
CNE's perspective on power	The CNE's perception of, and value placed on, the achievement of goals
Control of effects of environmental forces[a]	Effectively managing the potential negative consequences that result from the effect of changing health care trends on the ability of a hospital to achieve its goals (Evans [Sieloff], 1989)
Group goals	"Events that are valued, wanted or desired" (King, 1981, p. 145) by a group
Position[a]	"The centrality of [the] nursing department within the communication network of a [hospital]" (Sieloff, 1995, p. 57)
Power (actualized)[a]	Theoretical—implementation of the capacity of a group to achieve its goals (Sieloff, 1996)
Power (capacity)[a]	Capacity of a group to achieve its goals (Sieloff, 1996)
Power competence	Level of knowledge and skills in relation to the achievement of group goals
Power perspective	The perception of, and value placed on, the achievement of goals
Resources[a]	Any commodity that the nursing department can use for goal achievement (Maas, 1988)
Role[a]	"Degree to which the work of a [hospital] is accomplished through the efforts of [the] nursing department" (Sieloff, 1995, p. 58)

Note. CNE = chief nurse executive; SKADP = Sieloff–King Assessment of Departmental Power.
[a] Stable concept following statistical analysis (six of nine concepts—67%).

Table 12.2 includes the concepts and definitions as revised, following the initial research. Table 12.3 details the changes in the theoretical concepts that resulted from the psychometric testing of the revised SKADP, the SKAGPO. Table 12.4 provides the additional concepts, and related definitions, that were identified as a result of the confirmatory factor analysis.

Evolving Conceptualizations of the TGPO

Models shown in Figures 12.1 to 12.4 depict the evolution of the TGPO. Figure 12.1 presents the original conceptualization of the middle range theory, the TNDP.

Following the initial psychometric testing of the instrument, associated with the TNDP, the conceptualization of the TNDP changed to

Table 12.3. Theoretical Definitions of the Concepts of the Theory of Group Power Within Organizations: Following Psychometric Testing of the Revised SKADP or SKAGPO

Concept	Definition
CNE's power competency	The knowledge and skills of the nurse leader in relation to the achievement of group goals
Communication competency	The knowledge and skill related to the giving of information from one group to another group
Control of effects of environmental forces[a]	Effectively managing the potential negative consequences that result from the effect of changing health care trends on the ability of a hospital to achieve its goals (Evans [Sieloff], 1989)
Goal and outcome competency	The knowledge and skill of a group in relation to the process of achieving "events that are valued, wanted or desired" (King, 1981, p. 145) by a group
Position[a]	"The centrality of [the] nursing department within the communication network of a [hospital]" (Sieloff, 1995, p. 57)
Power (actualized)[a]	Theoretical—implementation of the capacity of a group to achieve its goals (Sieloff, 1996)
Power (capacity)[a]	Capacity of a group to achieve its goals (Sieloff, 1996)
Power perspective[a]	The perception and value regarding the achievement of goals
Resources[a]	Any commodity that the nursing department can use for goal achievement (Maas, 1988)
Role[a]	"Degree to which the work of a [hospital] is accomplished through the efforts of [the] nursing department" (Sieloff, 1995, p. 58)

Note. CNE = chief nurse executive; SKADP = Sieloff–King Assessment of Departmental Power; SKAGPO = Sieloff–King Assessment of Group Power Within Organizations.
[a] Stable concept following statistical analysis (7 of 10 concepts—70%).

the TGPO, based on theoretical consideration of the factor analysis. The variables contributing to a department's power capacity remained stable. However, the conceptualization of the variables proposed to intervene in the actualization of power were modified. Five intervening variables were collapsed into three intervening variables, and the variable labels were modified to reflect the conceptual basis of the loaded items.

Following the psychometric testing of the SKAGPO, the conceptualization of the TGPO was further refined. The items initially linked to the three variables, proposed to intervene in a group's ability to actualize its power capacity, were further reconfigured to comprise four variables, based on a theoretical consideration of the relevant items' factor loadings and their theoretical contribution to the proposed subscale.

Table 12.4. Theoretical Definitions of the Concepts of the Theory of Group Power Within Organizations: Following Confirmatory Factor Analysis of the SKAGPO

Concept	Definition
CNE's power competency[a]	The knowledge and skills of the nurse leader in relation to the achievement of group goals
Communication competency[a]	The knowledge and skill related to the giving of information from one group to another group
Control of effects of environmental forces[a]	Effectively managing the potential negative consequences that result from the effect of changing health care trends on the ability of a hospital to achieve its goals (Evans [Sieloff], 1989)
Goals/outcomes competency[a]	The knowledge and skill of a group in relation to the process of achieving "events that are valued, wanted or desired" (King, 1981, p. 145) by a group
Position[a]	"The centrality of [the] nursing department within the communication network of a [hospital]" (Sieloff, 1995, p. 57)
Power (actualized)[a]	Theoretical—implementation of the capacity of a group to achieve its goals (Sieloff, 1996)
Power (capacity)[a]	Capacity of a group to achieve its goals (Sieloff, 1996)
Power (capacity) mediated by CNE's power competency	Capacity of a group to achieve its goals (Sieloff, 1996) mediated by the knowledge and skills of the nurse leader in relation to the achievement of group goals
Power (capacity) mediated by communication competency	Capacity of a group to achieve its goals (Sieloff, 1996) mediated by the knowledge and skill related to the giving of information from one group to another group
Power (capacity) mediated by goals/outcomes competency	Capacity of a group to achieve its goals (Sieloff, 1996) mediated by the knowledge and skill of a group in relation to the process of achieving "events that are valued, wanted or desired" (King, 1981, p. 145) by a group
Power (capacity) mediated by power perspective	Capacity of a group to achieve its goals (Sieloff, 1996) mediated by the perception and value regarding the achievement of goals
Power perspective[a]	The perception and value regarding the achievement of goals
Resources[a]	Any commodity that the nursing department can use for goal achievement (Maas, 1988)
Role[a]	"Degree to which the work of a [hospital] is accomplished through the efforts of [the] nursing department" (Sieloff, 1995, p. 58)

Note. CNE = chief nurse executive; SKAGPO = Sieloff–King Assessment of Group Power Within Organizations.
[a] Stable concept following statistical analysis (nine of nine concepts—100%) plus mediated concepts.

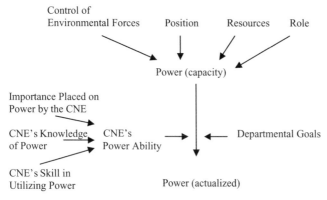

Figure 12.1. The theory of nursing departmental power. *Note.* Adapted from "Proposed Relationships of the Concepts Within the Theory of Departmental Power," C. L. Sieloff, 1995, *Advancing King's Systems Framework and Theory of Nursing*, p. 61, Thousand Oaks, CA: Sage. CNE = chief nursing executive.

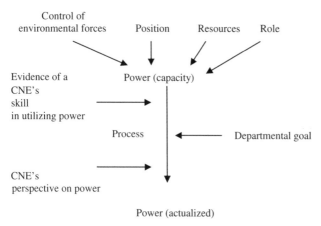

Figure 12.2. The theory of group power within organizations after initial psychometric testing of the Sieloff–King Assessment of Departmental Power.

Confirmatory factor analysis of the SKAGPO provided statistical support for the TGPO as previously proposed. However, further statistical clarification identified that each of the four intervening variables also mediated with the variable power capacity within the model. As a result, these four variables were integrated into the model of the theory.

Table 12.5 summarizes the current substruction, from concepts within King's conceptual systems (1981), of the TGPO.

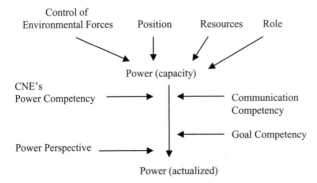

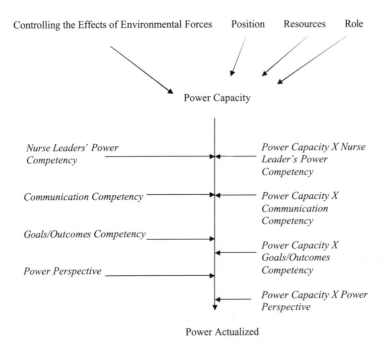

Figure 12.3. The theory of group power within organizations after psychometric testing of the revised Sieloff–King Assessment of Departmental Power or Sieloff–King Assessment of Group Power Within Organizations.

Figure 12.4. The theory of group power within organizations after confirmatory factor analysis of the Sieloff–King Assessment of Group Power Within Organizations.

Table 12.5. Current Substruction for the Theory of Group Power Within Organizations

Conceptual System Concept	Communication	Decision Making	Organization	Organization	Perception
Middle range theory concept	Communication competency	Goals/outcomes competency	Control of environmental forces	Resources	Power perspective
Empirical indicator	Designated items on the SKAGPO	Designated items on the SKAGPO	Designated items on the SKAGPO	Designated items on the SKAGPO	Designated items on the SKAGPO

Conceptual System Concept	Power	Power	Role	Self	Status
Middle range theory concept	Power (actualized)	Power (capacity)	Role	CNE's power competency	Position
Empirical indicator	SKAGPO	Items related to control of environmental forces, position, resources, and role	Designated items on the SKAGPO	Designated items on the SKAGPO	Designated items on the SKAGPO

Note. CNE = chief nurse executive; SKAGPO = Sieloff–King Assessment of Group Power Within Organizations.

STRENGTHS AND LIMITATIONS

In any theory development program of research, strengths and limitations must be identified. For the TGPO, a major strength is the development, and repeated psychometric testing of the related instrument, the SKAGPO. The demonstration of the instrument's consistent reliability and validity provide support for its use within other research not related to the TGPO.

However, because of the consistent emphasis on the psychometric testing of the instrument, a limitation in this program of research is the lack of empirical studies designed to test the TGPO. Additional research should be implemented to test hypotheses related to the TGPO.

Application to the Lack of Group Power Within Nursing

The theory of group power and its related instrument (the SKAGPO) can be used by all nursing groups to assess, develop plans, and act to improve their power levels. An initial completion of the SKAGPO identifies a group's power capacity as well as its level of actualized power. By identifying the items on which the group scored low, the group can then establish short and long-term plans to further improve both its power capacity and actualized power.

In addition, by using the TGPO, and focusing on further improving their levels of power, a nursing group will tend to decrease its oppressed group behaviors through an increased focus on the group's power. As a result, the visibility of nursing within the particular health care organization should also tend to increase. Increasing the visibility of nursing's contribution within health care organizations will enable nursing groups to change the organizational view of nursing from that of an expense to a revenue-producing group.

FUTURE RECOMMENDATIONS

Additional research is needed to provide empirical support, beyond the psychometric testing of the associated instrument, for the TGPO. Potential hypotheses that could be tested include the following: (a) The existence of clear group goals for a nursing group increases the group's actualized power, (b) an increase in the CNE's power competency will increase the actualized power of a nursing group, (c) an increase in a nursing group's communication competency will increase the actualized power of a nursing group, (d) an increase in a nursing group's goals and outcomes competency will increase the actualized power of a nursing group, (e) an increase in a nursing group's power perspective will increase the actualized power of a nursing group, and, (f) an increase in a nursing group's actualized power will result in increased nursing group satisfaction.

In addition to additional empirical tests of the TGPO, the SKAGPO can be used within other research to determine the effect of a nursing group's power levels on dependent variables. Such dependent variables could include (a) medication errors, (b) patient falls, (c) nosocomial infections, (d) retention of registered nurses, and (e) recruitment of registered nurses.

SUMMARY

In summary, the TGPO was initially developed to clarify why nursing departments seemed to lack sufficient power to achieve their goals. Through the repeated psychometric testing of the related instrument (the SKAGPO), this middle range theory has evolved into a more generalizable middle range theory that can assist any group to further improve its group's power within an organization. This process has also lent support to the perspective that King's conceptual system (1981) can have applicability within administrative situations beyond nursing.

REFERENCES

Ashley, J. A. (1973). This I believe about power in nursing. *Nursing Outlook, 21*(10), 637–641.

Ashley, J. A. (1975). Power, freedom and professional practice in nursing. *Supervisor Nurse, 6*, 12–14, 17, 19, 20, 22–24, 29.

Byrne, B. M. (2001). *Structural equation modeling with AMOS: Basic concepts, applications, and programming.* Mahwah, NJ: Erlbaum.

Chinn, P. L. (1995). *Peace and power: Building communities for the future.* New York: National League for Nursing.

Evans [Sieloff], C. L. (1989). Development of a departmental theory of power within Imogene King's framework. Unpublished manuscript, Wayne State University, Detroit, MI.

Farrell, T. A. (2001). From tall poppies to squashed weeds: Why don't nurses pull together more? *Journal of Advanced Nursing, 35*, 26–33.

French, J. R. P., & Raven, B. (1959). The bases of social power. In D. Cartwright (Ed.), *Studies in social power* (pp. 150–167). Ann Arbor: University of Michigan Press.

Hair, J. F., Anderson, R. E., Tathan, R. L., & Black, W. C. (1998). *Multivariate data analysis* (5th ed.). Mahwah, NJ: Prentice-Hall.

Hickson, D. J., Hinings, C. R., Lee, C. A., Schneck, R. E., & Pennings, J. M. (1971a). A strategic contingencies' theory of intraorganizational power. *Administrative Science Quarterly, 16*, 216–229.

Hickson, D. J., Hinings, C. R., Lee, C. A., Schneck, R. E., & Pennings, J. M. (1971b). *About your own and other departments.* Unpublished instrument, University of Alberta, Edmonton, Alberta, Canada.

Kerfoot, K. M. (1990). To manage by power or influence: The nurse manager's choice. *Nursing Economics, 8,* 117–118.

King, I. M. (1981). *A theory for nursing: Systems, concepts, process.* New York: Wiley.

Lynn, M. R. (1986). Determination and quantification of content validity. *Nursing Research, 35,* 382–385.

Maas, M. L. (1988). A model of organizational power: Analysis and significance to nursing. *Research in Nursing and Health, 11,* 153–163.

Reverby, S. M. (1987). *Ordered to care: The dilemma of American nursing.* Cambridge, England: Cambridge University Press.

Roberts, S. J. (1996). Point of view: Breaking the cycle of oppression: Lessons for nurse practitioners. *Journal of American Academy of Nurse Practitioners, 8,* 209–214.

Roberts, S. J. (2000). Development of a positive professional identity: Liberating oneself from the oppressor within. *Advances in Nursing Science, 22,* 71–82.

Sieloff, C. L. (1995). Development of a theory of departmental power. In M. A. Frey & C. L. Sieloff (Eds.), *Advancing King's systems framework and theory of nursing* (pp. 46–65). Thousand Oaks, CA: Sage.

Sieloff, C. L. (1996). *Development of an instrument to estimate the actualized power of a nursing department.* Unpublished doctoral dissertation, Wayne State University, Detroit, MI.

Sieloff, C. L. (1999). *Sieloff–King assessment of group power within organizations.* Unpublished instrument, Oakland University, Rochester, MI.

Sieloff, C. L. (2003). Measuring nursing power within organizations. *Journal of Nursing Scholarship, 35,* 183–187.

CHAPTER THIRTEEN

Further Exploration of Family Health Within the Context of Chronic Obstructive Pulmonary Disease

Mona Newsome Wicks, Muriel C. Rice, and Costellia H. Talley

Chronic obstructive pulmonary disease (COPD) is a major public health problem because of its worldwide prevalence and contribution to morbidity, mortality, disability, and health care cost (Murray & Lopez, 1996; Voelkel, 2000). An estimated 16 million people suffer from COPD, and by the year 2020, it will be the fifth leading cause of societal burden worldwide (Pauwels, Buist, Calverlye, Jenkins, & Hurd, 2001).

Chronic obstructive pulmonary disease affects both patients and families, particularly family caregivers. In the presence of inadequate resources, COPD likely contributes to disruptions in family functioning, which is an indicator of family health. As COPD progresses, family caregivers must adapt to patient's impaired physical functioning. Expressive and instrumental support is often necessary. The support needed varies but may include encouragement and assistance with disease management, activities of daily living (ADLs), and managing personal affairs. Breathing difficulty and associated airflow obstruction are progressive and pervasive because the disease is not reversible (Wouters, Creutzberg, & Schols, 2002). Depression and anxiety are common comorbidities (Light, Merrill, Despars, Gordon, & Mutalipassi, 1985; van Manen et al., 2002).

Because COPD impairs patients' physical, social, and emotional health, the disease likely influences dimensions of family health or functioning such as family communication within patient–family caregiver dyads. Other researchers have recognized the potential effects of obstructive lung diseases on family functioning and have examined this outcome in parents of children with cystic fibrosis (Spieth et al., 2001; Venters, 1981) and asthma (Gavin, Wamboldt, Sorokin, Levy, & Wamboldt, 1999) as well as in family members of individuals with COPD (Kanervisto, Paavilainen, & Astedt-Kurki, 2003). This chapter explores predictors of family communication as a dimension of family health for caregivers in general and wife caregivers in particular. The findings extend existing research by focusing on family communication as a dimension of family health and differences in the caregiving experience based on kinship. Spouse caregivers, particularly wives, often experience more negative outcomes such as more caregiver burden compared with other family members (McFall & Miller, 1992; Miller, McFall, & Montgomery 1991; Pruchno & Resch, 1989). The theory of family health described in this chapter was originally developed and tested between 1987 and 1992 during the first authors' dissertation research. Based on King's (1981) conceptual system, the theory was tested with patient–caregiver dyads (irrespective of caregiver kinship) of patients with COPD (Wicks, 1992). Additional testing was conducted to further establish its utility for research and practice by identifying predictors of general family health (Wicks, 1995). The current analysis expands previous testing by examining the degree to which the concepts within the theory explain *family communication* as a dimension of family health using the original study data. The clinical problems facing persons with COPD and their caregivers, strategies used to formulate and revise the theory, clinical applications, and future recommendations for theory testing and refinement are presented. Although the theory was developed to understand family health in the context of COPD, it may have broader utility with regard to understanding family health in the context of chronic caregiving.

THEORY FORMULATION STRATEGIES

Four strategies were used to formulate the middle range theory of family health in the context of COPD: systematic examination of clinical experiences from COPD patient–caregiver populations, review of nursing and nonjuring theories, synthesis of published research, and empirical tests of the theory (Smith & Liehr, 2004). Each strategy is briefly discussed to describe the evolution of the theory. Thus, the theory has both inductive and deductive roots. The focus is on the patient–caregiver dyad as a component of the family system because these individuals are most intimately involved in caregiving.

SYSTEMATIC EXAMINATION OF CLINICAL EXPERIENCES

Clinical experiences with and observations of this patient–caregiver population suggested families and family relationships are an important factor in the rehabilitation and care of patients with COPD. The American Association for Respiratory Care (2002) and clinicians who care for patients with COPD have recently confirmed these observations (Fahy, 2004; Penrod, Kane, Finch, & Kane, 1998). The first author of this chapter observed in clinical practice that some patients with severe airway obstruction displayed seemingly high levels of social and emotional functioning despite severe disease-imposed physical limitations. In contrast, there were other patients with similar levels of airflow obstruction who were less functional in all areas. Although the severity of airflow obstruction can be objectively measured using standard pulmonary function tests, the experience of disease severity varies between patients (Ferrer et al., 1997). Objective indicators such as pulmonary function tests may not accurately predict the severity of disease limitations (Leidy & Haase, 1996) or dependence on caregivers for assistance with ADLs (Ferrer et al., 1997). In addition, observations seemed to point to discernable differences in the support received by patients within their family systems and whether or not these family interactions seemed "healthy." Healthy families were those families that the first author perceived as facilitating patients' rehabilitation or care by encouraging independent and interdependent roles whenever possible and who communicated effectively, respectfully, and with clear messages. In less healthy families, caregivers, patients, or both often fostered dependence or battled with one another displaying tension or distress such as harsh language, angry verbal exchanges, or cold silence during patient–caregiver interactions. These observations led to an examination of theories that might capture *family health* as a key concept for understanding family interactions within the context of COPD and perhaps other chronic illnesses.

THE SEARCH FOR THEORY TO UNDERSTAND CLINICAL EXPERIENCES

Key concepts that emerged from the clinical observations just described included the patient and caregiver perceptions of illness severity, perceived caregiver stress, length of diagnosis, family stressors, and family functioning as an indicator of family health. The first author undertook a systematic review of published theories related to chronic illnesses and the experiences of family members, particularly family caregivers. Specific models that were examined included the McMaster Model of Family Health and T-Double ABCX Model of Family Adjustment and Adaptation (McCubbin & McCubbin, 1987; Westley & Epstein, 1969). Although these endeavors were fruitful, they failed to explain clinical observations fully, perhaps because the reviewed theories were not specific to the clinical problem, did not address the concepts of interest (i.e. family health), or were not in the nursing practice context that Meleis (1997) and others (Liehr & Smith, 1999) viewed as critical for theory development within a practice discipline. Thus, this family health theory emerged from efforts to explain and communicate the essence of family health within the context of an existing nursing conceptual framework. Exploration of existing nursing frameworks to understand this clinical phenomenon resulted in careful examination of the work of nurse theorists who viewed the *family* as client and a *family health* focus as relevant for clinical practice and research. This approach to theory development is consistent with Merton (1968) and Liehr and Smith's (1999) belief that middle range theory must fit within grand theories and be empirically based.

The review of nursing theories suggested that King's conceptual system (King, 1971, 1981, 1995) would provide a useful perspective to understand family health. The assumptions, concepts, and relationship among concepts in King's conceptual system are logically consistent with examining family health in the context of chronic illnesses such as COPD. The theory of family health within the context of COPD was formulated from King's concepts of perception, time, stress, and stressors. Each concept has been investigated in family caregiving research and to varying degrees found to be important across patient populations.

Influence of King's Framework

King's conceptual system influenced the development, theoretical definitions, and measures of key concepts and variables in the theory (Wicks, 1995). Optimizing family health, like individual health, is a key nursing function. King defined health as a process of continuous adjustment to internal and external environmental stressors through optimum resource use to achieve maximum potential for daily living (King, 1981). She also acknowledged that families require health for successful interpersonal and social role functioning and that culture influences health because social roles are embedded in cultural values and norms (King, 1981; Wicks, 1995). Because health is linked to functioning within King's framework, family functioning is an appropriate indicator of family health. King views families as social systems that translate cultural values and norms and interpersonal systems when the focus is on group interactions such as the patient–caregiver dyad. The theory of family health within the context of COPD specifically focuses on the patient–caregiver dyad as an interpersonal system. A true open systems perspective, however, recognizes that there are interactions among multiple systems. For example, other family members as personal systems influence patient–caregiver dyads or interpersonal systems that are also affected by social systems such as health care institutions. Thus, from King's perspective, the outcomes of patient–caregiver dyads within a systems perspective are linked to the dyad's interactions with personal, social, and other interpersonal systems. Consistent with this important point, the focus of this theory of family health is on the perceptions of personal systems such as patients and caregivers and interactions that occur within the patient–caregiver dyads as interpersonal systems. Accordingly, the logical congruence between this systems-based middle range theory and King's conceptual system supports the inclusion of patients and caregivers as well as families as the units of analyses (Wicks, 1995).

Description of the Theory of Family Health

Although the description and testing of the theory of family health has been reported in the literature (Wicks, 1995, 1997), both are briefly reviewed to give context to this discussion. The theory describes the factors associated with family health in the context of COPD. Concepts included in the theory are derived from King's personal and interpersonal systems. Perception and time are personal system concepts, whereas stress and stressors are derived from the interpersonal system. Variables derived from these concepts include patient and caregiver perceptions of symptom severity, time since diagnosis, caregiver stress, and family stressors. Family health is defined as family functioning. Empirical testing showed that patient and caregiver perceptions of symptom severity, time since diagnosis (duration of illness), caregiver stress, and family stressors influenced family health (Wicks, 1997).

Although families often adapt to patients' chronic illnesses, negative changes in health or functioning may occur. Whether families adapt to the illness may be linked to concomitant situational and developmental stressors such as deaths, births, child launching, and financial strain. Symptom progression over time likely contributes to stress for patients, caregivers, and the family system as a result of progressive patient dependence, loss of family resources, and altered emotional bonds. The theory of family health in the context of COPD acknowledges the importance of the perceptions

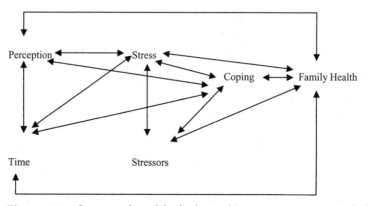

Figure 13.1. Conceptual model of relationships among concepts included in a study of family health in patients and family caregivers coping with the patient's chronic obstructive pulmonary disease.

Table 13.1. Summary of Theoretical Concepts, Variables, and Indicators

Concepts	Constructs	Variables	Empirical Indicators
Perception	Patient and caregiver perceptions	Patient and caregiver perceptions of patient's symptom severity	Bronchitis Emphysema Symptom Checklist
Time	Time since diagnosed	Time since diagnosis	Number of years with chronic obstructive pulmonary disease diagnosis
Stress	Caregiver stress	Subjective caregiver burden	Burden Interview
Stressors	Concurrent family stressors	Concurrent family stressors	Family Inventory of Life Events
Family health	Family health	Family functioning	Family Assessment Device

of caregivers and patients with regard to understanding family health. Figure 13.1 depicts the proposed concepts and relationships (Wicks, 1995). Perception of symptom severity, time since diagnosis, caregiver burden, and concurrent family stressors are independent variables and family health is the dependent variable. Table 13.1 provides a summary of concepts, constructs, variables, and indicators used to test the theory. Although King (personal communication, November 18, 1989) suggested that coping likely mediated the effects of these factors on family health, it was not measured in the original test of the formulation.

Many of the predictor variables were interrelated, with some predictor variables achieving correlations of .40 to .70 with other predictor variables. Within King's conceptual system are implicit as well as explicit statements indicating relationships among variables within and across the fluid boundaries of personal, interpersonal, and social systems as open systems (King, 1971, 1981, 1995). However, the direction and magnitude of these relationships are not specified, which is consistent with the nature of a conceptual frameworks (Fawcett, 2000) and the primary reason for theory testing in relation to specific clinical concerns and populations.

According to King (1983), stress is necessary for families to function in society. King (1981, 1983) suggests that the stressors (i.e., COPD and other concurrent family stressors), the time of the event (time since diagnosis), and individual perceptions (symptom severity) influence a family's stress response. King also contends that family members' perceptions of patients' illness are linked to the perceptions of the ill person (1983, p. 81). Thus, when there are disruptions in normal patterns of family interactions, family functioning is disrupted if resources and other coping mechanisms are inadequate. Some families may be significantly challenged by COPD as a situational stressor resulting in the need for professional support. Assessing family health provides important information about how families respond to catastrophic or stressful events and life changes (Bishop, Epstein, Keitner, Miller, & Srinivasan, 1986), such as the presence of a severe debilitating and progressive disease. COPD is a catastrophic disorder that alters the social, physical, and emotional functioning of individuals and has the potential to similarly affect family caregivers. Disease-related changes in interactions between the patient–caregiver dyad may alter family interactions such that family health or functioning is compromised. Chronic obstructive pulmonary disease is a disorder that progressively worsens over *time* and is associated with individual *stress*. The life-threatening and pervasive symptoms, progressive dysfunction and dependence, social isolation, unpredictable exacerbations, and impaired mood states associated with the disease act as situational *stressors*. These stressors likely affect family roles, communication, and behavior, which are key dimensions of *family health*. Thus, King's conceptual framework provides considerable direction for developing a theory of family health in the context of COPD.

Related Literature Supporting the Theory

Family caregivers could perceive chronic caregiving as an individual (personal) and family (interpersonal) system stressor with potentially positive consequences (Cohen, Colantonio, & Venich, 2002; Picot, 1995; Sterrit & Porkorny, 1998). For example, a positive consequence of chronic caregiving is the belief that caregiving is rewarding. Depression, anxiety, and subjective burden are negative consequences of chronic caregiving (Pearlin, Mullan, Semple, & Skaff, 1990; Picot, 1995). COPD potentially strains or strengthens marital relationships and interactions with children, other family members, and friends for the caregiver and patient. However, social withdrawal and resultant social isolation are common for patients with COPD, particularly if patients fear acquiring respiratory infections that further compromise their already challenged breathing. Depression and anxiety are also common in persons with COPD (Light et al., 1985; van Manen et al., 2002), which is further isolating. Caregivers are similarly affected. Researchers have found social isolation, anxiety, depression, and burden in family members of persons with COPD and other chronic diseases (Biegel, Sales, & Schulz, 1991; Braithwaite, 1996; Sexton & Munro, 1985; Teel, Duncan, & Lai, 2001). Russo and Vitaliano (1995) found that caregiver burden was significantly predicted by six concurrent family stressors or life events: being a victim of crime, experiencing age discrimination, having serious family arguments, a change in caregiver's health, trouble with Medicaid/Medicare or Social Security, and move to a retirement home. The move to a retirement home was the sole stressor associated with lower burden scores.

Several studies have targeted caregivers of persons with COPD (Cain & Wicks, 2000; Cossette & Levesque, 1993; Heru & Ryan, 2004; Kanervisto et al., 2003; Keel-Card, Foxall, & Barron, 1993; Sexton & Munro, 1985; Wicks, 1997). These studies demonstrated that wives experienced less life satisfaction and higher levels of subjective stress than comparison groups of noncaregivers. Greater subjective burden occurred in caregivers of patients with more frequent symptoms. Increased levels of subjective burden were associated with poorer general family health and family communication. Poor communication was one of the most impaired dimensions of family functioning in one study (Kanervisto et al., 2003). Moreover, family communication, particularly disagreements about communication, may be a significant and modifiable correlate of caregiver burden (Fried, Bradley, O'Leary, & Byers, 2005.). Family communication impairments have been identified in several small studies in other caregiver populations (Edwards & Forster, 1999; Payne, Smith, & Dean, 1999; Pecchioni, 2001; Zhang & Siminoff, 2003). None of the reviewed studies specifically examined the association between family communication and time since diagnosis, perception of illness severity, or concurrent family stressors. Thus, the associations among perception of illness severity, time since diagnosis, concurrent family stressors, caregiver stress, and family communication seemed warranted.

Initial Test of the Theory

Sample and procedure

The theory of family health was tested (Wicks, 1997) with a convenience sample of 140 patient–caregiver dyads coping with COPD. Participating caregivers were predominantly women (85%), White (84%), and the wives (65%) of men (78%) with COPD. Other caregivers included in the sample were husbands, daughters, sons, and other family members. Caregivers on average were 58.6 ± 13.64 (M ± SD) years of age and cared for patients who were diagnosed for 10.66 ± 8.80 years.

Measures

Each study instrument was selected because it was conceptually consistent with King's conceptual system. All study instruments and subscales had internal consistency reliabilities of .73 or greater in the study sample. Perception of symptom severity reflected the caregiver and patient's perception of symptom frequency and was measured using the Bronchitis Emphysema Symptom Checklist (BESC; Kinsman et al., 1983). The BESC is a 57-item self-report scale designed to elicit patient reports of 11 symptoms and experiences. Each symptom and experience reflected one subscale comprised of four to six items. Symptoms and experience assessed were dyspnea, fatigue, sleep difficulties, congestion, irritability, anxiety, decathexis, helplessness–hopelessness, poor memory, peripheral–sensory problems, and alienation. Subscale scores were used in the analysis. Instructions were changed, with permission from Kinsman et al., to elicit independent ratings of symptom frequency by the caregivers.

The Burden Interview (Zarit, Todd, & Zarit, 1980), completed by the caregiver, is a 22-item self-report measure that assesses caregiver stress. The instrument provides information on the subjective effects of caregiving. Likert-type scale item responses range from 0 (*never*) to 4 (*nearly always*) resulting in summative scores of 0 to 88 indicating low to high burden, respectively. Situational and family stressors were assessed using the 71-item Family Inventory of Life Events and Changes (FILE; McCubbin & Patterson, 1987). The FILE measures family stressors over the past year and was completed jointly by the patient–caregiver dyad. Respondents indicate either *yes* (1) or *no* (0) that an event occurred. Scoring reflects the sum of "yes" responses, with higher scores indicating more stressors. Family health was assessed with the Epstein, Baldwin, and Bishop (1981) Family Assessment Device, a 60-item self-report questionnaire that provides information regarding perceived family functioning. The instrument is based on the McMaster Model of family functioning, which indicates that families assist members with basic, developmental, and hazardous tasks. The six subscales included on the instrument and their respective numbers of items are as follows: problem solving (6), communication (9), roles (11), affective responsiveness (6), affective involvement (7), behavior control (9), and general functioning (12). The instrument has a family systems and transactional focus and includes communication, roles, behavior control, and problem solving as key concepts. Although neither health nor family health is specifically defined using these concepts within King's conceptual system, she made key statements suggesting the relevance of these concepts with regard to interpersonal systems such as families. Communication and roles are key interpersonal system variables, whereas problem solving and behavior are discussed in the context of communication and roles within her framework. King (1981) specifically asserted that *communication* is the vehicle by which human relations are developed and maintained and a fundamental process that facilitates ordered *functions* of human groups, such as families. Moreover, she asserted that all *behavior* is *communication* and *roles* are learned from *functioning* in social systems. Finally, she described transactions as goal-directed human behaviors and the process of interaction whereby persons communicate with the environment to achieve goals that are valued. Thus, problem solving is embedded in achieving goals because negotiation (i.e., problem solving) occurs as transactions are made to achieve shared goals. According to King, these transactions reduce *stress,* which could improve *health.* Thus, the FAD is derived from a conceptual formulation that shares key concepts with King's conceptual system. The general functioning subscale score of the FAD was used in the analysis. Time since diagnosis was quantified as patient-reported disease duration in years.

Analysis

Multiple regression analysis was used to determine the amount of variance explained by the proposed predictor variables. Although path analysis would have been a stronger analytic approach, it was not used because the sample size was less than the recommended 30 subjects per predictor variable suggested by Nunnally and Bernstein (1994). Although current modeling approaches permit the use of smaller samples, these approaches were not widely available when the original model was tested. Data were subjected to hierarchical multiple regression analysis. Time since diagnosis was entered into the regression analysis followed by symptoms, stressors, and stress (burden) scores, respectively. Because there were 22 possible symptoms (11 from both the caregivers and patients), symptoms were included in the regression equation if the bivariate correlation with family health approximated .30 or greater. This decision was critical because we found strong positive and significant correlations between and across patients' and caregivers' BESC (symptom) scores. Six symptom scores from patients and caregivers were entered into the analysis: patient perceived memory impairment, irritability, and alienation and caregiver-perceived patient irritability, alienation, and helplessness–hopelessness. Incremental increases in explained variance and level of significance were determined for each independent variable.

Results

Following regression diagnostics, multiple regression analysis indicated that 23% of the variance in general family health measured by the FAD was explained by time since diagnosis, perception of symptom severity, caregiver stress, and family stressors, $F(3) = 10.74$, $p = .001$. Patient perceived impaired memory remained in the model as the sole *symptom* significantly contributing to family health, $B = .33$, $SE = .21$, $t = 3.86$, $p = .0002$) along with subjective caregiver burden and concurrent family stressors. Time since diagnosis was not statistically significant at the .05 level. Impaired memory explained 13.9% of the variance in general family health, and concurrent family stressors explained 5.7% and subjective burden explained 3.7% of the variance. Regression diagnostics revealed significant multicollinearity in the original model, which included the six previously described patient and caregiver symptoms. Large correlation coefficients among symptom measures and suspicious variance inflation factor and variance proportion values suggested significant multicollinearity within the original model that was not present in the final model. Mean general family health scores were at the cut-off of normal ($M = 2.01$, $SD = .34$); however, 46% of the sample had unhealthy scores.

Significant bivariate associations among time since diagnosis and caregiver stress, symptom severity, and general family health were not found. There are several possible explanations for these unexpected findings: an unmeasured intervening variable may have suppressed these relationships, the predominantly male patient sample may have under-reported symptoms, and the symptom instrument did not fully capture symptom severity as it did not measure the intensity or intrusiveness of symptoms. The absence of significant relationships between time since diagnosis and family health may also in part reflect the use of a cross-sectional rather than longitudinal design. Moreover, time since diagnosis might not have been a significant predictor of family health because families may adapt to chronic illness over time. Zarit and colleagues (1986) found that caregivers of persons with Alzheimer's disease reported lower subjective caregiver burden scores over time. In contrast, Heru and Ryan (2004) reported that patterns of burden differed over 1 year by patient diagnosis in a sample that included caregivers of persons with major depressive disorder and bipolar depression. There may be critical time periods in the course of the disease that are more important predictors of family health than disease duration that were not captured in this cross sectional study. Overall, the findings suggest that the theory was partially supported by the data.

Reformulation and Retesting

We examined the amount of variance in family communication explained by time since diagnosis, perceived symptom severity, caregiver stress, and concurrent family stressors because King (1981) identified communication as a fundamental process that facilitates ordered *functions* of human groups like the family. This statement suggests that family communication is a relevant aspect of family health. Thus, we present the findings related to the degree to which the model explained family communication as dimension of family health. Mean family communication scores in this sample reflected the cutoff score for unhealthy communication, which is a score of 2.2. This finding is relevant because King asserted that it is difficult to stay healthy if information is withheld or inadequate (1981, p. 81). Moreover, nurses should assess communication between patients, their families, and self (p. 77) because communication is essential for effective care of patients. Communication between the family caregiver and patient would also be important to facilitate effective family caregiver administered care in the home environment. Thus, family communication was assessed using the communication subscale of the FAD. The scale includes nine items, which ask questions such as "when someone is upset others know why" and "people come right out and say things instead of hinting at them." Within this subscale, communication is defined as the exchange of information among individuals, which is consistent with King's definition of the concept. We have not previously published results of this regression analysis focused on family communication.

The formulation was retested using family communication as the dependent variable and time since diagnosis, perception of illness severity, subjective caregiver burden, and concurrent family stressors as predictor variables. We elected to limit symptoms used in this formulation to caregiver-perceived patient symptoms because we believed that their perceptions of the patient's symptoms were more likely predictive of caregiver perceptions of family communications. We previously reported that patient and caregiver perceptions of patient symptoms were not statistically significantly different for 7 of 11 symptoms (Wicks, 1997). Caregivers reported greater patient fatigue, irritability, helplessness–hopelessness, and alienation than reported by patients. Thus, no patient-perceived symptoms were included in this test of the model. Symptoms entered into this regression equation included caregiver-perceived patient dyspnea, congestion, helplessness–hopelessness, anxiety, and decathexis. Following regression diagnostics, caregiver perceived patient decathexis was the sole symptom remaining in the family communication model ($B = .82$, $SE = .26$, $t = 3.14$, $p = .08$). Findings indicated that 16% of the variance in family communication was explained by time since diagnosis, caregiver-perceived patient decathexis, caregiver stress, and family stressors, ($F(4) = 7.00$, $p < .0001$) for the entire sample ($N = 122$). Caregiver-perceived patient decathexis explained 6% of the variance, subjective caregiver burden explained 8%, and concurrent family stressors explained 2%. The contribution of time since diagnosis was not statistically significant at the .05 level, and decathexis approached significance ($p = .08$), while subjective caregiver burden and concurrent family stressors made significant contributions to the model ($p < .05$).

Analysis was then repeated using only responses of caregiver wives ($n = 72$) because several previous studies have suggested that kinship influences the caregiving experiences (McFall & Miller, 1992; Miller et al., 1991; Pruchno & Resch, 1989). In the wife-specific formulation, 17% of the variance ($F(4) = 4.65$, $p < .0022$) in family communication was explained. Perception of frequent patient decathexis approached significance ($B = .65$, $SE = .34$, $t = 1.94$, $p = .056$), and subjective caregiver burden significantly contributed to explained variance in family communication ($B = .007$, $SE = .003$, $t = 2.10$, $p = .04$). Time since diagnosis and concurrent family stressors, however, did not.

DISCUSSION

The findings of this study are important because they suggest that the proposed model has relevance for understanding general family functioning and family communication as dimensions of family health within the context of COPD. We previously reported our findings related to general family functioning; however, results related to family communication as an indicator of family health reflects an extension of our earlier work because these results have not been previously reported. Family communication was impaired in our study sample. King suggested that impaired communication is problematic because effective communication is necessary to achieve valued goals, such as the goal of staying healthy. King identified families as both interpersonal and social systems. A key responsibility of families as social systems is the transmission of social norms and values through communication, thus family communication has relevance within King's conceptual system. Other researchers have shown that family communication is associated with caregiver burden.

Our work supports this relationship and further shows that burden is correlated with both general family functioning and family communication as indicators of family health. Fried and colleagues (2005) have shown that a large proportion of caregivers of older persons coping with COPD, cancer, and congestive heart failure desired more frequent communication, reported communication difficulties, disagreed with the patient regarding the frequency of communication, and were significantly more burdened if they desired more frequent communication. Dissatisfaction with family communication reflects ineffective communication, which challenges the healthy functioning of social groups such as the family.

It is unclear whether King's framework supports the view that family communication is a dimension of family health. There are general statements within the discussion of interpersonal systems that provide some support for assessing family communication as a dimension of family health. King agreed with Kuhn, stating that "it would be difficult to achieve what one values, such as the goal to stay healthy, if information is withheld or inadequate" (1981, p. 81). Thus, inadequate information in the context of the family has the potential to influence family health and therefore family functioning, because communication is a fundamental social process that facilitates ordered functions of human groups (King, p. 83), such as the family.

All predictor variables except time since diagnosis were significantly correlated with both general family health and family communication. Although some predictor variables within the model failed to contribute significantly to the explained variance in family health and communication scores obtained by study participants, each model was significant. The lack of significance for some predictor variables may reflect methodological limitations related to sampling, instrumentation, and regression analysis procedures as well as the limited scope of the theory, as coping was not included in tests of the model. Each of these limitations along with strengths of the theory is discussed.

Strengths and Limitations of the Theory

This middle range theory of family health within the context of COPD was derived from a nursing conceptual framework, from published research, and from Wicks's clinical experiences with this population of patients and caregivers. Thus, both deductive and inductive processes were used to develop this theory of family health. The concepts perception, time, stress, stressors, and family health derived from King's conceptual system served as the organizing framework for this study. Model concepts were measured as perception of symptom severity, subjective caregiver stress or burden, concurrent family stressors, and general family functioning and family communication. Study findings provided support for the importance of variables derived from King's conceptual system with regard to explaining general family functioning as well as family communication as dimensions of family health in the context of COPD. Although each predictor variable did not significantly contribute to the family health and family communication models, most predictor variables were significantly correlated with the outcome variables and each model was statistically significant. Strengths of this theory include the significant associations among most predictor and outcome variables, the statistical significance of these theory-based models, and the congruence between the model concepts and King's conceptual system. There are five limitations associated with these tests of the theory: the small sample used to test the wife-specific model of family health; instrumentation issues, particularly with regard to the Bronchitis Emphysema Checklist, Family Inventory of Life Events and Changes, and the measurement of time since diagnosis; and the limited scope of the theory given that more than 70% of the variance in general family functioning and family communication scores was not explained by variables included in the theory as tested.

The power analysis performed before model testing suggested that we needed a minimum of 100 subjects to find an estimated explained variance of .30. Although the study was sufficiently powered to test both the general family health and family communication models for the entire sample of caregivers, the study was underpowered to assess the wife-specific multiple regression model of family health because only 76 wives were included in this analysis. This sample size is also less than the 20 subjects per predictor variable recommended by Tabachnick and Fidell (2000). The wife-specific test of the family communication model was significant despite this sampling limitation; however, the amount of explained variance was small. This small R^2 could reflect the generally moderate correlations found among predictor variables. It is uncommon to find predictor variables that are well correlated with the dependent variable but moderately associated with one another (Polit & Beck, 2004).

Time since diagnosis, perceived symptoms, and family stressors did not consistently and significantly contribute to the explained variance in general family health or family communication. As measured, time since diagnosis was not supported in either test of the theory, which suggests that as operationalized the concept of time was not relevant in the study population. The loss of *personal time,* which interferes in participation in hobbies and recreational activities, may be more important than the time since diagnosed. A loss in personal time significantly correlates with caregivers' emotional distress (Cameron, 2002) and may be associated with impaired family health.

Family stressors did not significantly contribute to family communication scores for the wife-specific formulation, perhaps because the measure of concurrent family stressors focused on the *number of stressors* patient–caregiver dyads reported rather than the *type of stressors* experienced by these families. Specific types of stressors have been shown to influence caregiver burden, and the same may be true for family communication (Russo & Vitaliano, 1995). For example, a negative change in caregiver health as a specific stressor may be more important than the total number of stressors experienced by the patient–caregiver dyad. Studies have shown that patients often avoid communication about issues of concern, in part to avoid emotional distress or if they have concerns about the patient's declining health. This pattern of communication may be worsened when caregivers and patients both have declining health. Caregivers in our sample were elderly, were sometimes frail, and many had multiple health problems.

Patient-perceived memory impairment was the sole symptom that explained a significant proportion of the variance in general family health. Although caregiver-perceived patient decathexis was included in the family communication model for the entire sample and wife-specific formulation, the contribution of this variable was not statistically significant. Both memory impairment and decathexis were measured using the BESC, which assesses symptom *frequency*. Perceived symptom severity is likely influenced by symptom frequency, intensity, and intrusiveness. Because of this limited focus on symptom frequency, the BESC was probably not an adequate indicator of perceived symptom severity.

Although each test of the model was statistically significant, explaining 16% to 23% of the variance in general family functioning and family communication scores, more than 70% of the variance in outcome scores was not explained. This is an important limitation, suggesting the need for further theory development.

Application of the Theory to Clinical Practice

This theory has relevance for practice because it can guide nurses to refocus their assessments to the patient–caregiver dyad rather than the patient alone. Specific interventions such as those that reduce burden, improve patient decathexis, and improve family functioning and communication could be beneficial.

Our study and two others specifically suggest that patient–caregiver dyads often experience impaired family health, particularly impaired communication (Heru & Ryan, 2004; Kanervisto et al., 2003). Although these impairments in family health cannot be directly attributed to the presence of the disease, COPD is probably an important stressor because of its progressively debilitating and frightening disease trajectory. Thus, nurses should consider the relevance of this disease for each patient–caregiver dyad as the presence of disease could be associated with impaired family functioning and family communication.

Theoretical relationships included within this family health theory could lead to nursing interventions focused on reducing burden because subjective caregiver burden significantly predicted this outcome. Moreover, caregiver burden also significantly predicted family communication. Previous research has shown that both group and individual interventions such as psychoeducational programs, support groups, counseling, and combined behavioral and cognitive educational programs can reduce subjective caregiver burden (Yin, Zhou, & Bashford, 2002). Reductions in burden as an indicator of caregiver stress could improve general family functioning and family communication.

Although caregiver-perceived patient decathexis approached significance in family communication models for the entire sample and wife caregivers, these symptoms were significantly correlated with family communication. Assessments should determine whether this perceived loss in the zest for life reflects patient depression. Clinical depression is common in persons who have COPD (Light et al., 1985; van Manen et al., 2002). Patients should be routinely evaluated for significant depressive symptoms because of this increased risk. Enhancing the mood of these patients through effective treatment, particularly if improved mood is perceived by the caregiver, could improve family communication in this population because social withdrawal often occurs in persons who are clinically depressed.

Recommendations for Future Testing and Theory Refinement

Although tests conducted to examine the statistical significance of this family health theory are promising, further testing is warranted. There is a need to explore whether specific types of concurrent family stressors are predictive of family communication because the number of stressors was not relevant in the wife-specific model. Moreover, time since diagnosis was not a relevant concept in the model; other time-related factors may be more relevant and should be explored. The time caregivers spend participating in personal interests or the time spent performing care-taking activities may be correlated with caregiver burden, family stressors, and family functioning.

Future development and testing of the theory should focus on more powerful statistical modeling strategies and the inclusion of a measure of coping; a more relevant measure of symptom severity that includes intensity, frequency, and/or symptom intrusiveness; and more relevant measures of time and concurrent family stressors in the model. The addition of these strategies might strengthen the explanatory power of the models. Also, the use of more powerful modeling approaches such as structural equation modeling could provide greater understanding of the causal patterns among predictor and outcome variables. These modeling approaches would help to determine the best fit between the model and the data. The hierarchical multiple regression approach that we used to test the model of family health and family communication may not have resulted in the best model for the data. In addition, testing the theory with other caregiver populations is appropriate because the theoretical concepts and relationships are relevant across caregiver populations. Finally, caregivers perceived that the patients in this study frequently seemed to have lost their interest in life. This disinterest could be a manifestation of depression, which is amenable to treatment. Future tests of the theory should determine whether depression, as an indicator of illness severity, exists in these patients and whether this depression is predictive of family functioning and family communication.

Summary

Middle range theory development significantly advances the knowledge of a discipline, transforms theories from an intellectual exercise to a useful way of understanding the phenomena of interest, and answers the questions relevant to a discipline (Liehr & Smith, 1999; Merton, 1968). In this middle range theory, a small but significant percent of the explained variance in general family functioning and family communication was predicted by perception, stress, and stressors but not by time. Although these findings are promising, further refinement and testing of the theory is warranted to optimize its explanatory power and therefore its relevance for nursing practice and research.

REFERENCES

American Association of Respiratory Care. (2002). AARC clinical practice guidelines. Pulmonary rehabilitation. *Respiratory Care, 47*, 617–625.

Biegel, D. E., Sales, E., & Schulz, R. (1991). *Family caregiving in chronic illness.* Newbury Park, CA: Sage.

Bishop, D. S., Epstein, N. B., Keitner, G. I., Miller, I. W., & Srinivasan, S. V. (1986). Stroke: Morale, family functioning, health status, and functional capacity. *Archives of Physical Medicine and Rehabilitation, 67*, 84–87.

Braithwaite, V. (1996). Between stressors and outcomes: Can we simplify caregiving process variables? *Gerontologist, 36*, 42–53.

Cain, C. J., & Wicks, M. N. (2000). Caregiver attributes as correlates of burden in family caregivers of persons with chronic obstructive pulmonary disease. *Journal of Family Nursing, 6,* 46–68.

Cameron, J. I., Franche, R. L., Cheun, A. M., & Stewart, D. E. (2002). Lifestyle inference and emotional distress in family caregivers of advanced cancer patients. *Cancer, 94,* 521–527.

Cohen, C. A., Colantonio, A., & Vernich, L. (2002). Positive aspects of caregiving: Rounding out the caregiver experience. *International Journal of Geriatric Psychiatry, 17,* 184–188.

Cossette, S., & Levesque, L. (1993). Caregiving tasks as predictors of mental health of wife caregivers of men with chronic obstructive pulmonary disease. *Research in Nursing and Health, 16,* 251–263.

Edwards, H., & Forster, E. (1999). Avoidance of issues in family caregiving. *Contemporary Nurse, 8,* 5–13.

Epstein, N. B., Baldwin, L. M., & Bishop, D. S. (1981). McMaster model of family functioning: A view of the normal family. In F. Walsh (Ed.), *Normal family process* (pp. 115–141). New York: Guilford Press.

Fahy, B. F. (2004). Pulmonary rehabilitation for chronic obstructive pulmonary disease: A scientific and political agenda. *Respiratory Care, 49,* 28–36.

Fawcett, J. (2000). *Analysis and evaluation of contemporary nursing knowledge: Nursing models and theories.* Philadelphia: Davis.

Ferrer, M., Alonso, J., Morera, J., Marrades, R. M., Khalaf, A., Aguar, M. C., et al. (1997). Chronic obstructive pulmonary disease stage and health-related quality of life. The Quality of Life of Chronic Obstructive Pulmonary Disease Group. *Annals of Internal Medicine, 127,* 1072–1079.

Fried, T. R., Bradley, E. H., O'Leary, J. R., & Byers, A. L. (2005). Unmet desire for caregiver–patient communication and increased caregiver burden. *Journal of the American Geriatric Society, 53,* 59–65.

Gavin, L. A., Wamboldt, M. Z., Sorokin, N., Levy, S. Y., & Wamboldt, F. S. (1999). Treatment alliance and its association with family functioning, adherence, and medical outcome in adolescents with severe, chronic asthma. *Journal of Pediatric Psychology, 24,* 355–65.

Heru, A. M., & Ryan, C. E. (2004). Burden, reward and family functioning of caregivers for relatives with mood disorders: 1-year follow-up. *Journal of Affective Disorders, 83,* 221–225.

Kanervisto, M., Paavilainen, E., & Astedt-Kurki, P. (2003). Impact of chronic obstructive pulmonary disease on family functioning. *Heart & Lung, 32,* 360–367.

Keel-Card, G., Foxall, M. J., & Barron, C. (1993). Loneliness, depression, and social support of patients with COPD and their spouses. *Public Health Nursing, 10,* 245–251.

King, I. M. (1971). *Toward a theory for nursing.* New York: Wiley.

King, I. M. (1981). *A theory for nursing: Systems, concepts, process.* New York: Wiley.

King, I. M. (1983). King's theory of nursing. In I. W. Clements & F. B. Roberts (Eds.), *Family health: A theoretical approach to nursing care* (pp. 178–188). New York: Wiley.

King, I. J. (1995). A systems framework for nursing. In M. A. Frey & C. L. Sieloff (Eds.), *Advancing King's framework and theory of nursing* (pp. 14–22). Thousand Oaks, CA: Sage.

Kinsman, R. A., Yaroush, R. A., Fernandez, E., Dirks, J. F., Schocket, M., & Fukuhara, J. (1983). Symptoms and experiences in chronic bronchitis and emphysema. *Chest, 8*, 755–761.

Leidy, N., & Haase, J. E. (1996). Functional performance in people with chronic obstructive pulmonary disease: A qualitative analysis. *Advances in Nursing Science, 18*, 77–89.

Liehr, P., & Smith, M. J. (1999). Middle range theory: Spinning research and practice to create knowledge for the new millennium. *Advances in Nursing Science, 21*, 81–91.

Light, R. W., Merrill, E. J., Despars, J. A., Gordon, G. H., & Mutalipassi, L. R. (1985). Prevalence of depression and anxiety in patients with COPD. Relationship to functional capacity, *Chest, 87*, 35–38.

McCubbin, H. I., & McCubbin, M. A. (1987). Family system assessment in health care. In H. I. McCubbin & A. I. Thompson (Eds.), *Family assessment inventories for research and practice* (pp. 53–78). Madison: University of Wisconsin Press.

McCubbin, H. I., & Patterson, J. M. (1987). FILE: Family inventory of life events and changes. In H. I. McCubbin & A. I. Thompson (Eds.), *Family assessment inventories for research and practice* (pp. 79–99). Madison: University of Wisconsin Press.

McFall, S., & Miller, B. H. (1992). Caregiver burden and nursing home admission of frail elderly persons. *Journal of Gerontology, 47*, S73–S79.

Merton, R. K. (1968). *Social theory and social structure*. New York: Free Press.

Meleis, A. (1997). *Theoretical nursing: Development and progress* (3rd ed.). Philadelphia: Saunders.

Miller, B., McFall, S., & Montgomery, A. (1991). The impact of elder health, caregiver involvement, and global stress on two dimensions of caregiver burden. *Journal of Gerontology, 46*, S9–19.

Murray, C. J., & Lopez, A. D. (1996). Evidence-based health policy—lessons from the Global Burden of Disease Study. *Science, 274*, 740–743.

Nunnally, J. C., & Bernstein, I. H. (1994). *Psychometric theory* (3rd ed.). New York: McGraw-Hill.

Pauwels, R. A., Buist, A. S., Calverlye, P. M., Jenkins, C. R., & Hurd, S. S. (2001). Global strategy for the diagnosis, management, and prevention of chronic obstructive pulmonary disease. NHLBI/WHO Global Initiative for Chronic Obstructive Lung Disease (GOLD) Workshop summary. *American Journal of Respiratory and Critical Care Medicine, 163*, 1256–1276.

Payne, S., Smith, P., & Dean, S. (1999). Identifying the concerns of informal carers in palliative care. *Palliative Medicine, 13*, 37–44.

Pearlin, L. I., Mullan, J. T., Semple, S. J., & Skaff, M. M. (1990). Caregiving and the stress process: An overview of concepts and their measures. *The Gerontologist, 30*, 583–94.

Pecchioni, L. L. (2001). Implicit decision-making in family caregiving. *Journal of Social and Personal Relationships, 18*, 219–237.

Penrod, J. D., Kane, R. L., Finch, M. D., & Kane, R. A. (1998). Effects of post-hospital Medicare home health and informal care on patient functional status. *Health Services Research, 33,* 513–529.

Picot, S. J. (1995). Rewards, costs, and coping of African American caregivers. *Nursing Research, 44,* 147–152.

Polit, D. F., & Beck, C. T. (2004). *Nursing research: Principles and methods.* Philadelphia: Lippincott, Williams, & Wilkins.

Pruchno, R. A., & Resch, N. L. (1989). Husbands and wives as caregivers: Antecedents of depression and burden. *The Gerontologist, 29,* 159–165.

Russo, J., & Vitaliano, P. P. (1995). Life events as correlates of burden in spouse caregivers of persons with Alzheimer's disease. *Experimental Aging Research, 21,* 273–294.

Sexton, D. L., & Munro, B. H. (1985). Impact of a husband's chronic illness (COPD) on the spouse's life. *Research in Nursing and Health, 8,* 83–90.

Smith, M., & Liehr, P. R. (2004). *Middle range theory for nursing.* New York: Springer Publishing Company.

Spieth, L. E., Stark, L. J., Mitchell, M. J., Schiller, M., Cohen, L. L., Mulvihill, M., et al. (2001). Observational assessment of family functioning at mealtime in preschool children with cystic fibrosis. *Journal of Pediatric Psychology, 26,* 215–224.

Sterritt, P. F., & Porkorny, M. E. (1998). African American caregiving for a relative with Alzheimer's disease. *Geriatric Nursing, 19,* 127–128, 133–134.

Tabachnick, B. G., & Fidell, L. S. (2000). *Using multivariate statistics* (4th ed.). New York: Harcourt College.

Teel, C. S., Duncan, P., & Lai, S. M. (2001). Caregiving experiences after stroke. *Nursing Research, 50,* 53–60.

van Manen, J. G., Bindels, P. J., Dekker, F. W., IJzermans, C. J., van der Zee, J. S., & Schade, E. (2002). Risk of depression in patients with chronic obstructive pulmonary disease and its determinants. *Thorax, 57,* 412–416.

Venters, M. (1981). Familial coping with chronic and severe childhood illness: The case of cystic fibrosis. *Social Science and Medicine, 15,* 289–297.

Voelkel, N. F. (2000). Raising awareness of COPD in primary care. *Chest, 117,* 372S–375S.

Westley, W. A., & Epstein, N. B. (1969). *The silent majority.* San Francisco: Jossey-Boss.

Wicks, M. N. (1992). *Family health in chronic illness.* (Doctoral dissertation, Wayne State University, 1992.) *University of Michigan Dissertation Services,* No. 9310756.

Wicks, M. N. (1995). Family health as derived from King's framework. In M. A. Frey & C. L. Sieloff (Eds.), *Advancing King's framework and theory of nursing* (pp. 97–108). Thousand Oaks, CA: Sage.

Wicks, M. N. (1997). Test of the Wicks family health model in families coping with chronic obstructive pulmonary disease. *Journal of Family Nursing, 2,* 189–212.

Wouters E. F., Creutzberg, E. C., & Schols, A. M. (2002). Systemic effects in COPD. *Chest, 121*(Suppl. 5), 127S–130S.

Yin, T., Zhou, Q., & Bashford, C. (2002). Burden on family members: Caring for frail elderly: A meta-analysis of interventions. *Nursing Research, 51,* 199–208.

Zhang, A. Y., & Siminoff, L. A. (2003). Silence and cancer: Why do families and patients fail to communicate? *Health Communication, 15,* 415–429.

Zarit, S. H., Todd, P. A., & Zarit, J. M. (1986). Subjective burden of husbands and wives as caregivers: A longitudinal study. *The Gerontologist, 26,* 260–266.

Theory of Social and Interpersonal Influences on Health

Tamara L. Zurakowski

Nearly 5% of all older adults and more than 18% of those aged over 85 years live in nursing homes (Administration on Aging, 2003). These numbers are somewhat misleading, however, because persons aged 65 and over have a lifetime probability of 44% of spending at least some time in a nursing home (Congressional Budget Office, 2004). The number of older adults who will be affected by nursing homes is huge and will grow larger as the baby boomers enter old age and experience the concomitant higher risk for health problems. A large portion of the services provided by long-term care facilities is nursing; hence, nurses must have the knowledge and skills that will allow institutionalized elders to enjoy optimal levels of health and well-being.

THE EFFECTS OF NURSING HOMES ON OLDER ADULTS

Nursing homes are intended to be therapeutic, supportive environments for older adults, yet research has consistently demonstrated that not all residents do well in them, particularly during relocation (Borup, Gallego, & Hefferman, 1980; Schulz & Brenner, 1977; Tobin & Lieberman, 1976). Nurses view admission to a nursing home as a stressor (Johnson & Tripp-Reimer, 2001; Kaisik & Cieslowski, 1996), and evidence supports this as a transcultural phenomenon (Johnson & Tripp-Reimer, 2001; Lee, Woo, & Mackenzie, 2002). Placement in a nursing home has even been likened to homelessness, with elders experiencing overwhelming loss of meaning in their lives (Carboni, 1990).

Some residents, on the other hand, thrive in the new environment. Older adults who participate in the decision to relocate demonstrate lower levels of morbidity and mortality (Davis, 1990), even though a full one third of elders say they were not involved in the decision to move (Reinardy, 1995). Various interventions have been made in an attempt to lessen the trauma of entering long-term care, including stress inoculation (Kaisik & Cieslowitz, 1996), provision of information (Johnson & Tripp-Reimer, 2001), social and instrumental support from caregivers (Patterson, 1995), strengthening the relationship between long-term care residents and their environments (Carboni, 1990), and including the older adult in the decision-making process (Reinardy, 1995). The effectiveness of these interventions have had mixed results, thus the problem of how and why some elders fare poorly in long-term care facilities remains. King's conceptual system (1981) provides a powerful framework for identifying the factors that influence the health status of older residents in either positive or negative ways. This framework, with its four universal ideas of social systems, health, perception, and interpersonal relationships (Fawcett, 2001) is ideally suited for considering the social system of the nursing home, the residents that live there, and how these interact to influence human health. The comprehensiveness of the three interacting systems guides the nurse to consider a wide range of causative and curative factors within the older adults, as well as in the social and physical environments (King, 1994, 1997). The use of a conceptual model of nursing helps ensure that a nursing perspective is brought to bear on the concerns of elders in long-term care and further assists nurses to identify their unique contributions (King, 2000; Gold, Haas, & King, 2000). This chapter explicates a middle range theory related to the roles of social support and the social environment of the nursing home as they affect the health of residents.

THEORY DEVELOPMENT APPROACH

General Approach

The deductive approach to theory development starts with an abstract set of relationships among concepts (Chinn & Kramer, 1999). Less abstract concepts are derived, bringing the relationships closer to phenomena that may be observed in the real world. If the theory is to be empirically tested, empiric indicators are selected for the concepts and a research methodology for testing relationships is selected. Concept analysis and clarification are critical steps in the process, particularly when dealing with abstract concepts, or constructs, such as the three interacting systems included in King's conceptual system. Each of the interacting systems includes many concepts. Within the interpersonal system are concepts that help explain interactions among two or more people, such as communication, interaction, stress, role, and transaction (King, 1995). The social system comprises decision making, organization, power, authority, and status—concepts that help explain the nature of large systems (King, 1995), such as health care institutions, both acute and long-term.

Social system

In the study described here, the social system of interest is the nursing home. Nursing homes are complex entities with a multitude of operant forces (Anderson, Issel, & McDaniel, 2003). The work of Emile Durkheim (1893/1933, 1897/1951) and the idea of anomie as a social factor that influences many aspects of human behavior are intriguing. Anomie is a lack of adequate social regulation. In Durkheim's conceptualization, regulation is an agreement among all members of a society, in which the expectations and prescribed manners of behaving are clearly delineated. Merton (1957) expanded the concept to include situations in which socially sanctioned goals are unattainable in socially approved ways, and Dudley (1978) added the presence of multiple normative systems as another aspect of anomie. Anomie, therefore, may be defined as a lack of clear, congruent, and predictable norms for daily life.

Some mistakenly define anomie as normlessness, but this is inaccurate. Durkheim (1897/1951) stated that anomie may be caused by anything that causes readjustment of the social order. This description seemed consonant with the literature on relocation to long-term care facilities, in which nursing home residents describe moving to a nursing home as becoming "homeless" (Carboni, 1990), traumatic (Tobin & Lieberman, 1976), and stressful (Patterson, 1995). New residents seem to face a total readjustment of their social order. Nursing home residents are faced with multiple informal rules, which may be contradictory to each other (Bennett & Nahemow, 1965) and may leave the resident feeling that the whole social environment is unintelligible. Anomie was selected as a concept, within the social system of the nursing home, to be studied in relationship to the personal and interpersonal systems of the residents. It is an indicator of the social organization of the nursing home and, viewed within King's concept of organization, a goal-directed system (King, 1981).

Interpersonal system

Interpersonal systems are also complex, with many applicable concepts. King (1981) identified interaction, communication, and coping as salient concepts. These concepts are also linked in the literature on social support. Social support is an asset in coping, in that social support helps the individual to deal with stressors. It is based on communication between the individual and others, and provides for interaction among the individual and people in the social environment. Social support provides for an individual's needs for intimacy, social integration, nurturing of others, reassurance of personal worth, steady source of alliance, and guidance (Weiss, 1969, 1974). It may have an important role in attenuating anomia by providing normative information (Moss, 1973). The role of social support in health is well accepted and has been found to be positively related to a number of health outcomes in the elderly (Johnson, 1998; Kim, 1999; Nicholas & Leuner, 1999; Ryan, 1998). Social support is viewed as being an indicator of King's concept of interaction.

Personal system

Humans, the recipients of nursing care, and their behavior, form the basis of King's (1995) conceptual system. Health is an outcome of the person's interactions with the environment (King, 1981), within a particular cultural and value system (Winker, 1995). This is a critical distinction—health is intimately tied to the social system that encodes values, norms, and beliefs. Winker elegantly phrased it thus: "health is defined as the ability of the individual to create meaningful symbols based on either biological or human values within his or her cultural and individual value systems" (1995, p. 42).

Health will change, or be affected by, the various contexts in which people find themselves. Furthermore, health is an intensely personal concept, and individuals may (will) define it for themselves and in a manner that may not coincide with professional appraisals of health. Nursing acts, however, are directed toward health (King, 1999).

Tobin and Lieberman (1976) and Chenitz (1983), among many others, asserted that admission to a nursing home requires constant adaptation by the resident. Older adults who do not "adapt" manifest a wide variety of negative outcomes, including withdrawal, hopelessness, abuse of staff, and refusal to accept assistance (Chenitz, 1983). These behaviors may be viewed as antithetical to any definition of health.

The theory derived from King's conceptual system seeks to explain the health of older residents of nursing homes as a function of the degree of anomie in the resident's interaction with the social system of the nursing home and the social support provided within the interpersonal system.

REVIEW OF THE LITERATURE

The Nursing Home as a Social System

Goffman (1961) was arguably the first researcher to study the nursing home as a context for aging adults. Tobin and Lieberman (1976) and Gubrium (1975) followed with their detailed accounts of life in a nursing home. It is noteworthy that so many scholars continue to cite these works, supporting the view of the nursing home as overwhelmingly negative. More recent conceptualizations, however, have identified nursing homes as complex systems, including positive *and* negative influences on residents (Anderson et al., 2003; Cox, 2003; Rantz et al., 1999; Riggs & Rantz, 2001). Berdes (2001) even suggested that the totality of the institution is on a continuum with *community,* a positively valued concept.

The management styles employed in the facilities are a factor in the social system of the nursing home, affecting both staff and resident outcomes (Anderson et al., 2003; Riggs & Rantz, 2001). The administrative staff and the management strategies they select create a system that supports (or inhibits) the staff behaviors that ultimately lead to selected resident outcomes.

Families are also an integral part of the nursing home social system and affect the staff and residents, even as the staff and residents affect the families (Rantz et al., 1999). These interactions are complicated by the fact that families and staff members have different expectations of the long-term facility, with families particularly valuing skilled and compassionate staff and quality care (Rantz et al., 1999).

One aspect of quality care is a recognition of the nursing home as being a home. Families described homelike feelings, privacy, and spaces for personal belongings as important to creating a home in a long-term care setting. This is a particularly salient finding when compared with Carboni's (1990) finding that nursing home residents consider themselves to be homeless and feel dependent and powerless, without decision-making ability.

Anomie and Anomia

Durkheim (1897/1951) empirically demonstrated that when the social order was disrupted, such as in financial upheavals, suicide rates increase. He attributed the suicides to anomie, when social life becomes unpredictable and therefore unbearable. Later researchers have linked anomie with psychiatric impairment (Srole, 1956) and hypertension (Walsh, 1980). Freidl (1997) studied a sample of Austrian adults and confirmed Durkheim's original assertion that anomie was inversely correlated with social connectedness, emotional support, and levels of education. Anomia was demonstrated to be a mediating variable among the variables of education, social connectedness, daily hassles, and emotional support, and the outcome variables of psychological quality of life and psychosomatic symptoms. Keyes (1998) also empirically validated Durkheim's study, linking social well-being with social integration, contribution, coherence, actualization, and acceptance.

Studies of anomia or anomie in older adults have tended to support Durkheim's early work. Widows and widowers were demonstrated to have higher levels of anomie than their married counterparts, and anomie levels rose with age (Wenz, 1977). Leonard (1977) hypothesized that the reason older adults are more anomic than younger adults is that they are blocked from societal goals. He supported the hypothesis in a study of middle-aged and older adults. Hendrick, Wells, and Faletti (1982) demonstrated that older Floridians living in "nonnormative" housing units were more anomic than those who lived in retirement complexes or who stayed in their preretirement homes.

Social Support and Older Adults

Social support has been positively linked to a number of health-related variables in the general population, as well as in older adults (Johnson, 1998; Kim, 1999; Nicholas & Leuner, 1999). Elders with higher levels of social support enjoy better psychological health and rate their own health as higher than their peers with lower levels of social support (Grundy & Sloggett, 2003). Bisconti and Bergeman (1999) examined the relationship among social support, social control, well-being, and self-reported health. The nature of the relationship was complex, and social control mediated the relationship between social support and health. In other words, having support is not sufficient to improve outcome; the older adult must have some control over the nature of the social interaction. The benefits of social support are most evident in the presence of a stressor, with stressed older adults with social support faring far better than those without social support (Johnson, 1998).

Social support for institutionalized older adults differed somewhat from that for community-dwelling elders. Sources of support in the nursing home include nursing staff, family members, other residents, and "others," such as housekeepers, dietary workers, therapists, and the family members of other residents (Patterson, 1995). Consistent with the findings of Bisconti and Bergeman (1999), not all behaviors are supportive, and residents are able to separate out the helpful from the nonhelpful. Length of stay in the nursing home did not change the types of support needed or provided but did alter the source of the support. Residents who had lived in the facility longer received more support from other residents than did newcomers.

DERIVATION OF A THEORY OF SOCIAL AND INTERPERSONAL INFLUENCES ON THE HEALTH OF ELDERLY NURSING HOME RESIDENTS

The theory of social and interpersonal influences on health (TSIIH) is a middle range theory that explains the relationships among anomie, social support, and health. The population of interest in this chapter is older adult residents of nursing homes, although the theory might also be used to examine health in other populations.

The literature related to the health of older adult residents of nursing homes was reviewed, and concepts that both demonstrated empirical connections to health and were consistent with King's conceptual system were selected. King's conceptual system was used as the overarching framework for understanding how the interpersonal and social system might affect the health of nursing home residents. The concepts found in the literature review were compared with those described by King, seeking conceptual fit and congruence. The interacting systems held forth the potential to explain and include the disparate research findings about older adults and their health status within nursing homes.

Social support and anomie are variables from the social and interpersonal systems that have theoretical and empirical effects on health. Anomie is an indicator of the organization of the nursing home, specifically how clear, congruent, and predictable the norms for behavior for residents are. Social support is an indicator of the interaction within the interpersonal system, providing a resident with a sense of belonging, integration, and a source of guidance and assistance. King's conceptual system is a powerful model for framing the relationships among the three levels of human systems. Exploration of the nature of the influences the social and interpersonal systems on health may lead to nursing interventions at either an interpersonal or social system level by strengthening social support or helping individuals understand the social environment of the nursing home. The purpose of this study, therefore, was to test a theory (TSIIH) that conceptually links anomie, social support, and health status in elderly nursing home residents. The theory was tested in its entirety for its fit to the data, using path analysis. The theory is displayed graphically in a path model in Figure 14.1. The relationships among the systems concepts, theory concepts, and empirical indicators are contained in Table 14.1.

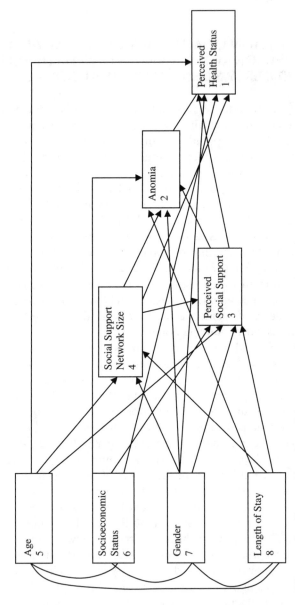

Figure 14.1. Proposed path model.

Table 14.1. Relationships Among Conceptual System and Theory Concepts, and Empirical Indicators

Conceptual system level	Social system	Interpersonal system	Interpersonal system	Personal system
Conceptual system concepts	Organization	Interaction	Interaction	Health
Theory concepts	Anomie	Social support	Social support	Perceived health status
Empirical indicators[a]	McCloskey and Schaar Anomy Scale (.70)	Network site	Weiner and Brandt PRQ, Part II (.84)	Cantril's Self Anchoring Ladders (.62)

Note. PRQ = Personal Resource Questionnaire.
[a] Figures in parentheses are Cronbach's alpha as calculated for this sample.

Method

Sample

A convenience sample of 91 residents of four nursing homes was obtained. All residents in each institution who were deemed by nursing staff to be sufficiently oriented to participate in the study were approached. Each potential subject was screened with the Short Portable Mental Status Questionnaire (Pfeiffer, 1975) and only those who scored as "intact" or "mildly impaired" were included. It was further stipulated that potential subjects had to speak English. Only White residents were solicited, because race is theoretically a factor in anomie (Srole, 1956). The sample consisted of 72 women (79.1%) and 19 men (20.9%). Their ages ranged from 42 to 99 years ($M = 79.4$ years, $SD = 16.22$). The residents had lived at their respective nursing homes an average of 2.5 years ($SD = 2.42$) and had a mean socioeconomic indicator (Hollingshead, 1957) of 3.49 ($SD = 1.021$), with 1 as the highest socioeconomic group and 5 as the lowest. Nearly 60% of the sample was widowed.

The sample was 79% female, average age was 79.4 years, and participants had been in residence at the nursing home for an average of 2.47 years. Compared with the national nursing home population (U.S. Department of Health and Human Services, 1989), this sample was not significantly different in terms of sex ($\chi^2 = 1.62$, $df = 1$, ns), age distribution ($\chi^2 = 3.24$, $df = 3$, ns), or length of stay ($\chi^2 = 4.96$, $df = 5$, ns). The exclusion of minority residents and moderately or severely cognitively impaired residents does make this sample significantly different from the national nursing home population. Measurement of functional status, using the Barthel Index (Mahoney & Barthel, 1965), indicated that most study participants were dependent in two or more activities of daily living (ADLs). The Barthel Index of ADL performance assesses feeding, transfer, grooming, toileting, bathing, ambulation, stair climbing, dressing, bowel continence, and bladder continence. The subject is given a score of 0 for *complete dependence* in ADLs, 5 for *partial independence,* and 10 for complete independence. The summed score, then, is from 0 to 100, with a mean in this sample of 49.6.

Procedures

Data were collected by graduate students in nursing, using a standard interview schedule. Each data collector had a list of those residents whom the nursing staff had identified as sufficiently oriented to participate. The study was explained, and verbal consent was obtained. Each participant was given a copy of the consent document. After consent was given, the potential subject was screened for cognitive intactness using the SPMSQ (Pfeiffer, 1975). If the resident met the requirement of fewer than five errors, the interview continued. The interview schedule contained measures of health status, social support, anomie, and demographic information. Measures are described in greater detail, below (see also Table 14.1). Standardized prompts were used when subjects had difficulty responding. For example, if a subject had difficulty answering the 3-point Likert scale, the interviewer asked: "Do you agree, or disagree, or have no opinion?" Prompts were printed on the interview schedule, so all interviewers used the same wording.

Measures

Health status was measured subjectively. Cantril (1965) ladders were used, and each question corresponded to a ladder with lowest, intermediate, and highest rung labeled with descriptive phrases. There were 10 rungs, and each was labeled with a number, from 1 to 10. Subjects were asked to rate their responses to the following questions: "How would you rate your health at the present time?," "How concerned do you feel about your health problems?" and "How much do your health troubles stand in the way of your doing the things you want to do?" (Fillenbaum, 1979). The score was calculated by averaging across the three ladders, yielding potential scores of 1 to 10. The Cantril ladder, combined with the language described, was selected because of King's (1981) assertion that individuals perceive their own health differently than others do. A self-appraisal, then, seems critical to measuring health within King's conceptual system. Winker (1995) stated that health within the conceptual system is defined as "the ability of the individual to create meaningful symbols based on either biological or human values within his or her cultural and individual value system" (p. 42), validating the self-appraisal approach. The Cronbach's alpha in this sample was .62.

Social support was measured in two ways: (a) quantitatively by ascertaining network size and (b) qualitatively by measuring the perception of social support. Subjects were asked to identify the size of their social support network by listing all significant persons in their life, after being given a list of types of resource persons (friend, relative, etc.). The measure of perceived social support was derived from the Personal Resource Questionnaire (PRQ), Part II (Brandt & Weinert, 1985). The original instrument consists of 25 statements responded to on 7-point Likert-type scales. A pilot study demonstrated that even cognitively intact elders had difficulty using these scales. Therefore, with permission of the authors (C. Weinert, personal communication, June 14, 1988), the statements were used with 3-point Likert scales (*agree, neutral, disagree*). The possible scores on the derived instrument ranged from 25 to 75, with 75 indicating the highest level of perceived social support. The instrument asked for the subject's perception of social supportive, compatible with King's emphasis on perception of social forces (King, 1981). It was validated with older adults by comparing scores on the PRQ, Part II, with those on measures of marital adjustment and family functioning (Weinert, 1985). Reliability in this sample was measured with Cronbach's alpha and equaled .84.

Anomie was assessed using the McClosky and Schaar Anomy Scale (McClosky & Schaar, 1965). Subjects responded to the nine statements in the scale with the same 3-point Likert scale described earlier. The Anomy Scale measured moral emptiness, wandering without clear rules, and without stable moral and normative moorings. Possible scores ranged from 9 to 27, with higher scores indicating higher levels of anomie. The Anomy Scale is compatible with King's description of the individual's perception of the organization in the social system. The instrument was originally validated on large national samples and was found to be unidimensional (Moore, 1980). In this sample, the Cronbach's alpha was .70.

Demographic data were collected from the face sheet in the subject's nursing home record, as well as through direct questions. Information gathered included gender, age, date of moving to the nursing home, marital status, highest level of education achieved, and usual career (or that of spouse, if subject was not employed).

Data Analysis

Data were analyzed using path analysis based on multiple regression analyses. Path coefficients were estimated with standardized regression coefficients and tested for significance. The statistical assumptions of path analysis were tested, and the only violation uncovered was that of measurement without error (Pedhazur, 1982). Two conceptual assumptions, however, are made in path analysis: Variables are related to each other in a causal relationship, and the relationships are recursive (unidirectional). These assumptions are discussed in more detail later in the chapter.

Path analysis is a statistical method for examining the relationship between a proposed theory and the data (Pedhazur, 1982). It also allows the investigator to determine direct and indirect paths among variables. As a multiple regression technique, sample size is determined based on power. The sample size of 91 was based on a desired level of power of .8 and anticipated moderate effect sizes.

RESULTS

As noted earlier, the sample was 79% female, average age was 79.4 years (range 42–99), and participants had been in residence at the nursing home for an average of 2.47 years (range, < 3 months to > 5 years, SD = 2.43 years). Although range was concatenated because of the eligibility requirements for the study, 62% were cognitively intact (as measured by the SPMSQ), and 38% were mildly cognitively impaired. Fifty-nine percent of the sample was widowed, and 86% were in the working or middle class, as determined by the Hollinsghead two-factor index of social position (Hollingshead, 1957). The mean perceived health status score was 4.8 (SD 2.2), slightly lower than the ladder rung labeled "average," with modes at 3.5 and 6.0. Eighty-six percent were not independent in bathing, 73.6% were not independent in personal grooming, and one third required at least some help with every ADL. The scores on the Anomy Scale in this sample included 34% in the low anomy range, 37% in medium anomy, and 29% in high anomy. The average social network size was 3.7 (SD = 2.4) and had a relatively high perception of their social support (M = 59.2, range 25–75, SD = 10.5).

Path Model

The path model tested has R^2 of .16 (adjusted R^2 = .09), which is statistically significant at p = .03. This indicates that 9% of the variance in health status was explained by the model and that the path coefficients may be interpreted with confidence. The calculated level of power is .81, indicating the results may be interpreted with less than a 20% chance of Type II error. The Q statistic was .95 (p < .30), indicating that the model does fit the data in comparison to a fully saturated model (i.e., no other paths should be added to the model).

Table 14.2. Path Coefficients, Predicted Directions, and p Values

Path Coefficient (standardized)		Predicted Direction	Significance
P_{12}	.22		.03
P_{13}	.21	+	.03
P_{23}	−.14		.10
P_{14}	.11	+	.30[a]
P_{24}	−.17		.06
P_{34}	.25	+	.01
P_{15}	−.11		.14
P_{35}	.00		.93[a]
P_{45}	.03		.79[a]
P_{16}	−.12[b]	+[b]	.15
P_{26}	.19[b]	−[b]	.04
P_{36}	−.11[b]	−[b]	.31[a]
P_{17}	.16	+	.07
P_{27}	.03	+	.39
P_{37}	−.27	+	.01[a]
P_{47}	−.09	+	.37[a]
P_{28}	.05		−.67[a]
P_{38}	.11	+	.13
P_{48}	−.03	+	.76[a]

[a] Two-tailed p values; all others are one-tailed.
[b] Socioeconomic status (SES) was coded in such a way that a low number corresponds to a high SES group. Therefore, signs that are opposite of the predicted direction are actually congruent with the prediction.

Path coefficients were tested for significance using one-tailed significance tests because the paths were hypothesized to be unidirectional. Alpha levels of .05 and .10 were used because the study was perceived to be at an early stage of theory development. The supported path model is depicted in Figure 14.2; path coefficients, predicted directions, and p values are shown in Table 14.2.

FINDINGS RELATED TO DEVELOPMENT OF THE TSIIH

The TSIIH proposed that factors in the interpersonal and social systems—namely, anomie and social support—would affect the personal system, that is, health. The model that was tested was conceptually derived from King's conceptual system, as descried earlier. Path analysis was chosen for statistical analysis of the data because of its ability to test empirically a model derived from a theory (Asher, 1983; Kerlinger and Pedhazur, 1973) to provide theoretical clarification (Cook & Campbell, 1973) or to examine the logical consequences of the model being tested (Kim & Kohut, 1975). (Note that, in this section, *model* is used in its statistical

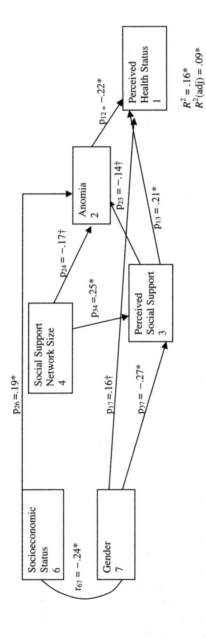

*The variables that did not demonstrate significant path coefficients have been deleted.

Figure 14.2. Supported path model. *Significant at $p < .05$ † Significant at $p < .10$

sense). Examination of the direction and statistical significance of the relationships among variables allows the investigator to evaluate whether the data support the theory. One of the main advantages of path analysis is the opportunity to delineate direct and indirect effects, as well as simple and compound links among concepts (Asher, 1983; Pedhazur, 1982). To put it simply, path analysis allows the theorist to see whether the theory fits the data and vice versa.

In general, the data supported the TSIIH. Using perceived social support, as measured by the PRQ, Part II, the concepts derived from the interpersonal system (social support) and social system (anomie) did, in fact, influence health. Furthermore, the interpersonal and social systems interact, with social support affecting anomie, as would be predicted from King's conceptual system. Theoretically, health would also affect social support and anomie, but path analysis did not allow testing of this relationship. Demographic factors reflect the social system-specific valuing of them, such as "isms" related to gender and social status in the wider society. Accordingly, their influence on health were also manifested as predicted.

Developing theory using empirical methods, however, is not without its problems. The assumptions of King's conceptual system are at variance with some of the assumptions of path analysis. The assumptions are discussed in detail, below. Suffice it to say here that the results of a path analysis are but one of the criteria used in evaluating the soundness of a developed theory.

STRENGTHS AND LIMITATIONS

The derived theory was partially supported in that testing more paths (in a fully saturated model) would not have yielded more explained variance. The theory, therefore, should not have included any further relationships among concepts.

Path analysis assumes that the relationships among variables are causal, additive, and recursive. King's conceptual system specifies that systems are open (King, 1981), suggesting that relationships among concepts might be nonrecursive, or bidirectional. The statistical method, then, may be inappropriate for use with King's model. Other techniques, such as LISREL, which can accommodate nonrecursivity, might be a better choice. Furthermore, this study employed a cross-sectional design, whereas King's model is dynamic. This may also contribute to the findings of this study.

Measurement is another source of concern in this study. The reliability coefficients, although respectable, are far from perfect. The amount of error introduced through instrumentation may have had an impact on the results.

The measures chosen may also have contributed errors by the manner in which they were conceptualized. The PRQ (Brandt & Weiner, 1985), which provided the basis for the instrument used in this study, is based on Weiss's (1969, 1974) work, which proposes six aspects of social support. The PRQ measures all six aspects, but it is possible that not all six are operant in the interpersonal system of nursing home residents or that not all six are important to health outcomes. It is also true that King (1981) did not specify provisions of social support nor how it affects health outcomes. Perhaps social support would be more accurately defined in this model as buffering the effects of stress, if stress were viewed as a force in either the social system of the nursing home or the interpersonal system. Health would then be viewed as the outcome of interactions between the interpersonal and social systems (i.e., stress and social support).

The expected link between anomie and health status was statistically significant, but the path coefficient was not large. The preponderance of theoretical and empirical evidence of the effects of anomie on health status in previous works (Durkheim, 1897/1951; Freidl, 1997; Srole, 1956; Walsh, 1980) leads one to consider a measurement problem in this study, which is then related to an underlying theoretical problem. The scale used in this study to measure anomie was not developed for use with institutionalized persons and therefore challenges the validity of its use in such populations. The questions, on reexamination, appeared to tap anomie as it is related to macrosociety, or the world outside the nursing home. For example, the stems of several questions included the phrase *in the world* or asked the respondent to comment on the pervasiveness of selected social values. This may not be nearly as important to the nursing home resident as anomie related to the microsociety of the nursing home.

The anomie instrument used in this study does not appear to address issues of microsocietal forces. King (1981) described social systems of varying sizes, each of which has a role in influencing the health of individuals. It seems possible that people may pass from one system into another, such as in nursing home admission. The nature of the nursing home, by its very nature, precludes significant interaction with the social system of the outside world. As one moves farther into the social system of the nursing home, one will become less aware of the norms and rules in the macrosociety, and, hence, more anomic in that social system. Conversely, though, it may be argued that although this more anomic interaction is occurring with the "world left behind," a less anomic interaction may develop with the nursing home environment.

King described health in a holistic fashion, but people tend to have very narrow views of what health means (Winker, 1995). In this study, therefore, the relationship between social support and health may not have been demonstrated because of differences in how health is defined. The measure of health used here directed subjects to consider their "health problems" and activities. This may have caused subjects to think about health in ways not consistent with their own definitions or with King's definition. Furthermore, assigning health as a variable of the personal system may not be consistent with King's conceptual system. It is clear that nursing acts are directed toward health and that health is an interaction, but perhaps it is not "owned" by the personal system.

APPLICATION TO THE CLINICAL PROBLEM

Many have described the relationship between nursing home environments and the residents of the facility. It is imperative that nurses understand these relationships to provide optimal nursing care. Social support may be strengthened, encouraged, or redirected to enhance health status. Anomie was present in the sample reported here and may be reduced by helping residents of nursing homes understand the social rules and regulations they face. The reality of a nursing home presents a nearly complete inversion of the norms, rules, and values found in the larger society. Nowhere else in the Western world do people spend months in nightgowns without backs, discuss bowel and bladder habits at the breakfast table, or receive visitors only with the permission of a person in authority. Yet these are common facts of life for the institutionalized elderly. Older adults in long-term care settings may have great difficulty detecting the subtlety of social norms, particularly if they are cognitively impaired. Social support systems are a valuable asset to the new resident because normative information is exchanged (Patterson, 1995). As nurses attend to the social environment of the nursing home, social support may be engendered, anomie reduced, and health status improved.

King's conceptual system is a powerful lens for examining social ecology in health care settings. Further investigation of the world of nursing homes, with more appropriate measures, will assist residents, as well as nurses, by strengthening the knowledge base for nursing practice.

REFERENCES

Administration on Aging. (2003). *A profile of older adults*. Retrieved January 10, 2005, from http://www.aoa.gov/prof/Statistics/profile/profiles.asp
Anderson, R. A., Issel, L. M., & McDaniel, R. R. (2003). Nursing homes as complex adaptive systems: Relationship between management practice and resident outcomes. *Nursing Research, 52*, 12–21.

Asher, H. B. (1983). *Causal modeling* (2nd ed.). Thousand Oaks, CA: Sage.

Bennett, R., & Nahemow, L. (1965). Institutional totality and criteria of social adjustment in residences for the aged. *Journal of Social Issues, 21*, 44–78.

Berdes, C. M. (2001). Sense of community in residential facilities for the elderly (Doctoral dissertation, Northwestern University, 2001). *Dissertation Abstracts International, 62*(4), 1586-A.

Bisconti, T. L., & Bergeman, C. S. (1999). Perceived social control as a mediator of the relationships among social support, psychological well-being, and perceived health. *The Gerontologist, 39*, 94–103.

Borup, J. H., Gallego, D. T., & Hefferman, P. G. (1980). Relocation: It's effect on health, functioning, and mortality. *The Gerontologist, 20*, 468–79.

Brandt, P., & Weinert, C. (1985). *Personal Resource Questionnaire.* Bozeman, MT: Montana State University, College of Nursing.

Cantril, H. (1965). *The pattern of human concerns.* New Brunswick, NJ: Rutgers University Press.

Carboni, J. T. (1990). Homelessness among the institutionalized elderly. *Journal of Gerontological Nursing, 16*, 32–37.

Chenitz, W. C. (1983). Entry into a nursing home as status passage: A theory to guide nursing practice. *Geriatric Nursing, 4*, 92–97.

Chinn, P. L., & Kramer, M. K. (1999). *Theory and nursing: Integrated knowledge development* (5th ed.). St. Louis: Mosby.

Congressional Budget Office. (2004). *Financing long-term care for the elderly.* Washington, DC: Author.

Cook, T. D., & Campbell, D. T. (1979). *Quasi-experimentation: Design and analysis issues for field setting.* Boston: Houghton Mifflin.

Cox, R. A. (2003). Using NANDA, NIC, and NOC with Levine's conservation principles in a nursing home. *International Journal of Nursing Terminologies and Classifications, 14*(Suppl. 4), 41.

Davis, R. E. (1990). *Effects of a forced institutional relocation on the mortality, morbidity and functional status of elderly residents.* Unpublished doctoral dissertation, University of Nebraska, Lincoln.

Dudley, C. J. (1978). The division of labor, alienation, and anomie: A reformulation. *Sociological Focus, 11*, 97–109.

Durkheim, E. (1933). *The division of labor in society* (G. Simpson, Trans.). Glencoe, IL: Free Press. (Original work published 1893)

Durkheim, E. (1951). *Suicide* (J. A. Spaulding & G. Simpson, Trans.). New York: Free Press. (Original work published 1897)

Fawcett, J. (2001). The nurse theorists: 21st century updates—Imogene M. King. *Nursing Science Quarterly, 14*, 311–315.

Fillenbaum, G. G. (1979). Social context and self-assessments of health among the elderly. *Journal of Health and Social Behavior, 20*, 45–51.

Freidl, W. (1997). The impact of anomia as a factor in a demand resource model of health. *Social Science and Medicine, 44*, 1357–1365.

Goffman, E. (1961). *Asylums.* New York: Anchor Books.

Gold, C., Haas, S., & King, I. (2000). Conceptual frameworks: Putting the nursing focus into core curricula. *Nurse Educator, 25*, 95–98.

Grundy, E., & Sloggett, A. (2003). Health inequalities in the older population: The role of personal capital, social resources and socioeconomic circumstances, *Social Science and Medicine, 56*, 935–947.

Gubrium, J. (1975). *Living and dying at Murray Manor.* New York: St. Martin's Press.

Hendrick, C., Wells, K. S., & Faletti, M. V. (1982). Social and emotional effects of geographical relocation on elderly retirees. *Journal of Personality and Social Psychiatry, 42*, 951–962.

Hollingshead, A. B. (1957). *Two-factor index of social position.* New Haven, CT: Author.

Johnson, J. E. (1998). Stress, social support, and health in frontier elders. *Journal of Gerontological Nursing, 24*(5), 29–36.

Johnson, R. A., & Tripp-Reimer, T. (2001). Relocation among ethnic elders: A review—part 2. *Journal of Gerontological Nursing, 27*, 22–28.

Kaisik, B. H., & Cieslowitz, S. B. (1996). Easing the fear of nursing home placements: The value of stress inoculations. *Geriatric Nursing, 17*, 182–186.

Kerlinger, F. N., & Pedhazur, E. J. (1973). *Multiple regression in behavioral research.* New York: Holt, Rinehart, & Winston.

Keyes, C. L. M. (1998). Social well-being. *Social Psychology Quarterly, 61*, 121–140.

Kim, J., & Kohout, F. J. (1975). Special topics in general linear regression. In N. H. Nie, C. M. Hull, J. G. Jenkins, K. Steinbrenner, & D. H. Bent (Eds.), *SPSS: Statistical package for the social sciences* (2nd ed., pp. 368–97). New York: McGraw-Hill.

Kim, O. (1999). Mediation effect of social support between ethnic attachment and loneliness in older Korean immigrants. *Research in Nursing and Health, 22*, 169–175.

King, I. M. (1981). *A theory for nursing: Systems, concepts, process.* New York: Wiley.

King, I. M. (1994). Quality of life and goal attainment. *Nursing Science Quarterly, 7*, 29–32.

King, I. M. (1995). A system framework for nursing. In M. A. Frey & C. L. Sieloff (Eds.), *Advancing King's systems framework and theory of nursing* (pp. 14–22). Thousand Oaks, CA: Sage.

King, I. M. (1997). King's theory of goal attainment in practice. *Nursing Science Quarterly, 20*, 180–185.

King, I. M. (1999). A theory of goal attainment: Philosophical and ethical implications. *Nursing Science Quarterly, 12*, 292–296.

King, I. M. (2000). Evidence based nursing practice. *Theoria: Journal of Nursing Theory, 9*, 4–9.

Lee, D. T. F., Woo, J., & Mackenzie, A. E. (2002). The cultural context of adjusting to nursing home life: Chinese elders' perspectives. *The Gerontologist, 42*, 667–678.

Leonard, W. M. (1977). Sociological and social–psychological correlates of anomia among a random sample of aged. *Journal of Gerontology, 32*, 303–310.

Mahoney, F. I., & Barthel, D. W. (1965). Functional evaluation: The Barthel Index. *Maryland State Medical Journal, 14*, 61–65.

McClosky, H., & Schaar, J. H. (1965). Psychological dimensions of anomy. *American Sociological Review, 30*, 14–40.

Merton, R. K. (1957). Social structure and anomie. In R. K. Merton (Ed.), *Social theory and social structure* (Rev. ed., pp. 131–60). Glencoe, IL: Free Press.

Moore, A. B. (1980). An instrument to measure anomie. *Adult Education, 30*, 80–92.

Moss, G. E. (1973). *Illness, immunity, and social interaction: The dynamics of biosocial resonation.* New York: Wiley.

Nicholas, P. K., & Leuner, J. D. (1999). Hardiness, social support, and health status: Are there differences in older African American and Anglo American adults? *Holistic Nursing Practice, 13*, 53–61.

Pedhazur, E. J. (1982). *Multiple regression in behavioral research: Explanation and prediction* (2nd ed.). New York: Holt, Rinehart & Winston.

Patterson, B. J. (1995). The process of social support: Adjusting to life in a nursing home. *Journal of Advanced Nursing, 21*, 682–689.

Pfeiffer, E. (1975). A short portable mental status questionnaire for the assessment of organic brain deficit in elderly patients. *Journal of the American Geriatrics Society, 23*, 433–441.

Rantz, M. J., Zwygart-Stauffacher, M., Popejoy, L., Grando, V. T., Mehr, D. R., Hicks, L. L., et al. (1999). Nursing home care quality: A multidimensional theoretical model integrating the views of consumers and providers. *Journal of Nursing Care Quality, 14*, 16–37.

Reinardy, J. R. (1995). Relocation to a new environment: Decisional control and the move to a nursing home. *Health and Social Work, 20*, 31–38.

Riggs, C. J., & Rantz, M. J. (2001). A model of staff support to improve retention in long-term care. *Nursing Administration Quarterly, 25*, 43–54.

Ryan, M. C. (1998). The relationship between loneliness, social support, and decline in cognitive function in the hospitalized elderly. *Journal of Gerontological Nursing, 24*, 19–27.

Schulz, R., & Brenner, G. (1977). Relocation of the aged: A review and thematic analysis. *Journal of Gerontology, 32*, 323–33.

Srole L. (1956). Social integration and certain corollaries: An exploratory study, *American Sociological Review, 21*, 709–16.

Tobin, S. S., & Lieberman, M. A. (1976). *Last home for the aged.* San Francisco: Jossey-Bass.

U.S. Department of Health and Human Services. (1989). *The National Nursing Home Survey: 1985 Summary for the United States.* Vital and Health Statistics, Series 13, no. 97 (Publication No. PHS 89-1758). Washington, DC: Author.

Walsh, A. (1980). The prophylactic effect of religion on blood pressure levels among a sample of immigrants. *Social Science and Medicine, 143*, 59–63.

Weinert, C. (1985). Internal consistency for PRQ—Part II. Unpublished data.

Weiss, R. S. (1969). The fund of sociability. *Transaction, 6*, 36–43.

Weiss, R. S. (1974). The provision of social relationships. In Z. Rubin (Ed.), *Doing unto others* (pp. 17–26). New York: Prentice Hall.

Wenz, F. V. (1977). Marital status, anomie, and forms of social isolation: A case of high suicide rate among the widowed in Flint, Michigan. *Diseases of the Nervous System, 83,* 891–95.

Winker, C. K. (1995). A systems view of health. In M. A. Frey & C. L. Sieloff (Eds.), *Advancing King's systems framework and theory of nursing* (pp. 35–45). Thousand Oaks, CA: Sage.

PART III

Post–Middle Range
Theory Development

If Goals Are Attained, Satisfaction Will Occur in Nurse–Patient Interaction

An Empirical Test

Tomomi Kameoka, Naomi Funashima, and Midori Sugimori

A theory is a set of interrelated concepts, definitions, and propositions that present a systematic view of essential elements in a field of inquiry by specifying relations among variables (King, 1997). Nursing theory is useful to describe, explain, and predict phenomena within nursing (Fawcett, 1999). The ultimate goal of theory development in professional disciplines such as nursing is the empirical testing of interventions that are specified in the form of predictive middle range theories (Fawcett, 1993). This suggests that, to develop propositions in nursing theory and test them empirically, it is important to improve the utilization of theory in nursing practice. That is because a proposition states the relation between concepts (Fawcett, 1999) and helps nurses to describe, explain, and predict phenomena.

This study had two purposes. The first was to test a proposition of King's theory of goal attainment. The proposition is, "If goals are attained, satisfaction will occur in nurse–patient interactions" (King, 1981). No previous study tested this proposition. If the adequacy of the proposition is confirmed by empirical data, it becomes the base of developing new propositions related to both goal attainment and satisfaction. Therefore, the second purpose was to explore the characteristics of nurses whose degree of goal attainment and satisfaction in interactions with patients were both high.

THEORY DEVELOPMENT APPROACH

Initial Constructive Processes

The theoretical framework was constructed through the following steps:

1. Determining the level and scope of the theory of goal attainment in the structural hierarchy of contemporary nursing knowledge (Fawcett, 2000)
2. Exploring approaches for testing theory
3. Selecting the most suitable instruments as empirical indicators of concepts

Level and scope

Theory is a component of the structural hierarchy of contemporary nursing knowledge that encompasses the metaparadigm, multiple philosophies, conceptual models and frameworks, theories, and empirical indicators (Fawcett, 1993). A theory is derived from a conceptual framework, reflects the philosophy of a theorist, and describes and explains the metaparadigm concepts in nursing. Theories are less abstract than conceptual frameworks but more abstract than empirical indicators. The concepts of a theory are more specific and concrete than those of a conceptual framework.

Theories are categorized into types by their breadth of scope (Fawcett, 1993). Theories that are broadest in scope are called grand theories, and those that are more circumscribed are called middle range theories (Fawcett, 1993). Middle range theories are substantively specific, encompassing a limited number of concepts and a limited aspect of the real world.

The theory of goal attainment is derived by King (1981) from her conceptual system for nursing. The theory is made up of nine major concepts and eight propositions relating humanistic interactions between nurses and patients. As such, the theory of goal attainment is positioned as a middle range theory in the structural hierarchy of contemporary nursing knowledge.

Approaches for theory testing

Theory testing in nursing is defined as "one or more processes through which one verifies whether what was purposed or experienced is indeed so, or whether what was purported or experienced solves problems of significance in one's discipline or practice" (Fawcett, 1993; Silva & Sorrell, 1992). There are four approaches to test nursing theories: traditional empiricism, description of personal experiences, problem-solving approaches, and critical reasoning (Fawcett, 1993; Silva & Sorrell, 1992). Among them, traditional empiricism is accepted as the best approach to test theory empirically and directly in the real world for middle range theories. Traditional empiricism is a quantitative approach, and the goal is to determine whether what is purported to be so is, in fact, so.

In traditional empiricism, selecting instruments as empirical indicators that fit the concepts of the theory is significant. Theoretical substruction helps to select instruments in theory testing research (Dulock & Holzmer, 1991; Gibbs, 1972; Hinshaw, 1979; McQuiston & Campbell, 1997). According to Hinshaw (1979), substruction includes identifying and isolating the major concepts or constructs under study, specifying the relationships between the concepts as given in the study of theoretical explanation, hierarchically ordering the concepts and relationships according to their level of abstraction, and portraying the identified concepts and relationships in a pictorial structure. In theoretical substruction, transformational statements explain the reason the instrument is suitable as an empirical indicator of the concept.

From 1981 to 1998, 120 articles that cited King's theory of goal attainment were searched by MEDLINE, CINAHL, and IGAKUCHUOZASSI (a database for searching Japanese literature related to medicine, nursing, and allied health care). Fifty-two of the articles used King's theory as the conceptual basis of the research (Kameoka, Sadahiro, & Funashima, 2000a). Not all of these were theory-testing research. Two articles were written by the authors of this chapter and are part of a series for this study. The first study clarified the attributes and requisites for *goal attainment* and *satisfaction* in King's *theory of goal attainment* using concept analysis (Kameoka, Funashima, & Sugimori, 2000). In the second study, the Nurse's Performance for Goal Attainment scale (NPGA; Kameoka, Funashima, & Sugimori, 1999) was used to measure the degree of goal attainment of nurses in interactions with patients.

Fourty-three focused on the adequacy, advantage, utility, and limitations of King's theory of goal attainment (Kameoka, Sadahiro, et al., 2000). These articles represent critical reasoning for theory testing. Many identified the need for empirical testing of King's theory of goal attainment because the theory development approach included deductive processes (Fawcett & Whall, 1995; Funashima, 1995). Twenty-four of the articles showed utilization of the theory in actual practice or education. These articles may represent the problem-solving approach for theory testing. Only three articles applied traditional empiricism and tested propositions of King's theory of goal attainment. Hence, the literature reviewed identified that five propositions of the theory had not been tested empirically. Therefore, it was clarified that empirical testing of King's theory of goal attainment was necessary. This study focused on the following untested

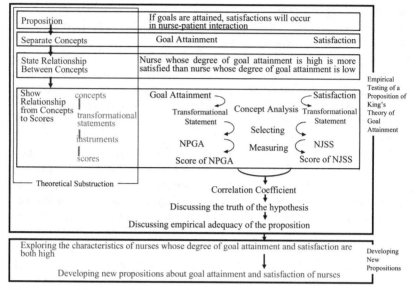

Figure 15.1. Theoretical framework.

proposition: If goals are attained, satisfaction will occur in nurse–patient interaction (King, 1981).

Selection of empirical indicators

The attributes of the two concepts, goal attainment and satisfaction, and the requisites for the instrument of each concept were clarified through concept analysis in previous studies (Kameoka, Funashima, et al., 2000). The NPGA (Kameoka et al., 1999) was designed to measure the degree of goal attainment of nurses in interactions with patients. Existing measures of nurses' job satisfaction were reviewed (Atwood & Hinshaw, 1986; Hinshaw & Atwood, 1984; Kramer & Hafner, 1989; Muller & McCloskey, 1990; Stamps & Eugene, 1986). Most of them measured nurses' job satisfaction with nonpatient care factors such as pay and career status. Only one, the Nursing Job Satisfaction Scale (NJSS), focused on nurses' satisfaction in interactions with patients (Atwood & Hinshaw, 1986). Thus, the NJSS was selected to test the proposition.

The literature was also reviewed to identify variables related to both goal attainment and satisfaction of nurses in interactions with patients. Few studies exploring this subject were located. Thus, the search was expanded to include studies on nurse performance, competence, attributes, and job satisfaction. As a result, 28 variables were identified that might relate to both goal attainment and satisfaction of nurses.

Theoretical substruction

Theoretical substruction for the study is shown in Figure 15.1. Two concepts, goal attainment and satisfaction in nurse–patient interactions, were identified and the relationship between the concepts was stated in the form of a hypothesis: A nurse whose degree of goal attainment is high is more satisfied than a nurse whose degree of goal attainment is low. The linkages among concepts, transformational statements, instruments, and scores on measures are also shown as recommended by Hinshaw (1979). The truth of the proposition, empirical adequacy of the proposition, and variables related to goal attainment and nurses' satisfactions will contribute to new propositions and nursing science based on King's conceptual system and theory of goal attainment.

Methods

Instrumentation

Three instruments were used in this study. The NPGA (Kameoka et al., 1999) measures the quality of nurses' performance that leads to goal attainment. The scale consists of 46 questions answered on a 5-point Likert-type scale. There are seven subscales: provide nursing care autonomously and support patients' attainment of goals, meet patients' individual needs with professional knowledge and skills, interact with other nurses and perform roles in the nursing unit, promote perceptual congruency with patients and involve patients in the nursing process, open and adequate communication, perform roles as a member of organization, use opportunity obtained in the organization, and respect the personality and individuality of patients. Satisfactory reliability and validity of the scale were reported previously (Kameoka et al., 1999). In this study, Cronbach's alpha of the NPGA was .965. The NJSS (Atwood & Hinshaw, 1986) was used to measure nurses' job and work satisfaction. The scale consists of 28 items answered on a 5-point Likert-type scale. Satisfactory reliability and validity were previously reported (Atwood & Hinshaw, 1986). The NJSS was translated into Japanese by applying the back-translation technique (Brislin, 1970; Brislin & Lonner, 1973). In this research, Cronbach's alpha of the NJSS was .874. Total scales scores were used in the analysis. Demographic and other data on the nurses were collected by an investigator developed scale. Responses were used as single item scales.

Sample and data collection procedure

To collect the data, nursing directors of 200 randomly sampled general hospitals in Japan were asked by mail whether they would participate in

Table 15.1. Demographic Characteristics of Nurses

Variable	N	%
Sex		
Male	9	1.7
Female		
Educational background in nursing	507	97.7
Diploma		
Associate degree		
Baccalaureate degree	443	85.3
Type of hospital		
National government	50	9.6
Prefecture or civic		
Private	6	1.2
	63	12.1
	137	26.4
	277	53.4

	Range	M	SD
Age	22–58	32.9	7.8
Length of working in clinical setting	1–37	10.4	6.9

the research. Forty-seven of the 200 nursing directors agreed to participate and instrument packets consisting of the three instruments described earlier were distributed to 1,180 nurses in those hospitals. Each nurse was asked to return the packet by mail. The data collection of the research was conducted from January to February in 1999.

Data analysis

Data were analyzed statistically by using SPSS 11.0 for Windows (SPSS Japan Inc., Tokyo, Japan). To test the research hypothesis, the correlation coefficient between the NPGA scores and the NJSS scores was calculated. To explore nurse characteristics related to both goal attainment and satisfaction, correlation coefficients, t tests, and analyses of variance were used.

Table 15.2. NPGA and NJSS Scores ($N = 519$)

	Range	M	SD
NPGA	52–213	149.4	20.4
NJSS	28–111	80.6	11.0

Note. NJSS = Nursing Job Satisfaction Scale; NPGA = Nurse's Performance for Goal Attainment scale;

Table 15.3. Relationships Between 28 Variables and Goal Attainment or Satisfaction of Nurses in Interactions With Patients

Variables (analysis method)	Goal attainment	Satisfaction
1. Age (correlation coefficient)	***	***
2. Marital status (ANOVA)		**
3. Responsibility for family members (t test)	**	
4. Family income (correlation coefficient)	***	***
5. Academic background in nursing (ANOVA)		
6. Who is research advisor (t test)		***
7. Experience of in-service education (t test)		
8. Experiences of continuing education (t test)	***	***
9. Activity at academic society in nursing (t test)		
10. Experience of preceptorship (t test)		
11. Feeling of being worthwhile to the job (ANOVA)	***	***
12. Perception of nursing as a job (ANOVA)	***	***
13. Reason for choosing nursing as one's career (ANOVA)	**	***
14. Reason for working as a nurse (ANOVA)	***	***
15. Intention to work continuously (ANOVA)	**	***
16. Intention to continue working at the present hospital (ANOVA)	*	***
17. Future goal as a nursing professional (ANOVA)	**	
18. Having role models (t test)	*	**
19. Years of clinical experience (correlation coefficient)	***	***
20. Experience of teaching students in clinical setting (ANOVA)	***	*
21. Location of hospital (ANOVA)		
22. Type of unit (ANOVA)		***
23. Nursing system of the unit (ANOVA)		
24. Distance to the hospital (correlation coefficient)		
25. Satisfaction for the unit (ANOVA)	**	***
26. Perception of one's contribution to the unit (ANOVA)	***	***
27. Shift system (ANOVA)	**	**
28. Frequency of night shifts per month (correlation coefficient)		

Note. ANOVA = analysis of variance.
$*p < .05.$ $**p < .01.$ $***p < .001.$

Results

Six hundred and fifty-five nurses, of the 1,180 nurses who received the instrument packets, participated in the research for a response rate of 55.5%. Of the 655 instrument packets, 519 were sufficiently complete to be analyzed.

Table 15.1 shows the demographic characteristics of the sample. Women comprised 97.7% of the participants. The mean age was 32.9 years old, with a range of 22 to 58 years old. The mean length of working in a clinical setting was 10.4 years, with a range of 1 to 37 years. The majority (85.5%) were diploma educated, 9.6% had associate degrees, and 1.2% had baccalaureate degrees. Approximately 53% were working in private hospitals. The hospitals were located all over Japan.

Descriptive statistics for the NPGA and NJSS are shown in Table 15.2. The mean score for each variable is above the midpoint of the score range. The Kolmogorov–Smirnov test indicated that the score distribution of each scale was normal. The correlation coefficient for the two scale scores was .395 ($p < .0001$). Thus, the primary hypothesis was supported. Nurses who reported higher professional goal attainment also reported significantly higher job and work satisfaction.

Next, the relationship between the 28 variables and both goal attainment and nurse satisfaction in interactions with patients were examined. The results (Table 15.3) showed that 15 variables were found to be significant to both goal attainment and job and work satisfaction. Nurses who reported a higher level of goal attainment and satisfaction in nurse–patient interactions were significantly older, had higher family income, had increased experiences with continuing education, had more positive perceptions of nursing as a job, perceived nursing as more worthwhile, had intrinsic motivation for choosing nursing as a career, experienced more enjoyment working as a nurse, had the intention to continue working at their current hospital of employment, had stronger role models, had more years of clinical experience and more experience teaching students in clinical settings, had higher satisfaction with their unit, and had higher perception of their aptitude for the unit.

DISCUSSION

This study was conducted to test a previously untested proposition from King's theory of goal attainment: If goals are attained, satisfaction will occur in nurse–patient interactions (King, 1981). It was hypothesized that a nurse whose degree of goal attainment is high is more satisfied than a nurse whose degree of goal attainment is low. The hypotheses were derived through theoretical substruction and the level of inquiry was association testing (Diers, 1979). The sample was determined to be representative of nurses in Japan (Kangomondaikenkyuukai, 1998).

Based on correlational analysis, the primary hypothesis was supported. Nurses whose degree of goal attainment was high were more satisfied than nurses whose degree of goal attainment was low. These results provide empirical support for King's theory of goal attainment in relation to goal attainment and satisfaction of nurses in interaction with patients.

Another purpose of this study was to explore characteristics of nurses whose degree of goal attainment and satisfaction in interactions with patients were both high, and to develop new propositions related to both goal attainment and satisfaction of nurses in interactions with patients. The relation-searching level of inquiry was used for this study (Diers, 1979). In relation-searching studies, interpretation of the results is in the form of hypotheses for further testing (Diers, 1979, p. 125). When the hypotheses generated by relation-searching studies are tested empirically, nurses can use them as propositions of theory to predict nursing phenomena.

The results of this study suggested 15 characteristics of nurses whose degree of goal attainment and satisfaction were both high. Four hypothesis were developed.

Hypothesis 1

A nurse whose degree of goal attainment and satisfaction are both high achieves his or her developmental tasks well. Of the 15 characteristics, being older and having a higher income occur along with human development, and they are important developmental tasks of adults (Havighurst, 1953). In addition, more years of clinical experience tend to lead to more experiences teaching students in a clinical setting, getting a job, and expanding social roles. These are also important developmental tasks of adults. Therefore, variables significantly related to goal attainment and satisfaction are also related to accomplishing developmental tasks.

Hypothesis 2

A nurse whose degree of goal attainment and satisfaction are both high has a strong career commitment in nursing. Career commitment is defined as attitude toward one's profession or vocation, and it is evidenced by intent to stay in the career, individual's value of the career choice, and willingness to invest and involve oneself in the profession (Gardner, 1992). Of the 15 characteristics, perceiving nursing as a worthwhile job, choosing nursing as one's job from intrinsic motivation, continuing nursing because one likes it as one's job, and having the intention to continue in nursing shows that the nurse has strong career commitment.

Hypothesis 3

A nurse whose degree of goal attainment and satisfaction are both high has strong goal directedness. When a person has a meaningful goal and knows the relationship between the goal and one's own daily experience, one's learning is related to the goal attainment. This is called goal-directedness (Chickering, 1972). Of the 15 characteristics, attending continuing education shows that the nurse has an active attitude about learning. Having role models shows that the nurse has ideal images of nurses as concrete goals. These suggest that the learning of the nurse is related to his or her own goals as a nursing professional.

Hypothesis 4

A nurse whose degree of goal attainment and satisfaction are both high is strongly empowered as a nurse. Empowerment is defined as intrinsic task motivation manifested in a set of four cognitions, reflecting an individual's orientation to his or her work role: meaning, competence, self-determination, and impact (Spreitzer, 1995; Thomas & Velthouse, 1990). Meaning is the value of a work goal or purpose, judged in relation to an individual's own ideals or standards. Competence is an individual's belief in his or her capability to perform activities with skill. Where competence is mastery of behavior, self-determination is an individual's sense of having choice in initiating and regulating actions. Self-determination reflects autonomy in the initiation and continuation of work behaviors and processes. Impact is the degree to which an individual can influence strategic, administrative, or operating outcomes at work. Of the 15 characteristics, perceiving nursing as a job that one can perform to the best of one's ability and through which one can further achieve personal development, having the intention to work continuously at the present hospital, being satisfied with the present work, and perceiving one's ward as a good place to work reflect the four concepts of empowerment.

SUMMARY

In summary, this study supported the empirical adequacy of one of the propositions of King's theory of goal attainment: If goals are attained, satisfaction will occur in nurse–patient interactions. In addition, four hypotheses were identified for future development and extension of King's theory of goal attainment.

REFERENCES

Atwood, J. R., & Hinshaw, A. S. (1986). *Anticipated turnover among nursing staff.* Research Grant U.S. D.H.H.S. #R01 NU00908, 1986.

Brislin, R. W. (1970). Back-translation for cross-cultural research. *Journal of Cross-Cultural Psychology, 1,* 185–216.

Brislin, R. W., & Lonner, W. J. (1973). *Cross-cultural research methods.* New York: Wiley.

Chickering, A. W. (1972). *Education and identity.* San Francisco: Jossey-Bass.

Diers, D. (1979). *Research in nursing practice.* Philadelphia: Lippincott.

Dulock, H. L., & Holzmer, W. L. (1991). Substruction: Improving the linkage from theory to method. *Nursing Science Quarterly, 4,* 455–461.

Fawcett, J. (1993). *Analysis and evaluation of nursing theories.* Philadelphia: Davis.

Fawcett, J. (1999). *The relationship of theory and research.* Philadelphia: Davis.

Fawcett, J. (2000). *Analysis and evaluation of contemporary nursing knowledge: Nursing models and theories.* Philadelphia: Davis.

Fawcett, J., & Whall, A. L. (1995). State of the science and future direction. In M. A. Frey & C. L. Sieloff (Eds.), *Advancing King's systems framework and theory of nursing* (pp. 327–334). Thousand Oaks, CA: Sage.

Funashima, N. (1995). King's theory of goal attainment and its further development. *Quality Nursing, 1,* 74–78 [in Japanese].

Gardner, D. L. (1992). Career commitment in nursing. *Journal of Professional Nursing, 8,* 155–160.

Gibbs, J. (1972). *Sociological theory construction.* Hinsdale, IL: Dryden.

Havighurst, R. J. (1953). *Human development and education.* New York: Longmans, Green, & Co.

Hinshaw, A. S. (1979). Theoretical substruction: An assessment process. *Western Journal of Nursing Research, 1,* 319–324.

Hinshaw, A. S., & Atwood, J. R. (1984). *Anticipated turnover among nursing staff.* Research Grant U.S. D.H.H.S. #R01 NU00908, 1984.

Kameoka, T., Funashima, N., & Sugimori, M. (1999). Development of an instrument of goal attainment in nurse-patient interaction for using in empirical testing of King's theory of goal attainment. *Journal of Chiba Academy of Nursing Science, 5,* 1–7 [in Japanese].

Kameoka, T., Funashima, N., & Sugimori, M. (2000). Concept analysis of "goal attainment in nurse-patient interaction" and "satisfaction in nurse-patient interaction": Toward to test King's theory of goal attainment. *Journal of Research for Nursing Education, 9,* 15–25 [in Japanese].

Kameoka, T., Sadahiro, W., & Funashima, N. (2000). Construction of theoretical framework for testing King's theory of goal attainment: Focused on the relationship between the degree of goal attainment and that of satisfaction of nurses in interactions with patients. *Journal of Chiba Academy of Nursing Science, 6,* 16–22 [in Japanese].

Kangomondaikenkyuukai (Ed.). (1998). *Statistical data on nursing service in Japan, 1998.* Tokyo: Nursing Association Publishing Company.

King, I. M. (1981). *A theory for nursing: Systems, concepts, and process.* Albany, NY: Delmar.

King, I. M. (1997). Knowledge development for nursing: A process. In I. M. King & J. Fawcett (Eds.), *The language of nursing theory and metatheory* (pp. 9–15). Indianapolis, Indiana: Sigma Theta Tau International Honor Society of Nursing.

King, I. M., & Fawcett, J. (1997). *The language of nursing theory and metatheory.* Indianapolis, IN: Sigma Theta Tau International.

Kramer, M., & Hafner, L. P. (1989). Shared values: Impact on staff nurse job satisfaction and perceived productivity. *Nursing Research, 38*(3), 172–177.

McQuiston, C. M., & Campbell, J. C. (1997). Theoretical substruction: A guide for theory testing research. *Nursing Science Quarterly, 10*(3), 117–123.

Muller, C. W., & McCloskey, J. C. (1990). Nurses' job satisfaction: A proposed measure. *Nursing Research, 39*, 113–117.

Polit, D. F., & Beck, C. T. (2004). *Nursing research: Principles and methods* (7th ed.). Philadelphia: Lippincott Williams & Wilkins.

Silva, M. C., & Sorrell, J. M. (1992). Testing of nursing theory: Critique and philosophical expansion. *Advances in Nursing Science, 14*, 12–23.

Spreitzer, G. M. (1995). Psychological empowerment in the workplace: Dimensions, measurement, and validation. *Academy of Management Journal, 38*, 1442–1465.

Stamps, P. L., & Eugene, B. P. (1986). *Nurses and work satisfaction: An index for measurement.* Ann Arbor, MI: Health Administration Press Perspectives.

Thomas, K.W., & Velthouse, B. A. (1990). Cognitive elements of empowerment: An "interpretive" model of intrinsic task motivation. *Academy of Management Review, 15*, 666–681.

Wilson, H. S. (1993). *Introducing research in nursing.* Boston: Addison-Wesley.

CHAPTER SIXTEEN

Testing Nursing Theory With Intervention Research

The Congruency Between King's Conceptual System and Multisystemic Therapy

Maureen A. Frey, Deborah A. Ellis, and Sylvie Naar-King

For nursing research to improve the quality of health care, it is imperative to increase the quality and quantity of intervention research. Important directions for nurse researchers include developing new intervention strategies, integrating interventions across individual and societal levels, conducting translational research, and enhancing multidisciplinary collaboration (Naylor, 2003). Multidisciplinary collaboration is especially important because it brings a broader perspective of skills and knowledge to the table and results in less compartmentalized approaches to improving the health of individuals, families, and communities.

An explicit theoretical framework is essential to an effective intervention (Gross, Fogg, & Conrad, 1993). The framework should provide a fairly explicit explanation as to how and why the intervention should work. Nursing theories, especially grand-level theories, also provide some direction for the content and expected outcomes of interventions. Interventions should also be consistent with descriptive data, have adequate specification so they can be replicated, and have processes in place to monitor and evaluate intervention fidelity, that is, determination that the intervention was delivered consistently as planned. Although these factors are important in designing new intervention strategies, they are critically important when using a nursing theoretical framework and an intervention developed by another discipline.

Over the past 5 years, our multidisciplinary research team has conducted clinical trials of multisystemic therapy (MST), an established evidence-based intervention developed in clinical psychology (Henggeler, Schoenwald, Borduin, Rowland, & Cunningham, 1998), to improve diabetes management and metabolic control in adolescents with Type 1 diabetes and chronically poor metabolic control (CPMC) (Ellis et al., 2004, 2005). King's conceptual system serves as the theoretical framework. Frey (1995) has demonstrated that middle range formulations can be derived and tested from King's conceptual system for this population. However, in moving to intervention research, it was essential to examine the correspondence between key elements of the intervention and King's conceptual system. This is especially important because the intervention was not uniquely developed to test King's theory and was developed outside of nursing. Accordingly, the purpose of this chapter is to describe the clinical problem of adolescents with Type 1 diabetes with CPMC and to examine the congruency between King's conceptual system and MST. The approaches used for intervention specification and fidelity are also described because they heavily influenced our decision to use MST and because both are critical to interpreting the findings in terms of theory testing.

ADOLESCENTS WITH TYPE 1 DIABETES AND CPMC

Type 1 diabetes is characterized by a demanding regimen that affects multiple aspects of daily functioning and requires many separate but related management behaviors to achieve good metabolic control. Metabolic control is important because of the well-established link between poor metabolic control and short-term complications, long-term complications, and excessive cost to the health care system (Diabetes Control and Complications Trial, 2000; Javor et al., 1997). Deterioration in metabolic control during adolescence is well documented in the literature (Anderson, Ho, Brackett, Finkelstein, & Laffel, 1997; Johnson, 1990). However, increasing evidence suggests that for some adolescents, poor metabolic control is not transient, that is, it continues into adulthood (Wysocki, Hough, Ward, & Green, 1992).

Although other factors may contribute to poor metabolic control, a significant factor is inadequate diabetes management (Orr, Golden, Myers, & Marrero, 1983). Kovacs, Goldston, Obrosky, & Iyengar (1992) followed a sample of 95 children with Type 1 diabetes from the time of diagnosis for an average of 6 years. Thirty percent of their sample developed "serious noncompliance" during the follow-up period. Children with severe adherence problems had significantly poorer metabolic control and significantly higher rates of avoidable postdiagnostic hospitalizations. Multiple studies of children, adolescents, and young adults with Type 1 diabetes have documented that postdiagnostic hospital admissions for diabetes ketoacidosis (DKA), a life-threatening condition characterized by a very high blood glucose level and poor metabolic control are related (Dumont et al., 1995; Kovacs, Charron-Prochownik, & Obrosky, 1994; Palta et al., 1997; Rewers et al., 2002). This relationship between poor metabolic control and DKA admissions is likely accounted for by inadequate diabetes management because the majority of postdiagnostic DKA admissions are caused by omission of insulin (Musey et al., 1995; Smith, Firth, Bennett, Howard, & Chisholm, 1998).

A substantial descriptive literature suggests that adolescents with CPMC are embedded within multiple systems that contribute to poor health outcomes. Individual risk factors that have been linked to diabetes management, poor metabolic control, or both for the general population of adolescents with diabetes are even more prevalent among high-risk adolescents. Such adolescents have been reported to have higher rates of behavioral and emotional problems and psychiatric disorders (Leonard, Jang, Savik, Plumbo, & Christensen, 2002; Orr et al., 1983; Rewers et al., 2002). Kovacs and associates (1992) reported that 60% of adolescents with Type 1 diabetes and severe management problems could be diagnosed with a formal psychiatric disorder. Family risk factors have been identified as well. For example, higher rates of general family dysfunction and psychopathology are related to postdiagnostic DKA admissions (Dumont et al. 1995; White, Kolman, Wexler, Ploin, & Winter, 1984), as are lower levels of parental support for diabetes care (Liss et al. 1998).

Examination of the broader social ecology of high-risk adolescents identifies many barriers to adequate diabetes management. For example, Orr and associates (1983) described excessive school absence beyond that accounted for by hospital stays. Whether such school absence occurs because of poor health status or other factors, school personnel are unlikely to manage adequately the diabetes care of children who are often not present and whose health care needs are therefore unclear. Poor metabolic control and postdiagnostic DKA admissions are also associated with poor interface with medical care providers, as indexed by irregular clinic attendance (Jacobson, Hauser, Willett, Wolfsdorf, & Herman, 1997; Kaufman, Halvorson, & Carpenter, 1999). Finally, high-risk adolescents are disproportionately likely to be from disadvantaged groups such as those of lower socioeconomic status, those who hold public insurance, single-parent-headed households, and members of minority groups (Auslander,

Thompson, Dreitzer, White, & Santiago, 1997; Delamater, Albrecht, Postellon, & Gutai, 1991; Harris, Greco, Wysocki, Elder-Danda, & White, 1999; Harris, & Mertlich, 2003). African American adolescents in particular have been found to be at significantly higher risk for problems with treatment adherence and metabolic control (Auslander et al., 1997; Delamater et al., 1999) and also for postdiagnostic DKA admissions (Delamater et al., 1991). Such outcomes may be accounted for by a clustering of risk factors among minority youth. These include higher numbers of single-parent families where parents must juggle diabetes care with multiple other demands and have fewer resources for supervising teens' diabetes care (Harris et al., 1999). Although several intervention approaches have been developed specifically to improve diabetes management and metabolic control in adolescence with varying degrees of success (Anderson et al., 2003; Grey, Boland, Davisdon, Li, & Tamborlane, 2000; Wysocki et al., 2000), very few intervention studies have focused on the subset of adolescents at highest risk for health complications. Very often, poor diabetes management or poor metabolic control (or both) are used as exclusion criteria for intervention trials that would benefit this high-risk population.

Although many have noted the need for interventions for high-risk youth with diabetes, the research base is highly limited and consists mainly of small sample ($N < 10$) studies that lack control groups (Francis et al., 1990; Silverman, Haines, Davies, & Parton, 2003; Steindel, Roe, Costin, Carlson, & Kaufman, 1995; Viinamaki & Niskanen, 1991). Couper, Taylor, Fotheringham, and Sawyer (1999) conducted one of the only randomized controlled trials for adolescents with CPMC using a home-based educational intervention with 69 adolescents. Although the intervention was found to be initially effective in improving metabolic control, results were not maintained 6 months after the completion of the intervention. Harris and Mertlich (2003) conducted a pilot study using 10 sessions of home-based behavioral family systems therapy to treat 18 adolescents with poor metabolic control. Pre–post improvements were reported for some aspects of diabetes management, although there were no significant improvements in either metabolic control or hospitalization rates. Limitations of these two studies include low recruitment rates (45% in the Harris study), short intervention periods, limited scope of intervention (i.e., no family intervention in the Couper study), failure to target diabetes management behaviors directly, which is the primary contributing factor to poor metabolic control, and lack of coordination of interventions between clinic-based medical providers and study interventionists.

In summary, adolescents with Type 1 diabetes and CPMC are at high risk for health complications and compromised quality of life. Research to date identifies that inadequate diabetes management is a major cause of poor metabolic control and that the barriers to inadequate diabetes management cross multiple systems. As such, interventions for adolescents with CPMC should target behavioral change and include multiple levels: family, school, community, and the health care system. In addition, a home-based, intensive approach by interventionists with mental health training is important to improve health outcomes for this population.

KING'S CONCEPTUAL SYSTEM AND MULTISYSTEMIC THERAPY

The areas selected to compare King's conceptual system and MST are the overall theoretical perspective, focus of intervention, and process for change. The presentation of each reflects their respective level of abstraction and language of the discipline.

Theoretical Perspective

Both King's conceptual system and MST are based in general systems theory. King (1981, 1995) characterized individuals as personal systems. Individuals interacting in groups form interpersonal systems. Larger groups with common goals form social systems. Relationships between and among systems are inherent in systems theory.

Concepts provide the knowledge and structure for understanding systems and interactions between systems. Individuals, as personal systems, are best understood by the concepts of perception, self, growth and development, body image, time, personal space, and coping. Concepts important for understanding interpersonal systems are interaction, communication, role, stress and stressors, and transactions. Concepts useful for understanding social systems are organization, authority, power, status, and decision making. Although grouped by system, concepts can be used and applied across systems. For example, health is a central concept in King's conceptual system and can be applied across personal, interpersonal, and social systems.

The treatment theory underlying MST draws on social–ecological (Bronfenbrenner, 1979) and family systems (Haley, 1976; Minuchin, 1974) theories of behavior. Extrafamilial systems, such as the health care system, school, work, peers, and community and cultural institutions, are seen as interconnected with the individual and his or her family. As a result, MST interventions are directed toward individuals, families, peers, schools, and other systems with which the child and family interact.

Focus of Intervention

According to King (1981), interactions between and among personal, interpersonal, and social systems influence human acts or behavior. Behavior, in turn, influences health and illness. Nurses deal with the behavior of individuals and groups in stressful situations pertaining to health and illness. Individuals and groups are active and responsible for their behavior. Often, however, individuals and groups need assistance in promoting health and managing illness. Understanding the ways that individuals and groups interact to promote health is critical to provide nursing care. For individuals with chronic conditions such as Type 1 diabetes, nurses help maintain a functional state of health and prevent complications. Multisystemic therapy has a strong behavioral focus because it was developed to treat antisocial behaviors of children and adolescents with severe mental health and addiction problems (Henggeler et al., 1998). The focus of MST is to improve diabetes management behavior and subsequently improve metabolic control. Problem behavior such as inadequate diabetes management may be a function of interactions within multiple systems or be due to difficulties that characterize the interface between these systems (e.g., family–health provider relations, family–school relations, child–peer relations). Feasibility and pilot studies were conducted to adapt MST for youth with Type 1 diabetes with chronically poor metabolic control (Ellis, Naar-King, Frey, Rowland, & Greger, 2003; Ellis et al. 2004).

Process of Change

King's (1981) theory of goal attainment, derived from selected personal and interpersonal system concepts, characterizes nursing as a process of human interaction and sets the standard of practice for nurse–patient interactions. Knowledge of interrelated concepts, the clinical population, and the clinical condition provide the substantive focus of nursing practice. King (1992) also linked the theory of goal attainment and the traditional nursing process: assess, plan, implement, and evaluate. Nurses conduct comprehensive assessments tailored to the patient's situation. Assessment is an ongoing process of communication and includes validation of perception, delineation and validation of patient concerns, and establishment of mutual trust. Developing a plan of care involves mutual goal setting and making decisions about means to achieve goals. Nurses and clients must both exhibit behavior that moves toward goal attainment. The final step is evaluation of goals attained. According to King, if goals are attained, health is improved. Unmet goals can result from incomplete data, incorrect interpretation of data, perceptual error, lack of knowledge, lack of commitment to goals, and patient nurse or system barriers.

In MST, the therapist begins by conducting a multisystemic assessment of the strengths and weaknesses of family members and their transactions with extrafamilial systems (e.g., peers, school, health care system). MST is not a typical, "one size fits all" intervention model in which the therapist follows a set of prearranged tasks in a time-limited sequence. The treatment plan is designed in collaboration with family members and is therefore family-driven rather than therapist-driven. Problems identified conjointly by family members and the therapist during the assessment phase are explicitly targeted for change during the treatment phase. Changes in specific targeted behaviors are called "overarching goals." Treatment is terminated when overarching goals are met.

Family interventions in MST attempt to provide the caregiver with the resources needed to achieve effective parenting and develop increased family structure and cohesion. Examples of family interventions include establishing systematic monitoring, reward, and discipline systems to increase parent involvement in diabetes management; developing family organizational routines such as regular meal times; prompting caregivers to communicate effectively with each other about adolescent problems; teaching strategies for problem solving day-to-day conflicts around diabetes; and developing supportive networks with friends, extended family, and church members.

Many adolescents and families have benefited from peer-level interventions directed toward decreasing the youth's involvement with peers who are not supportive of the diabetes regimen or who display oppositional or deviant behavior. At the same time, supportive peers and supportive activities through church youth groups, organized athletics, and after-school activities are actively encouraged. Other targets of intervention include the school and health care system. Optimally, interventions are conducted by the youth's caregivers with the guidance of the therapist. For example, caregivers are assisted to develop strategies to monitor diabetes management, peer contacts, and school performance. Developing a positive relationship with health care providers is critical for these families. Therapists consider such factors as the family's satisfaction with care, their communication with the diabetes treatment team, and their access to services, especially appointment keeping. Therapists also meet with members of the health care team to understand individualized treatment plans so that everyone is working on the same goals. To meet management goals, therapists can draw on a menu of evidence-based intervention skills such as cognitive–behavioral therapy, parent training, communication skills training, and strategic family therapy to assist families. For diabetes-specific interventions to address knowledge and skill deficits, the diabetes nurse educator from the clinic accompanies therapists into family homes.

INTERVENTION SPECIFICATION AND FIDELITY

Specification refers to the procedural aspects of the intervention. Interventions that are not sufficiently defined open the door to considerable bias, especially when interventions are socially complex (Lindsay, 2004). Inadequate intervention specification results in unreliable evidence for practice, severely limits replication research, and does not allow for interpretation of intervention result in terms of the theory. Specification of MST is based on the following nine core principles (Henggeler & Schoenwald, 1998):

1. The primary purpose of assessment is to understand the fit between the identified problems and the broader systemic context.
2. Therapeutic contacts emphasize the positive and use systemic strengths as levers for change.
3. Interventions are designed to promote responsible behavior and decrease irresponsible behavior among family members.
4. Interventions are present-focused and action-oriented, targeting specific and well-defined problems.
5. Interventions target sequences of behavior within and between multiple systems that maintain the identified problems.
6. Interventions are developmentally appropriate and fit the developmental needs of the youth.
7. Interventions are designed to require daily or weekly effort from family members.
8. Intervention effectiveness is evaluated continuously from multiple perspectives with providers assuming accountability for overcoming barriers to successful outcomes.
9. Interventions are designed to promote treatment generalization and long-term maintenance of therapeutic change by empowering caregivers to address family members' needs across multiple systemic contexts.

The MST principles are internally consistent with systems theory, King's focus on behavior, mutual goal setting, continuous evaluation of progress toward goals, accountability by providers, and the active role of the individual and family members. In addition, there is attention to the concept of development, an explicit concept in King's conceptual system. Of particular interest is the emphasis on sequences of behavior in MST. This is not unlike King's model of interactions leading to transactions and goal attainment.

Fidelity refers to whether the intervention was delivered as specified (Moncher & Prinz, 1991). Assessment of intervention fidelity is important in establishing the internal validity of a study by demonstrating that the intervention was delivered as intended (Hogue et al., 1998; Miller & Binder, 2002). Assurance of intervention fidelity is also critical in terms of interpreting a study's findings. Without evidence of treatment fidelity, the absence of significant findings could be due to ineffectiveness of the intervention or inadequate delivery of the intervention. Interpretation of significant findings are also jeopardized because they could result from variables other than those specific to the intervention, such as individual characteristics of the interventionist or variation in implementation between interventionists. Finally, strategies to assess adequate intervention fidelity play an important role in the effective translation and dissemination of research to real-world clinical settings compared with controlled trials in university settings. Potential barriers to implementation of evidence-based interventions in real-word settings are inadequate training of interventionists or inadequate time to do the intervention correctly (Bellg et al., 2004; McHugo, Drake, Teaugue, & Xie, 1999; Schoenwald & Hoagwood, 2001). Translation research, also called effectiveness studies, are of particular interest to nurse clinicians (Brown, 2002).

The evaluation of treatment fidelity is based on therapists' and family members' ratings of therapists' adherence to the core MST principles (Huey, 2001). Several prior studies have shown relationships between MST treatment fidelity and child and family treatment outcomes using self-report fidelity measures (Huey, Henggeler, Brondino, & Pickrel, 2000; Schoenwald, Henggeler, Brondino, & Rowland, 2000) in populations of adolescents with severe antisocial behavior. In these studies, higher ratings of treatment fidelity by parents, adolescents, or therapists were related to lower rates of psychiatric symptomatology and arrests and incarceration (Henggeler, Melton, Brondino, Scherer, & Hanley, 1997). In the current study of MST with adolescents who have Type 1 diabetes and CPMC, treatment fidelity was assessed through two methods: objective ratings of therapy sessions and questionnaires completed by caregivers and therapists. Relationships between fidelity measures and among fidelity, diabetes management, and metabolic control at the conclusion of the intervention were assessed. Objective ratings of treatment fidelity were significantly related to therapist-reported treatment fidelity. Therapist report and objective ratings of fidelity were the best predictors of diabetes management and metabolic control at the 7-month posttest, which corresponded to the end of treatment. As hypothesized, higher treatment fidelity was associated with improved blood glucose testing and metabolic control. The relationship between treatment fidelity and metabolic control was mediated by diabetes management (Ellis, Naar-King, Templin, Cunningham & Frey, in press).

SUMMARY

King's conceptual system provides the structure and function for understanding the complex factors that interplay and influence behavior and health outcomes. Multisystemic therapy provides an empirically supported intervention approach for improving diabetes management behaviors, the most likely route to improving metabolic control and, subsequently, health outcomes for adolescents with Type 1 diabetes and CPMC. The fit between the theoretical perspectives of MST and King's conceptual system is excellent. In addition, the multiple systems perspective is an excellent fit with the known etiology of CPMC in adolescents with Type 1 diabetes. Because King's conceptual system is a grand-level theory, MST is much more specific about mechanism for behavioral change. Nurses could provide MST with advanced practice preparation in mental health nursing. In addition, MST is consistent with King's perspective of goal setting and the active role of individuals to promote and maintain their own health. Finally, the mechanisms of intervention fidelity are sufficiently developed to interpret the findings relative to King's conceptual system.

REFERENCES

Anderson, B., Ho, J., Brackett, J., Finkelstein, D., & Laffel, L. M. (1997). Parental involvement in diabetes management tasks: Relationship to blood glucose monitoring adherence and metabolic control in young adolescents with insulin dependent diabetes mellitus. *Journal of Pediatrics, 130,* 257–265.

Anderson, B., Laffel, L. M., Vangsness, L., Connell, A., Goebel-Fabbri, A., & Burler, D. (2003). Impact of ambulatory, family focused teamwork intervention on glycemic control in youth with Type 1 diabetes. *Journal of Pediatrics, 142,* 409–416.

Auslander, W. F., Thompson, S., Dreitzer, D., White, N. H., & Santiago, J. V. (1997). Disparity in glycemic control and adherence between African American and Caucasian youths with diabetes. *Diabetes Care, 20,* 1569–1574.

Bellg, A. J., Borrelli, B., Resnick, B., Hecht, J., Minicucci, D. S., Ory, M., et al. (2004). Enhancing treatment fidelity in health behavior studies: Best practices and recommendations from the NIH Behavior Change Consortium. *Health Psychology, 23,* 443–451.

Bronfenbrenner, U. (1979). *The ecology of human development: Experiments by design and nature.* Cambridge, MA: Harvard University Press.

Brown, S. J. (2002). Nursing intervention studies: A descriptive analysis of issues important to clinicians. *Research in Nursing & Health, 25,* 317–327.

Couper, J. J., Taylor, J., Fortheringham, M. J., & Sawer, M. (1990). Failure to maintain the benefits of home-based intervention in adolescents with poorly controlled Type 1 diabetes. *Diabetes Care, 22,* 1933–1937.

Delamater, A. M., Albrecht, D. R., Postellon, D. C., & Gutai, J. P. (1991). Racial differences in metabolic control of children and adolescents with Type 1 diabetes. *Diabetes Care, 14,* 20–25.

Delamater, A. M., Shaw, K., Applegate, E. B., Pratt, I., Eidison, M., Lancelott, G., et al. (1999). Risk for metabolic control problems in minority youth with diabetes. *Diabetes Care, 22,* 700–705.

Diabetes Control and Complications Trial/Epidemiology of Diabetes Interventions and Complications Research Group. (2000). Retinopathy and neuropathy in patients with Type 1 diabetes four years after a trial of intensive therapy. *New England Journal of Medicine, 342,* 381–389.

Dumont, R. H., Jacobson, A. M., Cole, C., Hauser, S. T., Wolfsdorf, J. I., Willett, J. B., et al. (1995). Psychosocial predictors of acute complications of diabetes in youth. *Diabetic Medicine, 12,* 612–618.

Ellis, D. A., Frey, M. A., Naar-King, S., Templin, T., Cunningham, P., & Cakan, N. (2005). Use of multisystemic therapy to improve regimen adherence among adolescents with Type 1 adolescents in chronic poor metabolic control: A randomized controlled trial. *Diabetes Care, 28,* 1604–1610.

Ellis, D. A., Naar-King, S., Frey, M. A., Rowland, M., & Greger, N. (2003). Case study: Feasibility of multisystemic therapy as a treatment for urban adolescents with poorly controlled Type 1 diabetes. *Journal of Pediatric Psychology, 28,* 287–293.

Ellis, D. A., Naar-King, S., Frey, M. A., Templin, T., Rowland, M. D., & Cakan, N. (in press). Multisystemic treatment of poorly controlled Type 1 diabetes: Effects on medical resource utilization. *Journal of Pediatric Psychology.*

Ellis, D. A., Naar-King, S., Frey, M. A., Templin, T., Rowland, M., & Greger, N. (2004). Use of multisystemic therapy to improve regimen adherence among adolescents with Type 1 diabetes in poor metabolic control: A pilot study. *Journal of Clinical Psychology in Medical Settings, 11,* 315–324.

Ellis, D. A., Naar-King, S., Templin, T., Cunningham, P. B., & Frey, M. A. (in press). Improving health outcomes among youths with poorly controlled Type 1 diabetes: The role of treatment fidelity in a randomized clinical trial of multisystemic therapy. *Journal of Family Psychology.*

Francis, G. L., Grogan, D., Hardy, L., Jensen, P. S., Xenakis, S. N., & Kearney, H. (1990). Group psychotherapy in the treatment of adolescent and preadolescent military dependents with recurrent diabetic ketoacidosis. *Military Medicine, 155,* 351–354.

Frey, M. A. (1995). Toward a theory of families, children, and chronic illness. In M. A. Frey & C. L. Sieloff (Eds.), *Advancing King's systems framework and theory of nursing* (pp. 109–125). Thousand Oaks, CA: Sage.

Grey, M., Boland, E. A., Davidson, M., Li, J., & Tamborlane, W. V. (2000). Coping skills training for youth with diabetes mellitus has long lasting effects on metabolic control and quality of life. *Journal of Pediatrics, 137,* 107–113.

Gross, D., Fogg, L., & Conrad, B. (1993). Designing interventions in psychosocial research. *Archives of Psychiatric Nursing, 7*, 259–264.

Haley, J. (1976). *Problem solving therapy*. San Francisco: Jossey-Bass.

Harris, M. A., Greco, P., Wysocki, T., Elder-Danda, C., & White, N. H. (1999). Adolescents with diabetes from single-parent, blended, and intact families: Health related and family functioning. *Families, Systems, & Health, 17*, 181–196.

Harris, M. A., & Mertlich, D. (2003). Piloting home-based behavioral family systems therapy for adolescents with poorly controlled diabetes. *Children's Health Care, 32*, 65–79.

Henggeler, S. W., Melton, G. B., Brondino, M. J., Scherer, D. G., & Hanley, J. G. (1997). Multisystemic therapy with violent and chronic juvenile offenders: The role of treatment fidelity in successful dissemination. *Journal of Consulting and Clinical Psychology, 65*, 821–833.

Henggeler, S. W., & Schoenwald, S. K. (1998). *The MST supervisory manual: Promoting quality assurance at the clinical level*. Charleston, SC: MST Services.

Henggeler, S. W., Schoenwald, S. K., Borduin, C. M., Rowland, M. D., & Cunningham, P. B. (1998). *Multisystemic treatment of antisocial behavior in children and adolescents*. New York: Guilford Press.

Hogue, A., Liddle, H., Rowe, C., Turner, R. M., Dakof, G. A., & LaPann, K. (1998). Treatment adherence and differentiation in individual versus family therapy for adolescent substance abuse. *Journal of Counseling Psychology, 45*, 104–114.

Huey, S. J. (2001). *Adherence training manual for multisystemic therapy (MST): Anchors and guidelines for coding audiotaped sessions*. Los Angeles: University of Southern California.

Huey, S. J., Henggeler, S. W., Brondino, M. J., & Pickrel, S. G. (2000). Mechanisms of change in multisystemic therapy: Reducing delinquent behavior through therapist adherence and improved family and peer functioning. *Journal of Consulting and Clinical Psychology, 68*, 451–467.

Jacobson, A. M., Hauser, S. T., Willett, J., Wolfsdorf, J. I., & Herman, L. (1997). Consequences of irregular versus continuous medical follow-up in children and adolescents with insulin-dependent diabetes mellitus. *Journal of Pediatrics, 131*, 727–733.

Javor, K., Kostsanos, J. G., McDonals, R., Baron, A. D., Kesterson, J. G., & Tierney, W. (1997). Diabetic ketoacidosis charges relative to medical charges of adult patients with Type 1 diabetes. *Diabetes Care, 20*, 349–353.

Johnson, S. B. (1990). Adherence behaviors and health status in childhood diabetes. In C. S. Holmes (Ed.), *Neuropsychological and behavioral aspects of diabetes*. New York: Springer-Verlag.

Kaufman, F. R., Halvorson, M., & Carpenter, S. (1999). Association between diabetes control and visits to a multidisciplinary pediatric diabetes clinic. *Pediatrics, 103*, 948–951.

King, I. M. (1981). *A theory for nursing: Systems, concepts, and process*. New York: Wiley.

King, I. M. (1992). King's theory of goal attainment. *Nursing Science Quarterly*, *5*, 19–26.

King, I. M. (1995). A systems framework for nursing. In M. A. Frey & C. L. Sieloff (Eds.), *Advancing King's systems framework and theory of nursing* (pp. 14–22). Thousand Oaks, CA: Sage.

Kovacs, M., Charron-Prochownik, D., & Obrosky, D. S. (1994). A longitudinal study of biomedical and psychosocial predictors of multiple hospitalizations among young people with insulin-dependent diabetes mellitus. *Diabetic Medicine, 12*, 142–148.

Kovacs, M., Goldston, D., Obrosky, D. S., & Iyengar, S. (1992). Prevalence and predictors of pervasive noncompliance with medical treatment among youths with insulin-dependent diabetes mellitus. *Journal of American Academy of Child and Adolescent Psychiatry, 31*, 1112–1117.

Leonard, B. J., Jang, Y. P., Savik, K., Plumbo, P. M., & Christensen, R. (2002). Psychosocial factors associated with levels of metabolic control in youth with Type 1 diabetes. *Journal of Pediatric Nursing, 17*, 28–37.

Lindsay, B. (2004). Randomized control trials of socially complex nursing interventions: Creating bias and unreliability? *Journal of Advanced Nursing, 45*, 84–94.

Liss, D. S., Waller, D. A., Kennard, B. D., McIntire, D., Capra, P., & Stephens, J. (1998). Psychiatric illness and family support in children and adolescents with diabetic ketoacidosis: A controlled study. *Journal of American Academy of Child and Adolescent Psychiatry, 37*, 536–544.

McHugo, G. J., Drake, R. E., Teague, G. B., & Xie, H. (1999). Fidelity to assertive community treatment and client outcomes in the New Hampshire dual disorders study. *Psychiatric Services, 50*, 818–824.

Miller, S. J., & Binder, J. L. (2002). The effects of manual-based training on treatment fidelity and outcome: A review of the literature on adult individual psychotherapy. *Psychotherapy: Theory, Research, Practice, Training, 39*, 184–198.

Minuchin, S. (1974). *Families and family therapy*. Cambridge, MA: Harvard University Press.

Moncher, F. J., & Printz, R. J. (1991). Treatment fidelity in outcome studies. *Clinical Psychology Review, 11*, 247–266.

Musey, V. C., Lee, J. K., Crawford, R., Klatka, M. A., McAdams, D., & Phillips, L. S. (1995). Diabetes in urban African Americans: Cessation of insulin therapy is the major precipitating cause of diabetes ketoacidosis. *Diabetes Care, 18*, 483–489.

Naylor, M. D. (2003). Nursing intervention research and quality of care. *Nursing Research, 52*, 380–385.

Orr, D. P., Golden, M. P., Myers, G., & Marrero, D. G. (1983). Characteristics of adolescents with poorly controlled diabetes referred to a tertiary care center. *Diabetes Care, 6*, 170–175.

Palta, M., LeCaire, T., Daniels, K., Shen, G., Allen, C., & D'Alessio, D. (1997). Risk factors for hospitalization in a cohort with Type 1 diabetes: Wisconsin Diabetes Registry. *American Journal of Epidemiology, 146*, 627–636.

Rewers, A., Chase, H. P., Mackenzie, T., Walravens, P., Roback, M., Rewers, M., et al. (2002). Predictors of acute complications in children with Type 1 diabetes. *JAMA, 287,* 2511–2518.

Schoenwald, S., Henggeler, S. W., Brondino, M. J., & Rowland, M. D. (2000) Multisystemic therapy: Monitoring treatment fidelity. *Family Process, 39,* 83–103.

Schoenwold, S. K., & Hoagwood, K. (2001). Effectiveness, transportability, and dissemination of interventions: What matters when? *Journal of Psychiatric Services, 52,* 1190–1197.

Silverman, A. H., Haines, A. A., Davies, W. H., & Parton, E. (2003). A cognitive behavioral adherence intervention for adolescents with Type 1 diabetes. *Journal of Clinical Psychology in Medical Settings, 10,* 119–127.

Smith, C. P., Firth, D., Bennett, S., Howard, C., & Chisholm, P. (1998). Ketoacidosis occurring in newly diagnosed and established diabetic children. *Acta Paediatrica Scandinavica, 87,* 537–541.

Steindel, B. S., Roe, T. R., Costin, G., Carlson, M., & Kaufman, F. R. (1995). Continuous subcutaneous insulin infusion (CSII) in children and adolescents with chronic poorly controlled Type 1 diabetes mellitus. *Diabetes Research and Clinical Practice, 27,* 199–204.

Viinamaki, H., & Niskanen, L. (1991). Psychotherapy in patients with poorly controlled Type 1 (insulin-dependent) diabetes. *Psychotherapy and Psychosomatics, 56,* 24–29.

White, K., Kolman, M. L., Wexler, P., Polin, G., & Winter, R. J. (1984). Unstable diabetes and unstable families: A psychosocial evaluation of diabetic children with recurrent ketoacidosis. *Pediatrics, 73,* 749–754.

Wysocki, T., Harris, M. A., Greco, P., Bubb, J., Danda, C. E., & Harvey, L. M. (2000). Randomized controlled trial of behavior therapy for families of adolescents with insulin dependent diabetes mellitus. *Journal of Pediatric Psychology, 25,* 23–33.

Wysocki, T., Hough, B. S., Ward, K. M., & Green, L. B. (1992). Diabetes mellitus in the transition to adulthood: Adjustment, self-care, and health status. *Journal of Development and Behavioral Pediatrics, 13,* 194–201.

CHAPTER SEVENTEEN

Rethinking Empathy in Nursing Education

Shifting to a Developmental View

Martha Raile Alligood

Although empathy has been a consistent theme in the nursing literature for the last 50 years, it continues to be surrounded by concept confusion. The empathy literature reveals various definitions of empathy most often based on the theoretical perspectives of disciplines other than nursing. At the time of this writing, it has been nearly 25 years since Gagan (1983) declared that further research on nurses and nursing empathy should cease until conceptual clarity for the discipline of nursing could be developed. Alligood (1992) and the Empathy Research Team at the University of Tennessee (Alligood, Evans, & Wilt, 1995; Alligood & May, 2000; Evans, Wilt, & Alligood, 1998; Walker & Alligood, 2001) accepted Gagan's challenge and developed three theories of empathy from a nursing framework.

In this chapter, the theories of nursing empathy discovered in King's (1981) three systems and the educational application of the personal system theory in nursing education are presented. The shift to trait empathy from state empathy is vital for educators to recognize the importance of the human developmental empathy trait within nursing students and to revolutionize their teaching–learning activities for empathy in nursing curricula. The human developmental approach to empathy that is proposed requires educator recognition and valuing of the capacities the student brings to nursing. It also requires facilitating students' awareness

287

and valuing of their own individual empathic abilities throughout their nursing education program. Therefore, the role of the educator requires creative teaching in an empathic relationship with the student.

BACKGROUND

Nurse educators have included empathy in nursing education and their discussions of what makes a "good nurse" since the mid-20th century. Recently there has been increasing recognition by the general public media of the importance of empathy throughout our lives. In the area of child development, a national competition held to learn the secret of the "Strongest Kids in America" noted that compassion and the capacity to have empathy for others was among the common values in the 25 finalists.

At the other end of the life span, findings from a landmark study of aging suggested that aging is controlled by how we live. L. A. Walker (2001), writing about successful aging from a landmark study by Harvard researcher George Vaillant, noted that empathy and the capacity to imagine how others see their world is an essential attribute for living long, happy lives.

Similarly, the nature of empathy in business has been described in the best-selling psychology literature promoting emotional intelligence (Goleman, 1995). Empathy is one of 12 essential attributes listed to meet the challenges in the day-to-day process of succeeding in the business world. This being true, it is not surprising that empathic failure has also been noted in relation to the growing problem of violence in our society. Specifically, learning to be empathic has been proposed as a possible treatment for those with a history of violence (Simon, 2000). Indeed, empathy has been proposed as the best emotional antidote to anger because efforts to understand the other person and feel empathy assists those prone to anger to cool down rather than letting their anger escalate (Hales, 2001).

Finally, as the world shrinks and persons from various countries struggle to learn to live with each other, the importance of empathy surfaces yet again. When exposed to cultures other than ones' own, some people developed cultural competence through the experience of the culture they were visiting, and others, who chose to interact only with those of their own culture, failed to develop cultural competence (Meleis, 1999; Zorn, 1996). One of the personality factors found in those who developed cultural competence was empathy. Therefore, it was concluded that empathy facilitated the development of cultural competence.

Despite the interest in empathy among nurses and the inclusion of empathy in nursing education curricula, the problem of conflicting findings in nursing empathy studies was recognized and reported in 1983 in the nursing literature (Gagan, 1983). In addition, comprehensive reviews of the empathy literature have confirmed that empathy in nursing is not well understood (Alligood, 1992; Wheeler, 1990; Williams, 1990). Despite the importance of using nursing theory to guide nursing research, it was noted that researchers had predominately relied on empathy measurement instruments from other disciplines and that their instruments represented various theoretical perspectives of empathy, which were different from nursing. Gagan's (1983) call for an in-depth study of nursing empathy prior to further measurement of empathy in nurses, was answered by Alligood (1992) and the Empathy Research Team at the University of Tennessee.

It was noted that although some research instruments were designed to measure the trait of empathy and others were designed to measure the state of empathy, nurse researchers were seemingly using these instruments indiscriminately. This practice threatened the construct validity of the measurement of empathy in many nursing studies. Therefore, a proposal was put forth calling for the recognition of two types of empathy, basic (or trait) and trained (or state) to improve the conceptual–theoretical linkages between the empathy variable to be measured and the instrument selected to capture the variable operationally. The basic trait of empathy was defined as a human developmental feeling attribute of the person and environment process. Trained empathy state was defined as transient behaviors enacted to convey understanding of another person. Accuracy of the conceptual–theoretical–operational linkage in empathy research was proposed as yet another solution to the methodological problems that had been noted in empathy research (Alligood, 1992).

PURPOSE OF OUR PROJECT

The purposes of our project were to describe the nature of empathy within a developmental nursing framework (Alligood et al., 1995) and from this new perspective to discover theories of nursing empathy and explore new teaching–learning approaches and strategies. Another goal was to use these strategies to assist students to discover, value, and further develop their own innate human developmental ability to empathize.

THE RESEARCH APPROACH

A qualitative design based on Allen (1995) and Gadamer (1989), known as rational hermeneutic interpretation of nursing science text, was used to discover empathy within the three systems in King's (1981) conceptual system. The research study was carried out by the Empathy Research Team who formalized nursing theories of empathy in each of the systems. The team was made up of faculty and graduate students (mostly doctoral) who received credit for becoming oriented to research groups in the college of nursing, met regularly, and participated in the current research project of the team. The membership changed from semester to semester as students moved on to another research group; however, some remained active in the group they selected for a number of years. The members of the team contributed to all aspects of the research process, and as the leader of the Empathy Research Team for 10 years, I am indebted to those students and faculty colleagues for their contributions to the empathy projects.

THEORIES OF NURSING EMPATHY

A conceptualization of empathy in each of the three systems of King's framework was published and noted by reviewers of the work to contain an implicit middle range theory of empathy (Alligood et al., 1995; Fawcett & Whall, 1995). Based on the understanding of two types of empathy, it became clear that most of the teaching strategies and empathy content in nursing educational programs focused on behaviors and techniques reflecting the state of empathy rather than the basic human developmental empathy trait. Because nursing is a learned profession acquired through an educational process, the basic developmental type of empathy (trait) seemed a better fit for nursing education than empathy techniques and behaviors (state).

This led us to the next step, which was a test of the two types of empathy to determine whether our proposal for nurses to focus on the human developmental trait and foster the development of nursing students' empathy rather than continuing to emphasize behavioral techniques and the empathy state could be supported with research. This test was important also because the literature suggested that the training of behaviors and techniques for the empathy state were not sustained over time.

Therefore, a longitudinal study was carried out to measure the two types of empathy in nursing students in the College of Nursing at the University of Tennessee and test the premise that the human developmental trait of empathy was sustained over time and that the behavioral state was not. The findings of the study supported our premise (Evans et al., 1998). The Empathy Research Team then designed a project to formalize a theory of nursing empathy using a rational interpretive hermeneutic study of King's systematic human developmental conceptual system (Alligood & May, 2000; King, 1981; Walker & Alligood, 2001).

THE HEART OF THE PROBLEM

Although two types of empathy were noted in the nursing literature and the literature of related disciplines, little if any attention was being given to the developmental trait (basic type). Similarly, the teaching of empathy in nursing curricula seemed to be behaviorally based with emphasis on teaching of techniques and rote responses rather than the human developmental empathy trait each nursing student brings to the profession. This led us to a question: Has behaviorism functioned as an ideology and led us, as nurse educators, to believe that the human developmental capacities that nursing students bring to nursing are less valuable than the instruction they receive from us?

What did we learn? We found that the basic trait of human developmental empathy was sustained when the behavioral state was not. We also confirmed our belief that education in nursing empathy should be based on a theory of nursing empathy, and so we continued our work toward that goal.

The Empathy Research Team formalized a theory of nursing empathy in each system of King's conceptual system as noted in Table 17.1. Each of the theories in Table 17.1 is useful because it defines empathy with defining prepositional statements within that system and shows how empathy differs across the three systems. Review of these theories will help educators recognize the type of empathy they are using and make the shift from conceptualizing empathy behaviorally according to the trained type of empathy (state) to the developmental basic type of empathy (trait) in their nursing education curricula.

STRATEGIES FOR IMPLEMENTING A PERSONAL SYSTEM THEORY OF NURSING EMPATHY

The focus of this chapter is on the individual student and the personal system theory of nursing empathy as the place to begin. Suggestions in Table 17.2 are offered to assist the educator and the student with the implementation of the personal system theory of nursing empathy. The table is organized according to the defining prepositional statements for the personal system theory. Examples of activities for the student and the educator are given for each prepositional statement. For example, the prepositional statement that the human developmental trait of empathy "organizes perceptions" leads to a shift that places the emphasis on the development of the student rather than on the content being taught.

From the beginning, the emphasis is on what students bring to nursing and how to help them learn to use their individual strengths and

Table 17.1. Theories of Nursing Empathy Discovered in King's (1981) Three Systems

The personal system theory of nursing empathy	The interpersonal system theory of nursing empathy	The social system theory of nursing empathy
Proposes that empathy is a human developmental ability that	Proposes that empathy is a human developmental ability that	Proposes empathy is a human developmental ability that
• facilitates awareness of self and others	• defines the quality of the interaction	• contributes to the achievement of standards
• organizes perceptions	• organizes perceptions	• enhances the valuing of authority resulting in participation/contribution
• increases sensitivity	• creates understanding	• facilitates use of authority
• promotes shared respect, mutual goals, and social awareness	• acknowledges, respects, and values others	• empowers the nurse to make decisions and practice with authority
• affects learning	• guides the conceptualization of the role of the nurse	• promotes perceptions of professional and organizational status
		• contributes to the nurse's perception of alternatives, judgment, and decision making, and sensitivity as action is taken

Note. The content of this table was developed over time by the members of the Empathy Research Team in the College of Nursing at University of Tennessee in Knoxville.

abilities as they learn nursing. The curriculum framework takes on special importance for students as the internal system (context) for students to understand the knowledge of nursing (content) they are receiving. For the educator, the shift is from an emphasis on specific aspects of content to the content within the framework and the development of the student. Indeed, the educator understands that the framework is as important for learning, critical thinking, and decision making as is the knowledge that fits in the framework.

Similarly, the developmental approach takes learning beyond the memorization of facts to a level of understanding based on all of the senses and perceptions. Thinking of the learning of a student from the perspective of the students' human development rather than from the isolated

Table 17.2. Personal System Theory of Nursing Empathy and Implementation Suggestions

Personal system theory of nursing empathy	Suggestions for student learning based on the developmental view	Suggestions for nurse educators teaching based on the developmental view
Organizes perceptions	Curriculum begins with framework for students to develop an internal system (context) for knowledge (content) they are learning	Develops curriculum with framework and understands that framework is as important for learning and decision making as knowledge that fits in it
Facilitates awareness of self and others	Reflection emphasized in didactic and clinical learning for understanding of self, patients, and other students	Faculty focus on capacities students bring to nursing and facilitating their development. Teaching strategies include reflection on self and others for intrapersonal development
Increases sensitivity	Learning activities for self-understanding such as telling their stories and listening to stories of other students; students helped to recognize, value, and understand their reactions	Provides learning activities that emphasize student reactions and opportunities for expressions of what is being experienced
Values sensitivity and promotes shared respect, mutual goals, and social awareness	Students develop mutual goals with faculty and others, gain respect for intergenerational and cross-cultural differences and similarities, and develop goals for progressive personal growth	Educators ensure that faculty and student goals are mutual and clear, expect mutual respect in the classroom in clinical practice, offer progressive content and experiences for professional development
Affects learning	Students develop an understanding of own learning style; understand how own human capacities fit within context and practice of nursing	Recognize differences and requirements of varied learning styles; help students understand the demands of nursing so they see where their unique abilities fit in the profession

facts of content assists the educator to identify learning activities that connect with a broader range of perceptions. Activities such as having students push one another blindfolded in wheelchairs so they can experience being in a wheelchair moving at a fast pace when unable to see, lets them learn by experiencing what this feels like. Such an activity shifts the learning from cognitive knowing of a behavior to the human experience and developmental knowing.

Table 17.2 presents suggestions of more learning activities for students and teachers from the developmental view for each of the prepositional statements of the personal system. A characteristic of theory is that it proposes something that is measurable or testable. Therefore, activities are suggested for both students and educators based on the guidance of the theory to foster the development of the students' basic individual empathy trait.

The human development in the interpersonal system and social system are dependent on the development of the individual personal system and are specific to each person. Each of these theories (interpersonal and social system) may also be used to guide the educator in the development of student activities in the same way as the personal system theory in this chapter. The reader is referred to an earlier publication on King's interacting systems and empathy (Frey & Sieloff, 1995, chap. 6) for a description of the progression of a nursing student through the personal system, to the interpersonal system level, and finally to the profession of nursing where professional development is described at the social system level.

CONCLUSION

Student development is a vital aspect of nursing education. Empathy is essential for nursing communication, leadership, decision making, and cultural competence. Personal system development of empathy forms the basis for interpersonal system and social system development of empathy. Nurse educators may be at varying points with regard to shifting to a developmental view as they come to recognize the vital nature of the person of the student and their educational development. The research of the Empathy Research Team led to an awareness that challenged us to reconsider our educational approach in the area of empathy.

Shifting to a developmental theory of nursing empathy and nursing education increases the meaning of the learning experiences for the students and for the educators. Students develop a sense of who they are early in the nursing program and begin to understand what it means to be a nurse. As they learn the values inherent in the profession of nursing and clarify their own values, they experience progressively more caring, self-confidence, intuitive knowing, decision-making accuracy, satisfaction, and professionalism.

What does this mean for other educators in nursing? Faculty interested in shifting to a developmental view of empathy in nursing education should first examine the basis of the learning approach currently being used to determine whether they value or devalue the students' developmental abilities. If empathy techniques are being taught without first assessing the human developmental empathy ability of the student, this practice should be evaluated. Then faculty should examine the teaching–learning activities currently in use to determine whether the emphasis is on content or on the students' human development in learning. Finally, helping students discover and value the abilities they bring to nursing is a good way to begin the shift to a developmental view.

ACKNOWLEDGMENTS

Dr. Alligood acknowledges the faculty and students who contributed to the Empathy Research Team projects during her tenure at the University of Tennessee, Knoxville, and Dr. Carol Seavor for contributions to this work. An earlier version of this chapter was presented at the National League for Nursing 2002 Education Summit, Anaheim, California, September 2002.

REFERENCES

Allen, D. (1995). Hermeneutics: Philosophical traditions and nursing practice research. *Nursing Science Quarterly, 8*, 174–182.

Alligood, M. R. (1992). Empathy: The importance of recognizing two types. *Journal of Psychosocial Nursing, 30*(3), 14–17.

Alligood, M. R., Evans, G., & Wilt, D. (1995). King's interacting systems and empathy, In M. A. Frey & C. L. Sieloff (Eds.), *Advancing King's systems framework and theory of nursing* (pp. 66–78). Thousand Oaks, CA: Sage.

Alligood, M. R., & May, B. (2000). A nursing theory of empathy discovered in King's personal system. *Nursing Science Quarterly, 13*, 243–247.

Evans, G., Wilt, D., & Alligood, M. R. (1998). Empathy: A study of two types. *Issues in Mental Health Nursing, 19*, 453–479.

Fawcett, J., & Whall, A. (1995). State of the science and future directions. In M. A. Frey & C. L. Sieloff (Eds.), *Advancing King's systems framework and theory of nursing* (pp. 327–324). Thousand Oaks, CA: Sage.

Frey, M. A., & Sieloff, C. L. (Eds.). (1995). *Advancing King's systems framework and theory of nursing*. Thousand Oaks, CA: Sage.

Gadamer, G. (1989). *Truth and method* (2nd rev. ed., J. Weinshieimer & D. G. Marshall, Trans.). New York: Crossroad.

Gagan, J. (1983). Methodological notes on empathy. *Advances in Nursing Science, 5*, 65–72.

Goleman, D. (1995). *Emotional intelligence.* New York: Bantam Books.

Hales, D. (2001, September 2). Why are we so angry? *Parade Magazine,* 10–11.

King, I. (1981). *A theory for nursing: Systems, concepts, process.* New York: Wiley.

Meleis, A. (1999). Culturally competent care. *Journal of Transcultural Nursing, 10,* 12.

Simon, R. I. (2000). Serial killers, evil, and us. *Phi Kappa Phi Forum, 80*(4), 23–28.

Walker, K. M., & Alligood, M. R. (2001). Empathy from a nursing perspective: Moving beyond borrowed theory. *Archives of Psychiatric Nursing, 15,* 140–147.

Walker, L. A. (2001, September 16). We can control how we age. *Parade Magazine,* 4–5.

Wheeler, K. (1990). Perception of empathy inventory. In O. L. Strickland & C. F. Walker (Eds.), *Measurement of nursing outcomes* (Vol. 4, pp. 181–197). New York: Springer Publishing Company.

Williams, C. (1990). Biopsychosocial elements of empathy: A multidimensional model. *Issues in Mental Health Nursing, 11,* 155–174.

Zorn, C. (1996). The long-term impact on nursing students of participating in international education. *Journal of Professional Nursing, 12,* 106–110.

CHAPTER EIGHTEEN

Development of Middle Range Theories Based on King's Conceptual System

A Commentary on Progress and Future Directions

Jacqueline Fawcett

PROGRESS

This book is outstanding testimony to the way in which a nursing conceptual model is used as the starting point for middle range theory development. As such, this book represents a major contribution to distinctive nursing knowledge that goes far beyond other books addressing middle range theories by including only theories derived directly from one conceptual model of nursing—Imogene King's conceptual system.

Two other recently published books devoted exclusively to middle range theories certainly contribute to knowledge development, although that knowledge is not in every case distinctive nursing knowledge (Peterson & Bredow, 2004; Smith & Liehr, 2003). For example, social support theory, self-efficacy theory, and the theories of reasoned action and planned behavior were developed by social psychologists to explain social psychological phenomena, and any test of those theories in nursing situations contributes primarily to the advancement of knowledge in the field of social psychology, not to the advancement of nursing discipline-specific knowledge (Fawcett, 2004; Fawcett & Alligood, 2005).

In contrast, the authors of the chapters in this book about the development of middle range theories derived their theories directly from King's conceptual system, which is widely recognized as a major conceptual model of nursing. King (1981) paved the way and set the standard for the work included in this book when she presented the theory of goal attainment and explained how she linked concepts from her abstract and general conceptual system (known earlier as the open systems model, the interacting systems model, and the general systems framework) with the more concrete and specific concepts of the middle range theory of goal attainment. Readers can appreciate the rich potential for even more middle range theory development as they read King's chapter in this book.

The approach to middle range theory development taken by King (1981) and followed by the authors of chapters in this book ensures logical congruence between the conceptual model and derived middle range theories. The logic is ensured because the same worldview undergirds both the conceptual model and the theories (Fawcett, 2004). The reciprocal interaction worldview undergirds King's conceptual system, which means that the conceptual system directs scholars to view human beings as holistic and active participants in their interactions with the environment. That worldview also directs scholars to study both objective and subjective phenomena by means of either or both qualitative and quantitative methodologies (Fawcett, 2005).

Whelton's chapter (chap. 2), an excellent example of metatheoretical work, focuses on the philosophic underpinnings of King's work. The content of her chapter holds even greater promise for assuring logical congruence between King's conceptual system and derived middle range theories than does the identification of the relevant worldview alone. Her chapter, along with her earlier work (Whelton, 1996, 1999), extends more simplistic analyses of King's philosophic claims and identification of the relevant world view (Fawcett, 1984, 1989, 1995, 2000, 2005). Whelton's more detailed analysis of King's philosophic orientation greatly facilitates the work of scholars who are committed to the derivation of middle range theories from King's conceptual system. With Whelton's work as an aid, theory derivations can proceed with a comprehensive understanding of what is required to ensure logical congruence between the conceptual system and middle range theories.

Review of the chapters in Part I of this book reveals careful and systematic derivation of middle range theories from King's conceptual system. Several of these scholars began their theory development work with their doctoral dissertations (Doornbos, 1994; du Mont, 1998; Ehrenberger, 2000; Fairfax, 2003; Frey, 1987; Fries, 1998; Killeen, 1996; May, 2000; Sieloff, 1996; Wicks, 1993; Zurakowski, 1991), which attests to their and their faculty advisors' commitment to advancing nursing-discipline-specific knowledge.

A hallmark of most of those chapters is the inclusion of a diagram or an explicit narrative explanation of the conceptual–theoretical–empirical (CTE) structure for the research that was designed to test the theory empirically. In those chapters, relevant concepts from King's conceptual system are clearly linked to the concepts of each middle range theory, which in turn are clearly linked to empirical indicators that measure the middle range theory concepts. These CTE structures summarize the profound intellectual and empirical efforts that are required to derive and test a middle range theory. What may appear relatively simple and straightforward to the reader actually reflects a major investment of time and a firm commitment to achieving logical congruence between the conceptual, theoretical, and empirical components of the work.

Noteworthy is the slight difference in the presentation of the CTE structures across chapters. Some authors used a relatively simple structure made up of conceptual model concepts, middle range theory concepts, and empirical indicators, which follows the schema put forth by Fawcett (1999; Fawcett & Downs, 1986, 1992). Other authors used a somewhat more complex structure made up of constructs, concepts, subconcepts, and empirical indicators, which is a component of Dulock and Holzemer's (1991) approach to theoretical substruction. The constructs in the Dulock and Holzemer type of CTE structure are analogous to conceptual model concepts in the Fawcett structure, and the concepts and subconcepts in the Dulock and Holzemer structure are analogous to middle range theory concepts and concept dimensions of the Fawcett structure.

Just as the approach to construction of CTE structures differ, chapter authors also adopted different approaches to theory development for derivation of their theories from King's conceptual system. Killeen (chap. 9) used Walker and Avant's (1983) theory derivation approach to develop her theory of satisfaction with patient care. Her application of that approach involved linking concepts from King's conceptual system with Eagly and Chaiken's (1993) attitude model and then deriving middle range theory concepts and propositions. Doornbos (chap. 3) used Walker and Avant's (1995) iterative process of induction and deduction to derive her family health theory. Wicks and colleagues (chap. 13) also used inductive and deductive processes to derive the theory of family health, but they did not provide a citation to a particular approach. Zurakowski (chap. 14) used Chinn and Kramer's (1999) theory deduction approach to derive her theory of social and interpersonal influences on health.

Sharts-Hopko (chap. 11) employed Walker and Avant's (1995) theory synthesis approach to derive her theory of health perception. Du Mont (chap. 4) explained how she derived the theory of asynchronous development from a synthesis of King's conceptual system and Peplau's (1952) theory of interpersonal relations. She did not, however, cite a particular approach to theory synthesis. Sieloff (chap. 12) used reformulation and synthesis to derive her theory of group power within organizations. In doing so, she linked concepts from King's conceptual system with concepts from the strategic contingencies theory of power (Hickson, Hinings, Lee, Schneck, & Pennings, 1971). Although Sieloff did not cite a particular reference for reformulation and synthesis, she may have drawn from Whall's (1980) discussion of reformulation of theories that are not completely logically congruent with a conceptual model.

Other chapter authors (Ehrenberger et al., chap. 5; Frey et al., chap. 16; May, chap. 10) described the development of the middle range theory without reference to inductive or deductive processes or any other approach. Still others (Fairfax, chap. 8; Fries Reed, chap. 6) cited Dulock and Holzemer's (1991) theoretical substruction approach.

Hernandez (chap. 7) explained how she situated her theory of integration, developed by means of the qualitative grounded theory method, within the context of King's conceptual system. The approach she used, which typically is referred to as secondary analysis, is proving to be an informative and productive strategy for conceptualizing and expanding a scholar's previous theoretical and empirical work within the context of a particular conceptual model of nursing (Radwin & Fawcett, 2002).

With the exception of Fairfax, the chapter authors discussed not only the derivation of the middle range theory but also the results of one or more empirical tests of the theory. Fairfax (2003) did, however, present the results of the test of her theory in her dissertation.

Some authors traced the evolution of the theory over time. For example, Doornbos provided an excellent discussion of the refinement of middle range theory concepts and the definitions of those concepts in response to the findings of the first empirical test of her theory of family health.

The chapters by Killeen and Sieloff are noteworthy for the descriptions of new research instruments they developed to measure middle range theory concepts derived directly from King's conceptual system. The authors of other chapters elected to use existing instruments to measure the concepts of their theories.

Kameoka and colleagues' chapter (chap. 15), in Part III of this book on post–middle range theory development, is an important example of how middle range theories can be tested empirically through careful selection of empirical indicators. Rather than derive a middle range theory from King's conceptual system, she elected to test a proposition of King's theory of goal attainment. Kameoka explained how her review of instruments designed to measure nurses' job satisfaction led her to select the one instrument that measures nurses' satisfaction with interactions with patients, which is much more in keeping with King's theory than other measures of nurses' job satisfaction.

FUTURE DIRECTIONS

The authors of the chapters of this book have accepted the challenge issued by Fawcett and Whall (1995) to move from implicit middle range theories to the formal derivation of explicit middle range theories derived from King's conceptual system. The acceptance of that challenge is especially evident in May's chapter in this book and in her earlier coauthored journal article (Alligood & May, 2000). Readers who have been conducting research but not formalizing their findings can use her description of explicit formalization of a theory of empathy as a template for progression from an implicit middle range theory of empathy (Alligood, Evans, & Wilt, 1995) to an explicit one.

A major relational proposition of King's conceptual system asserts that the personal, interpersonal, and social systems are interrelated. Several authors of chapters in this book have derived middle range theory propositions from that conceptual system proposition. For example, Fries Reed, Doornbos, Fairfax, and Hernandez linked concepts derived from the personal and interpersonal systems, whereas du Mont linked concepts derived from the personal and social systems, and Ehrenberger and Zurakowski linked concepts derived from the personal, interpersonal, and social systems. A meta-analysis or other integrative review of the results obtained from empirical tests of those propositions would provide valuable evidence regarding the credibility of King's conceptual system (Fawcett, 1999).

Additional metatheoretical work is needed to specify the relations between the concepts within the personal, interpersonal, and social systems. To date, King has been silent on those relations. Thus, for example, it is unclear how perception is related to self or growth and development or body image; how interaction is related to communication or stress; or how organization is related to authority or power or decision making. Consequently, scholars must rely not on the conceptual system but rather on theoretical and empirical literature based in other sometimes implicit conceptual models to specify and justify middle range theory relational propositions that link the concepts so carefully derived from the conceptual model concepts of the personal, interpersonal, or social system. Some chapter authors have proposed relations between middle range theory concepts derived from concepts within one of the three systems. Both Sharts-Hopko and May, for example, proposed relations between concepts derived exclusively from the personal system; the rationale for the proposed relations came from the literature beyond that guided by King's conceptual system.

Additional empirical work also is needed. Fawcett and Whall (1995) pointed to the need for continued empirical testing of middle range theories derived from King's conceptual system:

> The fact that the theory of goal attainment has been tested and found to be empirically adequate is significant. Additional tests of the theory of goal attainment, as well as the other middle range theories that have been derived from [King's conceptual system], would add to the evidence regarding the empirical adequacy of the theories and their generalizability across various situations and client populations. Furthermore, the credibility of [King's conceptual system] requires continuous investigation by means of systematic tests of conceptual–theoretical–empirical structures derived the [conceptual system], the theory of goal attainment or other relevant theories, and appropriate empirical indicators. (pp. 332–333)

The need for additional empirical testing extends to all of the theories included in this book. Thus, chapter authors and other scholars who are interested in any one or more of the middle range theory derived from King's conceptual system are strongly encouraged to repeatedly test the theories in diverse situations and to refine the theories on the basis of the research findings.

Empirical tests of the theories that already have been conducted have involved statistical techniques ranging from descriptive statistics to zero-order coefficients of correlation to path analysis. Zurakowski (chap. 14) raises a particularly salient issue when she points out that structural equation modeling (SEM) techniques should be used to test any propositions that are derived from King's conceptual system proposition asserting that the personal, interpersonal, and social systems are interrelated. Whether just two or all three of the systems are included, SEM allows tests of the reciprocal relations specified by the assertion that the systems are interrelated (Norris, 2005).

Not all theories included in this book have been found to be empirically adequate, which raises a question about the credibility of some aspects of King's conceptual system. Ehrenberger and colleagues' (chap. 5) theory of decision making, for example, was not supported by empirical research findings. Although she and her colleagues did not question the credibility of King's conceptual system, they did provide a thorough discussion of the findings and called for a revision of the theory of decision making. It is important that scholars raise questions about the credibility of the conceptual model from which their middle range theories are derived. Conceptual models are most valuable to scholars and practitioners when they are dynamic, that is, when they change in response to results of tests of logically derived and rigorously tested middle range theories. In other words, conceptual models must not take on the characteristics of dinosaurs (Fawcett, 2003).

The contents of this book reflect nursing's clarion call for middle range theories that have a closer connection to practice than do the more abstract conceptual models of nursing. Yet although "the most important influence on practice is theory" (Kerlinger, 1979, p. 296), and "nothing is quite so practical as a good theory" (Van de Ven, 1989, p. 486), we must keep in mind that theories, whether grand, middle range, or situation-specific practice level (Fawcett, 2005; Im, 2005), cannot be used directly in practice. Rather, theories are indirectly used when assessment tools and intervention protocols are devised from the content of the theories. Consequently, a time lag occurs between the development of a theory and its indirect use in practice.

Chapter authors have taken the first step in reducing that time lag by disseminating their theories (Funk, Tornquist, & Champagne, 1995) in this book and other publications. The next step, which involves changing fixed sets of beliefs about how practice is conducted (Funk et al., 1995), may be taken by the authors themselves as well as by other nurses who are committed to the use of theory-guided, evidence-based practice (Hinton Walker & Redman, 1999). As fixed sets of beliefs about practice are changed, new theory-guided, evidence-based assessment tools and intervention protocols can be introduced to practicing nurses and become the standards for practice.

Most of the middle range theories included in this book are descriptions of phenomena or explanations of the relation among phenomena. Accordingly, those theories can be used to devise targeted assessment tools that can be applied in specific practice situations to better understand clients' perceptions of their health-related experiences and, therefore, provide a comprehensive basis for nursing interventions. Intervention protocols can be devised after predictive middle range theories are derived from King's conceptual system and tested empirically. When applied, the protocols for nursing interventions should help individuals, families and other groups, and communities to attain, maintain, and restore their health, so that they can function in their respective roles or should help individuals to die with dignity (King, 1981, 1997).

Killeen (chap. 9) and Sieloff (chap. 12), in the course of testing their middle range theories, developed new instruments to measure theory concepts. The decision to develop a new instrument rather than use existing instruments reflects a commitment to a rigorous and time-consuming endeavor. It is far easier to select an existing instrument. Selecting an existing instrument, which most likely was developed within the context of some other implicit or explicit conceptual model, however, may compromise its validity when used in the context of King's conceptual system-based theory testing research. For example, Ehrenberger and colleagues (chap. 5) used existing instruments to measure the concepts of the middle range theory of decision making. One of those instruments, the Inventory of Functional Status–Cancer (Tulman, Fawcett, & McEvoy, 1991) was developed within the context of the role function mode of Roy's (1984) adaptation model. Clearly, an instrument developed to measure a middle range concept associated with one conceptual model may not be valid when used to measure a middle range concept—even if the concept has the same label—associated with another conceptual model.

Killeen and Sieloff have not only ensured a logical connection between King's conceptual system and their instruments but also moved their theories a step closer to practice in that the instruments used for research purposes can now be evaluated for use in practice situations. The use of research instruments as practice tools is a major component in the integration of research and practice and a practical approach to closing the so-called theory–practice gap (Fawcett, 2005). Other chapter authors and other scholars can extend that pioneering work by developing research instruments that measure concepts of the various King conceptual system-based middle range theories and then evaluating the utility of those instruments as practice tools.

Fitzpatrick (2005) pointed out that the "process of knowledge development leads nurses to discover new ideas and potential applications of knowledge" (p. 1). This book is the embodiment of new ideas and applications of knowledge in the form of elucidation of the philosophic underpinnings of King's conceptual system and the derivation and testing of middle range theories derived from King's conceptual system in diverse situations and populations. The chapter authors have provided pathways for their own further theory development work. Readers may follow the same paths or create new pathways to middle range theory development using King's conceptual system or any one of the many other conceptual models of nursing.

CONCLUSION

The large number of middle range theories that have been derived from King's conceptual system attest to the broad utility of that conceptual model of nursing as a guide for theory development. The large number of theories also attests to the commitment of many nurse scholars to engage in the critical thinking and rigorous research required to develop and refine middle range theories.

Clearly, much very fine work related to King's conceptual system already has been accomplished. But much remains to be done. The many nurses throughout the world who are interested in King's conceptual system are urged to undertake that work. The many nurses throughout the world who are interested in other conceptual models of nursing are urged to use this book as a template for their theoretical and empirical work and, ultimately, for their practical work. The benefits to those individuals, families and other groups, and communities who become participants in nursing are potentially enormous in terms of enhanced health-related quality of life. Certainly those benefits far outweigh the costs of theoretical and empirical work.

REFERENCES

Alligood, M. R., Evans, G. W., & Wilt, D. L. (1995). King's interacting systems and empathy. In M. A. Frey & C. L. Sieloff (Eds.), *Advancing King's systems framework and theory of nursing* (pp. 66–78). Thousand Oaks, CA: Sage.

Alligood, M. R., & May, B. A. (2000). A nursing theory of personal system empathy: Interpreting a conceptualization of empathy in King's interacting systems. *Nursing Science Quarterly, 13,* 243–247.

Chinn, P. L., & Kramer, M. K. (1999). *Theory and nursing: Integrated knowledge development* (5th ed.). St. Louis: Mosby.

Doornbos, M. M. (1994). Family health in the families of the young chronically mentally ill. *Dissertation Abstracts International, 55,* 820B.

Dulock, H. L., & Holzemer, W. L. (1991). Substruction: Improving the linkage from theory to method. *Nursing Science Quarterly, 4,* 83–87.

du Mont, P. M. (1998). The effects of early menarche on health risk behaviors. *Dissertation Abstracts International, 60,* 3200B.

Eagly, A. H., & Chaiken, S. (1993). *The psychology of attitudes.* Orlando, FL: Harcourt Brace Jovanovich.

Ehrenberger, H. E. (2000). Testing a theory of decision making derived from King's systems framework in women eligible for a cancer clinical trail. *Dissertation Abstracts International, 60,* 3201B.

Fairfax, J. (2003). Theory of quality of life of stroke survivors. *Dissertation Abstracts International, 63,* 5156B.

Fawcett, J. (1984). *Analysis and evaluation of conceptual models of nursing.* Philadelphia: Davis.

Fawcett, J. (1989). *Analysis and evaluation of conceptual models of nursing* (2nd ed.). Philadelphia: Davis.

Fawcett, J. (1995). *Analysis and evaluation of conceptual models of nursing* (3rd ed.). Philadelphia: Davis.

Fawcett, J. (1999). *The relationship of theory and research* (3rd ed.). Philadelphia: Davis.

Fawcett, J. (2000). *Contemporary nursing knowledge: Analysis and evaluation of nursing models and theories.* Philadelphia: Davis.

Fawcett, J. (2003). On bed baths and conceptual models of nursing [Invited guest editorial]. *Journal of Advanced Nursing, 44,* 229–230.

Fawcett, J. (2004, October). *Middle-range nursing theories are necessary for the advancement of the discipline.* Paper presented via video for a conference sponsored by Universidad de LaSabana Facultad de Enfermeria, Chia, Cundinamarca, Colombia.

Fawcett, J. (2005). *Contemporary nursing knowledge: Analysis and evaluation of nursing models and theories* (2nd ed.). Philadelphia: Davis.

Fawcett, J., & Alligood, M. R. (2005). Influences on advancement of nursing knowledge. *Nursing Science Quarterly, 18,* 227–232.

Fawcett, J., & Downs, F. S. (1986). *The relationship of theory and research.* Norwalk, CT: Appleton-Century-Crofts.

Fawcett, J., & Downs, F. S. (1992). *The relationship of theory and research* (2nd ed.). Philadelphia: Davis.

Fawcett, J., & Whall, A. L. (1995). State of the science and future directions. In M. A. Frey & C. L. Sieloff (Eds.), *Advancing King's systems framework and theory of nursing* (pp. 327–334). Thousand Oaks, CA: Sage.

Fitzpatrick, J. J. (2005). Nursing knowledge development: Relationship to science and professional practice. In J. J. Fitzpatrick & A. L. Whall, *Conceptual models of nursing: Analysis and application* (4th ed., pp. 1–4). Upper Saddle River, NJ: Pearson/Prentice Hall.

Frey, M. A. (1987). Health and social support in families with children with diabetes mellitus. *Dissertation Abstracts International, 48,* 841A.

Fries, J. E. (1998). Health and social support of older adults. *Dissertation Abstracts International, 59,* 6262B.

Funk, S. G., Tornquist, E. M., & Champagne, M. T. (1995). Barriers and facilitators of research utilization. *Nursing Clinics of North America, 30,* 395–407.

Hickson, D. J., Hinings, C. R., Lee, C. A., Schneck, R. E., & Pennings, J. M. (1971). A strategic contingencies theory of intraorganizational power. *Administrative Science Quarterly, 16,* 216–229.

Hinton Walker, P., & Redman, R. (1999). Theory-guided, evidence-based reflective practice. *Nursing Science Quarterly, 12,* 298–303.

Im, E-O. (2005). Development of situation-specific theories: An integrative approach. *Advances in Nursing Science, 28,* 137–151.

Kerlinger, F. N. (1979). *Behavioral research: A conceptual approach.* New York: Holt, Rinehart and Winston.

Killeen, M. B. (1996). Patient-consumer perceptions and responses to professional nursing care: Instrument development. *Dissertation Abstracts International, 57,* 2479B.

King, I. M. (1981). *A theory for nursing: Systems, concepts, process.* New York: Wiley.

King, I. M. (1997). Knowledge development for nursing: A process. In I. M. King & J. Fawcett (Eds.), *The language of nursing theory and metatheory* (pp. 19–25). Indianapolis: Sigma Theta Tau International Center Nursing Press.

May, B. A. (2000). Relationships among basic empathy, self-awareness, and learning styles of baccalaureate pre-nursing students within King's personal system. *Dissertation Abstracts International, 61,* 2991B.

Norris, A. E. (2005). Structural equation modeling. In B. H. Munro, *Statistical methods for health care research* (5th ed., pp. 405–434). Philadelphia: Lippincott Williams and Wilkins.

Peplau, H. E. (1952). *Interpersonal relations in nursing.* New York: G. P. Putnam's Sons.

Peterson, S. J., & Bredow, T. S. (2004). *Middle range theories: Application to nursing research.* Philadelphia: Lippincott Williams and Wilkins.

Radwin, L., & Fawcett, J. (2002). A conceptual model-based programme of nursing research: Retrospective and prospective applications. *Journal of Advanced Nursing, 40,* 355–360.

Roy, C. (1984). *Introduction to nursing: An adaptation model* (2nd ed.). Englewood Cliffs, NJ: Prentice Hall.

Sieloff, C. L. (1996). Development of an instrument to estimate the actualized power of a nursing department. *Dissertations Abstracts International, 57,* 2484B.

Smith, M. J., & Liehr, P. R. (Eds.). (2003). *Middle range theory for nursing.* New York: Springer Publishing Company.

Tulman, L., Fawcett, J., & McEvoy, M. D. (1991). Development of the Inventory of Functional Status–Cancer. *Cancer Nursing, 14,* 254–260.

Van de Ven, A. (1989). Nothing is quite so practical as a good theory. *Academy of Management Review, 14,* 486–489.

Walker, L. O., & Avant, K. C. (1983). *Strategies for theory construction in nursing.* Norwalk, CT: Appleton Century Crofts.

Walker, L. O., & Avant, K. C. (1995). *Strategies for theory construction in nursing* (3rd ed.). Norwalk, CT: Appleton and Lange.

Whall, A. L. (1980). Congruence between existing theories of family functioning and nursing theories. *Advances in Nursing Science, 3,* 59–67.

Whelton, B. J. B. (1996). A philosophy of nursing practice: An application of the Thomistic–Aristotelian concept of nature to the science of nursing. *Dissertation Abstracts International, 57,* 1176A.

Whelton, B. J. B. (1999). The philosophical core of King's conceptual system. *Nursing Science Quarterly, 12,* 158–163.

Wicks, M. L. N. (1993). Family health in chronic illness. *Dissertation Abstracts International, 53,* 6228B.

Zurakowski, T. L. (1991). Interpersonal factors and nursing home resident health (anomia). *Dissertation Abstracts International, 51,* 4281B.

Index